Paradigm Freeze

WHY IT IS SO

HARD TO REFORM

HEALTH-CARE

POLICY IN

CANADA

D1607497

Edited by
Harvey Lazar
John N. Lavis, Pierre-Gerlier Forest, and John Church

Institute of Intergovernmental Relations
Queen's Policy Studies Series
School of Policy Studies, Queen's University
McGill-Queen's University Press
Montreal & Kingston • London • Ithaca

The Institute of Intergovernmental Relations

The Institute is the only academic organization in Canada whose mandate is solely to promote research and communication on the challenges facing the federal system.

Current research interests include fiscal federalism, health policy, the reform of federal political institutions and the machinery of federal-provincial relations, Canadian federalism and the global economy, and comparative federalism.

The Institute pursues these objectives through research conducted by its own associates and other scholars, through its publication program, and through seminars and conferences.

The Institute links academics and practitioners of federalism in federal and provincial governments and the private sector.

The Institute of Intergovernmental Relations receives ongoing financial support from the J.A. Corry Memorial Endowment Fund, the Royal Bank of Canada Endowment Fund, the Government of Canada, and the governments of Manitoba and Ontario. We are grateful for this support, which enables the Institute to sustain its program of research, publication, and related activities.

L'Institut des relations intergouvernementales

L'Institut est le seul organisme universitaire canadien à se consacrer exclusivement à la recherche et aux échanges sur les enjeux du fédéralisme.

Les priorités de recherche de l'Institut portent présentement sur le fédéralisme fiscal, la santé, la modification des institutions politiques fédérales, les mécanismes des relations fédérales-provinciales, le fédéralisme canadien dans l'économie mondiale et le fédéralisme comparatif.

L'Institut réalise ses objectifs par le biais de recherches effectuées par ses chercheurs et par des chercheurs de l'Université Queen's et d'ailleurs, de même que par des congrès et des colloques.

L'Institut sert de lien entre les universitaires, les fonctionnaires fédéraux et provinciaux et le secteur privé.

L'Institut des relations intergouvernementales reçoit l'appui financier du J.A. Corry Memorial Endowment Fund, de la Fondation de la Banque Royale du Canada, du gouvernement du Canada et des gouvernements du Manitoba et de l'Ontario. Nous les remercions de cet appui qui permet à l'Institut de poursuivre son programme de recherche et de publication ainsi que ses activités connexes.

Library and Archives Canada Cataloguing in Publication

Paradigm freeze : why it is so hard to reform health-care policy in Canada / edited by Harvey Lazar, John N. Lavis, Pierre-Gerlier Forest, and John Church.

(Queen's policy studies series)
Includes bibliographical references.
Issued in print and electronic formats.
ISBN 978-1-55339-324-5 (pbk.)—ISBN 978-1-55339-338-2 (ebook).
  ISBN 978-1-55339-339-9 (pdf).

1. Health care reform—Canada. 2. Medical policy—Canada. 3. Medical care—Canada. I. Forest, Pierre-Gerlier, editor of compilation II. Lazar, Harvey, editor of compilation III. Lavis, John, editor of compilation IV. Church, John, 1961-, editor of compilation V. Queen's University (Kingston, Ont.). Institute of Intergovernmental Relations, issuing body VI. Queen's University (Kingston, Ont.). School of Policy Studies issuing body VII. Series: Queen's policy studies series

RA395.C3P36 2013   362.10971   C2013-904389-6
                                             C2013-906525-3

CONTENTS

LIST OF TABLES AND FIGURES

FOREWORD

The Institute of Intergovernmental Relations is pleased to publish this book on health-care policy reform. It continues a collaboration between Harvey Lazar and me on health policy that started in the 1990s when we worked together on an Institute book on health and federalism. Harvey was then the director of the Institute and I was head of policy at Health Canada.

This is, of course, not the main reason that the Institute of Intergovernmental Relations agreed to publish this book. Health care remains a major issue in Canadian federalism, even though a key finding of the authors is that federalism has not been a major factor in explaining the success or failure of reform in the 30 case studies presented in this book. I strongly believe that this is a useful and important clarification that should not, however, be interpreted as supporting or opposing even a modest federal role in Canadian health care. There remain many areas where the nature of a federal role is worthy of a serious discussion.

In the editor's preface, Harvey Lazar acknowledges the work of his fellow editors as well as of the authors of individual chapters. He also notes the support he has received from the publishing staff of the School of Policy Studies. I wish to add my own appreciation for their contribution to this important book. I do want to single out and thank Valerie Jarus, the person responsible for typesetting. I also thank Mary Kennedy, the Institute's administrative assistant, who can always help me to figure out what I am supposed to do.

André Juneau
Director, Institute of Intergovernmental Relations

PREFACE

This book originates with a question that troubled me toward the end of my tenure as director of the Institute of Intergovernmental Relations, School of Policy Studies at Queen's University. To what extent was the federal government the *problem* and to what extent the *solution* to the seemingly never-ending challenge of health-care policy reform in Canada? I had no illusions that the answer would be simple. The size and complexity of the health-care world made it highly unlikely that any answer would apply to all aspects of health-care policy.

My research colleagues and I rapidly decided that the research question should be formulated at a more general level than the federal-provincial relationship. Why was it so difficult to reform health-care policy? We adopted a case study method that involved 30 cases and several roll-up studies. The case studies or proxies for them will be available at http://www.queensu.ca/iigr/apps/secure/index.php later this year (2013).

For Canadians, what came to be known as "medicare" serves three broad purposes. First and foremost is the provision of medically necessary hospital and medical services based on the urgency of need, not income. A second has to do with social values embedded in the arrangements. Payment for medicare is mainly through the consolidated revenues of provinces. On the whole, this involves redistribution from higher-income persons to lower-income persons. Third, medicare has also been about nation building. The fact that Canadians are able to travel, study, work, or retire in all parts of Canada without jeopardizing their hospital and medical insurance speaks to the social rights of Canadians.

Most Canadians had a passionate love affair with medicare for the first three to four decades of its existence. They received timely, high-quality services in the egalitarian "Canadian way." The early to mid-1990s was a period of "retrenchment and disinvestment" (in the words of the Canadian Institute for Health Information) that affected health-care services adversely. Canadians nonetheless remained attached to their distinctive program although some of the ardour may have dissipated.

There was no shortage of diagnoses about the nature of the problem or about reform solutions. These could be found in reports of the numerous commissions, task forces, and advisory committees that provincial and federal governments appointed to help deal with the challenges of health-care reform. There were also many proposals by think tanks and individual researchers, with seemingly meagre follow-up by governments.

There have already been many health-care reform proposals from all points on the political spectrum. Whether the proposals favoured the market or the state, whether they were centralizing or non-centralizing, too often they seemingly led to a blind alley. Was policy reform in fact as sparse as other researchers had concluded? If so, why? What explained the apparent rigidity in the health-care reform decision process? This book explores the space between policy diagnosis and policy treatment. What happened to policy ideas? What factors helped to explain the policy reform decisions that were taken and not taken? Were there patterns associated with different kinds of reform? What factors facilitated reform?

Our research method was executed systematically and is reported herein transparently. Readers who wish to use our methodology to study additional policy reform issues will find it laid out in considerable detail, especially in chapter 2 and annexes 1 and 2. Readers who doubt the validity of our conclusion in a specific case will be able to locate the factors that we considered to be relevant to our assessment. They can pinpoint the discrepancy and weigh their assessment against ours. The reader may give different factors more or less weight than we do.

This book was a long time in coming. The blame is mine. The result is not, I hope, any worse for the wear. We extended the main case study period 1990–2003 both backward and forward. These analyses helped to illuminate the trajectory that health-care reform has followed and provide some hints of what may lie ahead.

I have tested the patience of many people including my co-editors and co-authors. I thank them all for sticking with this project. The editorial team at the Publications Unit, Queen's School of Policy Studies, has been very supportive, beyond the call of duty. I thank Ellie Barton, Val Jarus, and Mark Howes. I also wish to thank Institute director André Juneau for reviewing and commenting on all of the chapters.

This project received most of its funding from the Canadian Institutes of Health Research and Health Canada. In addition, the Canadian Foundation for Healthcare Improvement provided funding for the final analysis and publication of this book. The research team thanks these three bodies for their support.

Harvey Lazar
October 2013

Glossary

3I framework. An approach to analyzing the influences on policy choices that focuses on the role of institutions, interests, and ideas

anti-reform. A position taken against consensus reforms that reflects attachment to the status quo (compare *consensus* and *counter-consensus* reforms below)

capitation. A payment made to health-care providers (typically individual practitioners but potentially also organizations) that is based on the number of patients to whom they provide care (with or without adjustments for factors such as the age and sex distribution of the patients)

consensus reforms. Decisions that are directionally consistent with what is recommended by the grey literature

counter-consensus reforms. Decisions that go in a different direction from what is recommended by the grey literature

dependent variable. The outcome being explained, which is typically the nature and extent of reform that actually occurred

endogenous variables. Factors influencing a dependent variable that are from within the policy sector, for example, insider interests

exogenous variables. Factors influencing a dependent variable that are from outside the policy sector, for example, the media

extra-billing. The practice of a doctor charging patients fees in excess of what provincial health insurance will pay

factor. Used interchangeably with the terms *independent variable* and *influence*

fee-for-service. A payment made to health-care providers (typically individual practitioners but potentially also organizations) that is based on the number and type of services they provide

first dollar coverage. An insurance provision under which the insured person pays no deductible; that is, the person is covered from the first dollar of expenses incurred

for-profit delivery. Provision of care by private, for-profit organizations

global funding. A payment made to health-care providers (typically organizations but potentially also individual practitioners) that is expected to fully cover the services they provide to patients

grey literature. Reports that are not indexed in the peer-reviewed literature and that are typically prepared by commissions and task forces appointed by provincial and federal governments

ideas. Knowledge or beliefs about "what is" (i.e., research knowledge) and views about "what ought to be" (i.e., values); knowledge and values combined

independent variable. Factors influencing a dependent variable such as the nature and extent of reform; the 3I's—institutions, interests, and ideas—are independent variables

influence. Used interchangeably with the terms *independent variable* and *factor*

institutions. Government structures, policy legacies, and policy networks; that is, the "rules of the game" within which decisions are made

interests. Various types of actors—such as elected officials, public servants, societal interest groups (e.g., physician, hospital, pharmaceutical, and other private interests), researchers, and policy entrepreneurs (called "insider champions") if they are directly involved in the policy-making process—who may influence or seek to influence policy outcomes

large reforms. Those assessed as "comprehensive" and "significant" as defined in annex 1; compare *substantial reforms* below

macro-policy framework. Refers to the factors that help determine "who" does "what" and under "what conditions" in the provision of health care. In this book it generally refers to the criteria and conditions specified in the *Canada Health Act* and provincial legislation that determine whether an expenditure is insured. It also includes alternatives to the *CHA* provisions that operate at the same level of generality

major factors. Independent variables that were the most important in determining policy outcomes

meso-level reforms. Reforms that touch the major components of a subsector, such as the hospital sector or physician sector; for example, the manner in which physicians are remunerated

New Public Management. Refers to government policies since the 1980s that have aimed to modernize and render the public sector more effective

not-for-profit health care. Care that is provided by private, not-for-profit organizations

palliative care. Medical care for people who are terminally ill

population-based funding. A payment made to health-care organizations that is based on the number of patients for whom they are accountable (with or without adjustments for factors such as the age and sex distribution of the patients)

primary health care. "First contact, continuous, comprehensive, and coordinated care provided to populations undifferentiated by gender, disease or organ system." (Starfield 1994, 1129)

privatization. Privatization in the health-care debate can refer either to the introduction of for-profit *funding* of health-care services that were previously financed publicly (e.g., user charges at point of delivery) or to *delivery* by private-for-profit organizations of health-care services that were historically provided by not-for-profit or public organizations. For-profit delivery is one of our six policy reform issues (see chapters 3–7), whereas for-profit funding is not a separate case study. In the later chapters (8–12), however, for-profit funding garners more attention. References to "privatization" in those chapters refer mainly to those financing questions

pro-reform. A position taken in favour of consensus reforms

regionalization. Decentralization of decision-making authority from provincial governments to subprovincial authorities

substantial reforms. Include comprehensive, significant, and moderate reforms

ABBREVIATIONS

AHS: Alberta Health Services

AMA: Alberta Medical Association

APP: alternative payment plan

BC: British Columbia

CCF: Co-operative Commonwealth Federation

CHA: *Canada Health Act*

CHC: Canadian Health Coalition

CHSLD: Centre d'hébergement et de soins de longue durée

CHST: Canada Health and Social Transfer (1996–2003)

CHT: Canada Health Transfer (since 2004)

CIHI: Canadian Institute for Health Information

CLSC: Centre local de services communautaires (local community service centre)

CMA: Canadian Medical Association

EPF: Established Programs Financing

FMG: family medicine group

FMOQ: Fédération des médecins omnipraticiens du Québec (Quebec Federation of General Practitioners)

FPT: federal/provincial/territorial

FFS: fee-for-service

GDP: gross domestic product

HFLA: *Health Facilities Licensing Act*

HSSCs: health and social services centres (Quebec)

IHF: independent health facilities

IHFA: Independent Health Facilities Act

LHIN: Local Health Integration Network

MLA: Member of the Legislative Assembly (Alberta)

MOHLTC: Ministry of Health and Long-Term Care (Ontario)

NAFTA: North American Free Trade Agreement

NCB: National Child Benefit

NDP: New Democratic Party

NHS: National Health Service (United Kingdom)

NLHBA: Newfoundland and Labrador Health Boards Association

NLMA: Newfoundland and Labrador Medical Association

NPM: New Public Management

ODB: Ontario Drug Benefits

OECD: Organization for Economic Co-operation and Development

OMA: Ontario Medical Association

PC: Progressive Conservative

PNBF: population needs-based funding

PQ: Parti Québécois

P/T: provincial/territorial

RAMQ: Régie de l'assurance maladie du Québec

RHA: regional health authority

SGAS: Système de gestion de l'accès aux services (service access management system)

SMA: Saskatchewan Medical Association

SSCN: Saskatchewan Surgical Care Network

CHAPTER 1

WHY IS IT SO HARD TO REFORM HEALTH-CARE POLICY IN CANADA?

HARVEY LAZAR

Democratically elected governments pay attention to the opinions of their citizens. Sometimes they are able to act on citizen demands in a timely fashion. Sometimes they do so with a time lag. When governments lack an adequate response, they may attempt to redefine the issue in a way that fits with what is achievable and convince the citizenry that it should accept the result and move on.

Paying attention to public opinion is a two-way street. Governments also try to manage the expectations of the public. When economic hard times are ahead, government leaders often try to precondition citizens to the future difficulties. When a military mission encounters unanticipated difficulties on the ground, it is not unusual for governments to redefine the mission to fit with what is achievable.

Due to the ongoing interaction between governments and citizens, it is rare that a single issue remains the leading concern of the public for an extended period. Yet, this has been the situation in Canada. Almost continuously since the late 1990s, Canadians have pointed to health care as their largest "national concern" or the issue that "should receive the greatest attention from Canada's leaders."[1] A 2002 poll found that, among 19 issues, "health care was both the highest priority and the one for which the federal government received the lowest ratings" (cited in Soroka 2007, 5 and Figure 5). In 2005, another pollster (Decima) surveyed opinion on 18 issues and again showed health care as the one in which the public was least satisfied by federal government performance (ibid., 9 and Figure 17).

Less than a decade earlier, in the 1980s, worries about health care had barely registered in public opinion data (Mendelsohn 2002, 31). In fact, since the introduction of countrywide hospital insurance in the late 1950s, Canadians have been smitten by that part of their health systems that provided universal, first-dollar, publicly financed hospital and medical services.[2] The public happily received this government program, eventually called medicare, as a way of enabling Canadians in each province and territory to access hospital and medical services on the basis of the urgency of their health needs, not their income. Subsequently, publicly financed health care evolved into something more—an embodiment of Canadian values.

No health system is problem-free. In the 1980s in Canada there were serious political tensions around the right of physicians to charge patients a fee for their services above the amount specified in the provincial and territorial fee schedules. These schedules had been negotiated between physicians' bargaining agents (medical unions in Quebec and provincial medical associations in all other provinces) and provincial governments. This dispute was eventually settled, but the political dynamics of the decision process were nasty and, among other things, included a strike by Ontario physicians. Equally if not more salient to this story were cost considerations. Between 1975 and 1990, total health expenditure in Canada grew from 7 to 9 percent of gross domestic product (CIHI 2012, 114). The public sector as a source of funds for health care was equal to 5.2 percent of GDP in 1975, and 6.3 percent in 1990. The governments of provinces and territories accounted for 93 percent of the public sector. By the late 1980s, public finances of the provinces and territories were in dreadful shape and then made worse by recession.

A series of decisions by provincial governments beginning in 1991/92 signalled a period of "retrenchment and disinvestment" in health care (CIHI 2012, 3). Over the next five years, some provinces tightened health-care expenditures more than others but the broad effects were similar across the country. The growth of health-care supply was constrained but demand was not. A supply-demand gap resulted. Although there was little or no scientific data on wait times then, by the mid-1990s Canadians sensed that they were encountering longer wait times than they had hitherto experienced or that were appropriate to their circumstances. This was especially the case for appointments for specialized procedures and diagnostic imaging. Emergency rooms were frequently overcrowded. Evidence of the supply-demand gap showed up in several ways: public opinion data, findings of the plethora of reports commissioned by governments, statements by interest groups, and articles written by the research community.

There was no shortage of policy proposals to fix the problem. In fact, a first wave of provincially commissioned reports landed on government desks around the time that provincial governments undertook their expenditure freezes. Provincial governments had commissioned these reports in the late 1980s in their search for ways to control costs and better integrate services. A second wave of provincially commissioned reports followed in the second half of the 1990s. The federally appointed National Forum on Health undertook a large research effort in the 1990s, and various think tanks contributed as well. At least 18 major reports published between 1988 and 2002 focused broadly on the issue of health-care policy reform (see annex 1 for a list and discussion of these reports).[3] A larger number were commissioned to deal with a specific issue or narrow range of issues.

Numerous calls for policy reform emanated from these generally well-researched reports.[4] Yet most reform proposals have not been acted on in a substantial way. The architecture of the health system was not much different in 2013 than it had been before all these reports were delivered to governments and made available to the public.

In a 2002 submission to the Commission on the Future of Health Care in Canada (Romanow Commission), the Canadian Medical Association wrote, "Over the past decade there have been countless studies on what is wrong with Canada's health care system. However, very little action has been taken to solve the problems identified in the reports" (CMA 2002, v). Eight years later the CMA (2010, 31) stated,

> In 2001 the Honourable Roy Romanow was tasked by the federal government to study and make recommendations in order to "ensure over the long-term the sustainability of a universally accessible, publicly funded health system." The Romanow Commission put forward 47 recommendations in 2002 with a view to "buying change." Similarly, the Kirby ... review of the Canadian health care system recommended an additional $5 billion of federal funding per year to restructure and renew Medicare. These reports were followed by additional federal funding in the amounts of $34.8 billion and $41.3 billion in the 2003 and 2004 First Ministers' Accords respectively. Eight years later it is evident that, for the most part, these Accords bought time, not change.

So many recommendations from so many reports have been set aside that we judged that it was important to understand why this was so. The reports were written by highly competent individuals with strong research teams available to them. Moreover, the authors of the reports were not at the political fringes. Governments rarely select people to head such bodies if they are hostile to the government's ideological stance.

This book is the product of a research project that began with an interest in why it is so hard to reform health-care policy in Canada and whether Canadian federalism in general or the federal government in particular was contributing more to the *problem* or to the *solution*. As we considered this matter, we translated that interest into a more precise set of objectives which are set out in chapter 2.

VERIFYING ASSUMPTIONS

Asking the question why it has been difficult to reform Canadian health-care policy involves two assumptions: that there was not much policy reform and that policy reform was desirable. In fact, much of the literature assumed or asserted that reform was sparse without providing systematic evidence that the assumption or assertion was valid. The starting point for this book was to determine whether the assumption of little reform could be verified.

The details of the methodology are discussed in chapter 2. Here it is sufficient to note that we use a case study approach to examine six representative health policy issues: regionalization, needs-based funding, alternative payment plans for primary care physicians, for-profit delivery, waiting lists, and prescription drug insurance coverage. The six issues span four policy domains: governance, finance, delivery, and program content. Each case was studied over the period 1990–2003 in five representative provinces: Alberta, Saskatchewan, Ontario, Quebec, and Newfoundland and Labrador. Thus, this book is based on 30 case studies.

To determine the nature and extent of reform, a benchmark was needed. The consensus position set out in the government-commissioned reports referred to above (sometimes called "grey literature") for each of the six policy issues was selected as the benchmark. The consensus position itself was assumed to be the highest level of reform that it was politically practicable for any government to achieve. We then analyzed and graded each of the 30 cases on the basis of how close it came to satisfying the benchmark. This method of analysis verified the starting assumption: taking the five provinces as a whole, there was in fact *meagre* policy reform (chapter 8). In chapter 10, we employed alternative methods of "measuring" policy reform. The alternatives did not alter our assessment of meagre reform.

The governments that commissioned these reports were generally centre or centre-left in their political orientation. Not surprisingly, therefore, the proposals from the literature tended to lean toward government as the optimal mechanism for responding to perceived shortcomings in the health systems. Decisions taken that were directionally consistent with the proposals in these reports are referred to as "consensus reforms" or, for ease of reading, just "reforms." Decisions that privileged the market or private for-profit sector, whether for the delivery or the financing of health services, are referred to as "counter-consensus reforms."

Although values influence policy choice in decision-making, the research program that led to this book made no assumptions about what is "good" policy reform. Big and small policy reforms that contemplated an enhanced role for markets in resource allocation (such as competition among imaging labs or surgical clinics) are equated with government-oriented reforms of equal magnitude. Thus, the fact that the Saskatchewan New Democratic government led by Premier Roy Romanow from 1991 to 2001 and the Alberta Progressive Conservative government led by Premier Ralph Klein from 1992 to 2006 had different ideological orientations does not matter for the purposes of determining the magnitude of their policy actions. The analysis similarly does not assess the appropriateness of reforms. This book is focused on understanding what makes policy reform, whether consensus or counter-consensus, so difficult to achieve.

In general, and not referring to health care in particular, the years from 1990 to 2003 were characterized by a shift to the political left whereas the years since 2003 have involved a shift toward the political right—toward conservatism and a larger role for markets. For this reason, in chapter 11 we re-examine and update the 30 cases for the 2004–2011 period. We want to determine whether the change in political stripe of governments in four of the five provinces and in Ottawa altered the finding of meagre policy reform.

The second starting assumption was that policy reform was desirable during the years from 1990 to 2003. Policy reform is neither a good nor a bad idea on its own. Context matters. If a health system is working well, lack of reform may constitute a form of desirable stability. If the system is under stress or worse, lack of reform may reflect an undesirable rigidity. During the study period, Canada's health systems were under stress and at times extreme stress. Government after government appointed commissions, task forces, or advisory committees to provide advice on what could be done to fix the situation (annex 1). Of equal interest for purposes of this study, the data on public opinion support the assertion of a system under stress. Matthew Mendelsohn (2002) undertook an analysis for the Romanow Commission "based on all available Canadian public opinion polls" on health care between 1985 and 2002.[5] He found that "while 61 percent of Canadians thought the system was excellent or very good in 1991 … only 29 percent shared that view in 2000" (1). A citizens' dialogue undertaken by Judith Maxwell and colleagues yielded similar findings (Maxwell, Rosell, and Forest 2003). In short, the weak reform record paralleled a period of stress when reform was perceived as desirable by many. The meagre outcomes are explained more by health system rigidities than a societal wish to protect a health-care system that was firing smoothly on all cylinders.

POLITICAL ECONOMY

In 2012, Canadians spent an estimated $207 billion on health care, or $5,948 per person, an amount equal to 11.6 percent of forecasted gross domestic product (CIHI 2012, xiii). To put that number into perspective, it is triple the amount Canadians spend on all levels of education (4 percent of GDP, OECD 2011) and an even larger multiple of what is expended on public pensions (3.5 percent of GDP, ibid). Canada has on occasion been referred to as an "energy superpower," and yet as a share of GDP, the entire energy industry—including oil, gas, and electricity—is a little over half the size of health care.

Of the more than 17 million Canadians employed in Canada in 2012, close to one in ten were working in the health care and social assistance sectors (Statistics Canada 2012). A large majority of the 1,651,000 people employed in these two sectors worked in health care. In 2009, this included 68,000 physicians, almost 350,000 nurses, and over 240,000 other health-care professionals, including dentists, pharmacists, midwives, and dietitians (CIHI 2011a, 2). That's around 650,000 professional jobs.

In 2009/10, the health-care industry was a high-paying, high-value-added industry. The "average gross fee-for-service payment per full-time equivalent physician was $293,000" (CIHI 2011c, 32). Registered nurses earned on average $28 to $36 per hour in the 2008–2010 period, depending on location, and licensed practical nurses $22 to $25 per hour (Living in Canada 2012).

The United States spent 17.6 percent of GDP on health in 2010. Canada was one of a grouping of ten OECD countries that came next, spending between 10 and 12 percent of GDP on health in that year. At 11.4 percent, Canada was fourth highest in this grouping and almost 2 percentage points over the OECD average of 9.5 percent (cited in CIHI 2012, 64).[6]

What do Canadians get for their money? In 2010 the *Commonwealth Fund International Health Policy Survey* compared how people in 11 countries assessed their health systems.[7] The Health Council of Canada used this report to discuss how Canada rated. The Council also compared the 2010 results for Canada with the results from 2004 and 2007 Canadian surveys. The Health Council (2010, 3-5) concluded,

> Canadians' confidence in their health-care system is related to many complex factors including their personal experiences within the system, including stories from friends and acquaintances, and articles in the news. This confidence has been steadily improving since 2004. However it is still below average compared with the other countries surveyed; almost two-thirds of Canadians think the system needs fundamental changes to make it work better.

Of the persons in the countries surveyed, Canadians had the greatest difficulty accessing care in the evenings, on weekends, and on holidays—anywhere other than in hospital emergency rooms (Health Council 2010, 5). Canada ranked lowest of all the countries when it came to the possibility of booking an appointment for the same day or the next day (4). Canadians also fared poorly, compared to others, in how long they had to wait for an appointment with a specialist or to get a diagnosis (5). The difficulties Canadians were experiencing with their health systems at the time Romanow reported had not disappeared eight years later.

Viewing these health system concerns and the relatively high cost of care in Canada through an economic lens provides a further perspective on the price Canadians are paying for system deficiencies. From a public finance perspective, realizing efficiencies equal to 1 percentage point of GDP (and still coming in nearly a point above the OECD average) would free up resources sufficient to increase education spending by more than 25 percent. Alternatively, these efficiency gains could go a long way in alleviating provincial fiscal challenges.

The impact of efficiency gains also has implications for jobs and the economy. With ongoing global economic development and the pace of technological change, health care is almost certain to become a larger part of the world economy and increasingly traded as a high-value-added service. Whether Canada becomes a net exporter of such services or a net importer is another reason to focus on reform.

EXPLAINING REFORM DECISIONS

The explanations for the reform decisions in each of the five provinces are set out in chapters 3 to 7. Some provinces accomplished more than others. Chapter 8 provides a single five-province assessment of the factors associated with reforms. Chapter 9 analyzes the data from cross-province and cross-policy issue perspectives. Foreshadowing these analyses, three themes are highlighted below: the extent of reform, barriers to reform, and factors that facilitated reforms.

Extent of Reform

No province attempted a "big bang"—a major set of reforms—in one fell swoop. Nonetheless, there were substantial differences among the governments in their broad approaches to reform that led to some variation in achievement. To emphasize the degree of difference, the provinces that undertook the most, Saskatchewan, and the least, Newfoundland and Labrador, are discussed first.

The 1991 general election saw the New Democratic Party (NDP) come to power in Saskatchewan with a large majority. It had made election commitments to "develop a healthcare system based on the 'wellness' model" (NDP 1991, 12). Once in office, the new government discovered that provincial finances were in deep trouble. Motivated by fiscal pressures on the one hand, and its commitment to a wellness-based reform on the other, the government quickly rationalized its hospital system (closing many small hospitals and amalgamating others, for example), integrated acute care hospitals and other institutions (like nursing homes) on a regional basis, and introduced a needs-based system of funding regions and hospitals. Tom McIntosh and Michael Ducie (chapter 4) attribute the speed of government action to a strong partnership between the premier, the minister of health (who had served as health critic for the NDP while it was in opposition), and senior officials in the health ministry. The pace of change inevitably led to resistance. By mid-term, the reform process began to lose steam.

The next planned reform in Saskatchewan was in primary care. Primary care reform was thought to be easier and more effective if physicians were paid through some alternative to the prevailing fee-for-service basis, such as capitation or salary. However, suggestions that the government might impose an alternative method of paying physicians led to stiff resistance from the Saskatchewan Medical Association. The NDP government "took its foot off the political accelerator." Although the NDP was re-elected three times (1995, 1999, and 2003), the first half of the first mandate was its period of greatest achievement.

Another noteworthy reform was introduced in 2003. After several years of trial and error, in response to the growth of wait times for surgical procedures and diagnostic imaging services, the Saskatchewan Surgical Care Network was established. It employed standardized assessment tools with the aim of consolidating and managing access to surgical procedures and diagnostic services across the province. Saskatchewan made this program mandatory for surgeons.

By contrast, in Newfoundland and Labrador health reform was not a political priority. Stephen Tomblin and Jeff Braun-Jackson (chapter 7) emphasize that the agenda of Premier Clyde Wells, whose Liberal party had been elected to office in 1989, was dominated by the moratorium and then closure of the cod fishery and the consequential adjustment process for fishers. Of the six policy issues studied in this book, Newfoundland and Labrador acted only on regionalization. Its motivation in introducing regionalization was principally cost containment. The Liberals did not increase the political priority attached to health care in the three subsequent general elections that they won. When the Conservative party toppled the Liberals in 2003, its party platform made no firm commitments on health care.

Turning to the other three provinces, Ralph Klein campaigned for the leadership of the Progressive Conservative Party in Alberta with the promise to swiftly balance the provincial budget. John Church and Neale Smith (chapter 3) note that this required that he rein in the provincial health budget. Beginning with a plan to reduce annual health spending by around 18 percent over a four-year period, the Klein government consolidated acute care, home care, continuing care, and public health services under a new regional structure, and introduced a needs-based system of regional and hospital funding. The Alberta government also slashed physician compensation as part of its fiscal plan (Church and Smith 2007,

5-9). In the government's give and take on physician compensation with the Alberta Medical Association, the latter floated the idea of encouraging alternative payment plans for primary care physicians but on a non-mandatory basis. This began a process, still underway, of encouraging alternative payment plans for primary care physicians. Premier Klein's successes in these areas were, however, overshadowed by his personal advocacy of for-profit delivery. The Friends of Medicare, made up of local activists, resisted fiercely.

As premier from 1992 to 2006, Klein secured only a modest fraction of what he aimed for, and it has not proven lasting. As with the NDP in Saskatchewan, most of his reforms were crowded into the early years of his first electoral mandate. In these key years, Klein made special use of legislative committees on some issues, purposively bypassing the public service. On other issues, particularly needs-based funding and wait times, he received strong support from the public service.

At the outset of the 1990s, unlike in other provinces, health services in Quebec had been regionalized for close to two decades. In the early 1990s, authority was moved downward from the provincial to regional level and from the regional to local level. In the 2003 general election, the Quebec Liberal Party campaigned in favour of eliminating regional boards. Once elected, the Liberal government moved swiftly to implement its platform but encountered stiff resistance and eventually adopted a compromise which saw the boards become regional agencies with a narrower role than they had previously enjoyed.

On most other issues, Pomey and co-authors (chapter 6) observe that Quebec commissioned numerous reports that led to little or no reform. The one exception, however, was important. In the 1994 general election, the opposition Parti Québécois (PQ) committed to drug reform. The prescription drug policy then in place insured against the costs of drugs for some illnesses and not others and thus insured some people and not others. The PQ acted during the first half of its mandate. Since the PQ was also committed to a balanced budget, it chose not to rely exclusively on public insurance. Instead it created a new universal and mandatory program of drug insurance financed partly through the private sector and partly through the public sector. This was the largest single reform among the 30 cases studied.

The Ontario NDP government (1990–1995) led by Bob Rae had not expected to win office and was not as prepared to take the reins of power as it might have been in other circumstances. It decided not to undertake the kind of regionalization already implemented or in the process of being implemented in other provinces. As for other issues, some of which arose in the Rae years and others during the subsequent premierships of Mike Harris and Ernie Eves (1995–2003), the assessment showed moderate reform. Acting under great pressure from civil society groups, the Rae government's most significant initiative among the six policy issues we studied was in improving access to some of the then new and expensive "breakthrough" drugs. The Harris government also chose not to create regional health authorities, but it introduced a program of hospital rationalization (closures and amalgamations) through an arm's-length Health Services Restructuring Commission. John Lavis and co-authors (chapter 5) describe the Ontario performance during these years as more like the tortoise in Aesop's fable than the hare.

Barriers to Reform: Insiders and Outsiders

The factors that explain the reform decisions depended on the policy domain. In the governance and financial arrangements domains, issues were influenced heavily by elite interaction, often with little transparency. The delivery and program content domains involved the public and civil society groups, often with media coverage, as well as elites.

In the discussion that follows, authoritative decision makers, generally a minister or ministers of the governing party, are considered as endogenous variables that we call "insider interests." It is not only their legal authority but the act of deciding itself that makes them endogenous to the decision process. Their advisors from the public service and elsewhere and those with relatively easy access to deciders or advisors are also viewed as having insider interests and thus endogenous influence. Provider associations generally meet this test. A crucial exception to this definition is that newly elected first-time governments may, depending on their behaviour, be considered outsiders in the early period of their first mandate. This is consistent with the idea of an opposition party running against the "powers that be" or the "establishment" and bringing in its outsider view to "clean house." It is analogous to candidates in federal elections in the United States running against Washington. Other endogenous variables discussed in the chapters that follow include ideas or institutions when they influence the behaviour of political actors who are insiders.

Variables that are not endogenous are referred to as exogenous and actors that are not insiders as outsiders. Opposition parties are typically outsiders, even if they engage on an issue. The media are outsiders. Even the public is an outsider. As patients, members of the public are not represented by provincial associations of patients that have either the power base or access to the decision process that provincial medical or hospital associations enjoy. As citizens and taxpayers, people do exercise some influence by electing government, but this does not make them insiders. Other exogenous variables include inanimate forces like fiscal crises and certain kinds of technological changes that affect behaviours.

To the extent that insiders saw their interests as potentially vulnerable, they constituted a major barrier to consensus reforms in two of the four policy domains: governance arrangements and financial arrange-ments. Provincial medical associations were the quintessential insiders in protecting their interests. Over the 1990–2003 period of study and the update to 2011, their relationships with provincial health ministries became progressively more intertwined. Other provider groups sought, often less successfully than medical associations, to protect their interests in the status quo. Outsiders played a similar blocking role in respect of consensus and counter-consensus reform proposals in the other two domains, delivery arrangements and program content.

In the case of provincial medical associations, much of their influence was taken for granted and in some sense barely noted, not only by the public but even by physicians. This was especially so for some non-decisions. For example, almost every commission and task force that proposed regionalization of health-care delivery insisted that the regional authorities should be responsible for medical budgets. Governments knew that medical associations would strongly oppose the transferring of medical budgets to regional authorities. They therefore chose to ig-nore these proposals, and the idea disappeared as an issue. In speaking of the power of the Alberta Medical Association (AMA), its executive director has stated, "It's not so much what we can do on our own, which is minimal actually, but it's what we can stop, which is a lot" (cited in Archibald and Jeffs 2004).

Delivery arrangements touched Canadians directly. When concerned about developments, the public found a way of communicating with government, albeit not necessarily directly. Civil society groups were, however, quick to draw attention to delivery issues. A majority of Canadians also showed strong support for the values embedded in univer-sal, pan-Canadian, publicly administered and publicly financed hospital and medical services. That politicians took this attachment seriously was reflected in the behaviour of federal and provincial political parties. All parties that aspired to form a government consistently declared their fealty to the *Canada Health Act* or its values. This federal statute set out the broad criteria and conditions that provincial health insurance law was required to meet in order for provincial health services to qualify for federal financing (discussed further below). Polling data showed that this program, medicare—in essence a provincially administered and financed insurance program, within a framework set by the federal government and with some federal government financial support—was seen by a large majority of Canadians as "embracing Canadian values" (Mendelsohn 2002, 27-28) and as "fundamental to the nature of Canada" (Soroka 2007, 5). Public opinion resisted counter-consensus reform propos-als that threatened to weaken the medicare legacy, as seen in the for-profit delivery case. Beyond our six policy reform issues, any proposals that brought into question the first-dollar coverage of hospital and medical services were quickly countered by civil society groups.

Insiders and outsiders did more than fend off reforms they disliked. They also urged reforms that promoted their values or enhanced their interests. But all political actors were better at defending turf than expanding it. The net effects of their efforts tended to cancel out one another. Insiders made it difficult to achieve consensus reforms in the governance and financial arrangements domains, and also exerted considerable influence on delivery and program content issues. Public opinion and civil society groups made it difficult to achieve consensus and counter-consensus reform proposals in the delivery and program content domains. Together, insiders and outsiders posed major barriers to most reforms.

Factors That Facilitated Reforms

Yet some reform did occur. Given the widespread resistance to governance and financial reforms from within the health sector, for those two domains it took factors exogenous to the decision process to force open the windows of opportunity and allow in the reform winds. Fiscal crisis was one such factor on some issues. Fiscal crises obliged governments to contemplate reforms that were politically difficult but that had the potential to make health care more efficient and help contain costs. For the delivery and program content domains, the exogenous pressures for change were more varied, ranging from values that contested the prevailing dominant values (as reflected in the medicare legacy) to technological change.

A further factor associated with reform applied to all four policy domains. It was political change. Of the 30 cases analyzed for this book, the largest reforms typically involved an opposition party attaching priority to health care, campaigning on the issue in a general election, and winning the election. The incoming premier then gave political priority to health care (often through appointing a political champion) and took swift action (in the first half of a first mandate). In order to act swiftly, the incoming government had to know what it wanted to achieve and be well prepared organizationally to fulfill its goals. In some situations, knowing how to use the existing public service was sufficient, in others changes in key public servants were required, and in others still mobilizing political staffers or backbenchers was part of the game plan. The alternative political route was through a leadership campaign within a governing party with the successful candidate making health-care reform commitments and acting on them quickly.

The keys to success were thus mainly exogenous. Political commitment was found to be necessary, but not sufficient, for substantial reform to occur in all four policy domains. Organizational preparedness was also needed to make reform happen. Values were not associated with more or less reform among the 30 cases.

Legacies and Lessons from the Past, 1945–1989

The past always influences the present and future. In the final section of this introduction, we note five factors associated with the years from 1945 to 1989 that cast light on or had implications for the period we studied (1990–2003) and the update (2004–2011). First is the broad consensus that health insurance was the priority issue for the health sector during the earlier period. Second, there was the clarity of policy choice associated with the insurance priority. It was possible to articulate the policy options in a manner that enabled people to understand trade-offs. The third relates to the impact of federalism on reform. The next is the *Canada Health Act* as symbol, and the last the relationship between provincial governments and provincial medical associations.

Health Insurance: The Priority Issue

During the years from 1945 to 1985, health insurance was the priority health policy issue for Canadians. While there were divergent views about how to achieve insurance coverage, there was little disagreement on its importance.

This consensus was a legacy of the 1930s and Second World War. Many Canadians had endured years of penury and desperation during the Great Depression of the 1930s. During the war years, they had paid even more dearly in lives lost, ruined health, and fiscal resources. As the war drew to a close the public mood, in Canada and other democracies, was one that demanded a better world. Individuals and families had done their fair share, and often vastly more, for society. Now it was society's turn to reward the individuals who had given so much for their country.

The Dominion had prepared for the postwar world. In its White Paper on Employment and Income (Canada 1945) and Green Book on Reconstruction (Dominion-Provincial Conference 1946), the federal Liberal government outlined a new social contract for Canadians. To achieve high and stable levels of employment and income, the government committed to facilitate private enterprise as an engine for job growth, to use public enterprise where the public interest required it for national economic development, and to offset periods of weak labour markets through macroeconomic counter-cyclical policy (fiscal and monetary policy), automatic stabilizers (unemployment insurance), and trade liberalization. A second set of commitments was directed at war veterans to help their integration into society. A third focus was on social insurance. To avoid a return to the social insecurity that had prevailed in the 1930s, the Dominion government further undertook to protect individuals against the contingencies of unemployment, sickness, and old age (Dominion-Provincial Conference 1946, 59). With respect to sickness, in particular, the vast majority of Canadians had no hospital or medical insurance, private or public. Given the constitutional division of powers that assigned the lion's share of law-making authority on illness and injury to the provinces, the Dominion's plans on health were predicated on provincial agreement. Fulfilling the part of that commitment that involved hospital and medical services took a quarter century and then some additional time when the bargain was subsequently challenged. It required deep commitment to achieve what was done.

Compared to the 1945–1989 years, during the period we studied there was less societal consensus about health priorities. It had taken cataclysmic change to facilitate the priority-setting in the post–Second World War years. The absence of clear priorities in the 1990s and beyond was thus not so much a character flaw as a sign of the times. But it affected the record of achievement.

Competition of Ideas and Interests, and Policy Choice

During the decades after the war, there was a competition of ideas and interests about how to act on the insurance priority. It can be thought of in terms of two axes of policy choice that sometimes intersect and sometimes do not. On one axis were a range of possibilities from the idea that health insurance should be mainly a matter of personal responsibility and individual choice to the opposite view that it should be mainly universal and mandatory as a matter of law. What were the trade-offs? Was the answer the same for all health services?

A second axis related to the role of government. Was this a matter for each province to decide alone within its own legislative jurisdiction? Or should the decision-making involve the federal government in partnership with the provinces? The implication of federal-provincial partnership was that the federal government would pay a share of the costs.

In practice, the intersection of these two axes created three policy paradigms. One is described as the "Canada-wide public payment/private delivery" paradigm, the "Canada-wide public payment" paradigm or just the "Canada-wide" paradigm. This paradigm, reflected in the Green Book on Reconstruction (Dominion-Provincial Conference 1946, 86-93), had government as the single payer but variation in delivery. In everyday language this is what Canadians now call "medicare." For medical services, the Canada-wide paradigm contemplated a continued large role for fee-for-service physicians and close to an exclusive role for private not-for-profit corporations in the delivery of hospital services.

A second paradigm favoured "private payment/private delivery." It reflected the view that individuals should be responsible for their health-care costs and that the market would provide a choice of competing insurers. For-profit delivery would be common, including in the hospital sector. Provincial governments would play a residual role by subsidizing the insurance of the poor. The federal government had no status in this paradigm.

"Provincial payment/private delivery" was the third paradigm. It involved the individual province as payer with delivery as in the Canada-wide paradigm. Like the Canada-wide paradigm, it too contemplated a continued large role for fee-for-service physicians and close to an exclusive role for private not-for-profit corporations in the delivery of hospital services.

In some provinces the governmental axis (exclusively provincial versus provincial/federal cooperation) was dominant. For example, the government of Quebec has consistently objected to any role for the federal government, whether the government in power leaned to private payment or public payment (Quebec 1998). The government of Alberta has traditionally leaned in that direction also. Conversely, in some other provinces, more weight was assigned to the payment axis. The government of Saskatchewan argued for a Canada-wide public payment arrangement for hospital services in the mid-1940s. But when it was not forthcoming, the government undertook its own hospital insurance plan. A similar set of events accompanied Saskatchewan's introduction of medical insurance.

The three paradigms reflected well the competing ideas and interests that were current and made it relatively easy to understand policy choices and their consequences.

Impact of Federalism on Reform

In the above discussion of barriers to reform and factors that facilitated reform, there is no mention of the "federal government" or "federal-provincial relations." Does this mean that Canada's federal system was a relatively small factor in explaining outcomes?

Federalism may have made a difference in two ways. One was by acting directly on the dependent variables (that is, the actual decision to be made). The second was through indirect routes. With respect to direct effects, the analysis will show that the federal government and federal-provincial relations had a small (barely perceptible) influence on the reform outcomes in the 30 cases taken as a whole.

Yet the history of medicare in Canada prior to 1990 is untellable without an understanding of federalism. At different points along the road different actors prevailed: a single province (Saskatchewan) blazed a trail twice; Ottawa led on several occasions, pulling recalcitrant provinces along; groups of provinces led, dragging Ottawa and other provinces forward on hospital insurance; and all jurisdictions agreed to the creative use of ambiguity (conditional opting out) to sustain harmony in a federation with much diversity. Put simply, when reform is attempted at the Canada-wide level, whether successfully or not, federalism is a major factor shaping reform decisions. When reform is not countrywide, it follows that federal-provincial relations and the federal government are less visibly engaged. But federalism may be influencing events or non-events in other indirect ways.

For example, the policy agenda of the federal Liberal government of Jean Chrétien, during its first five-to-six years in office (1993 to 1998/99), was quite different from that of most provinces. It emphasized divisive issues in federal-provincial relations, drawing the attention of the media and the public away from important reform issues that were within provincial jurisdiction. A second and closely related example stems from one of those divisive issues. We are referring here to the large cut in federal cash transfers to the provinces announced in 1995 and implemented in part beginning in the 1996/97 fiscal year. With a time lag, provincial premiers decided to give the restoration of these fiscal transfers top billing in their relations with Ottawa. In so doing, they diverted energy that might have been directed to health reform.

The *Canada Health Act* as Symbol

The *Medical Care Act, 1966* required that provincial medical insurance plans provide, as a condition of federal matching grants, for the furnishing of "insured services upon uniform terms and conditions" and that the compensation arrangements for physicians "not impede or preclude, either directly or indirectly whether by charges made to insured persons or otherwise, reasonable access to those services by insured persons" (section 4). "Reasonable access" was not defined. By the late 1970s, six provinces allowed extra-billing as part of their accommodation of the medical profession (Tuohy 1999, 93). Physicians in some of the permissive provinces began to step up "extra-billing," and their freedom to do so was supported by their provincial governments (Taylor 2009, 428-62; Tuohy 1999, 93-95). This triggered a series of responses in Ottawa that led ultimately to the enactment in 1984 of the *Canada Health Act* (CHA) with all-party support. The CHA authorized the federal government to impose financial penalties on provinces to the extent of extra-billing by physicians or user charges by hospitals and clinics. The aim of the penalty provisions was to discourage provinces from allowing these charges. It is the symbolic aspect of the CHA and the politics of the process that led to it, however, that are of interest here.

By restating and clarifying the broad principles of the old hospital and medical insurance legislation, the CHA gave enhanced profile to the overarching health "rights" of Canadians within the Canadian social contract.[8]

The process leading up to the *CHA* involved much acrimony between the federal government and several provincial governments and between the federal government and medical associations. In separate actions, the Canadian Medical Association and the Ontario Medical Association (OMA) unsuccessfully challenged the constitutionality of the *CHA* (dealt with together by the court). Physicians in Ontario went on strike. The last recourse for the OMA was public opinion. The language it used was seemingly intended to bring the public to see the *CHA* as threatening the quality of medical care (Taylor 2009, 455-60).

Public opinion polls helped settle the matter. An Environics Poll in 1977 had asked the following question: "Should medical care be guaranteed by the government?" The answer "yes" was given by 72 percent of respondents. The question was repeated in 1985, the year after the *Canada Health Act* was enacted, and again in 1991. The percentages answering "yes" were 95 and 96 (cited in Mendelsohn 2002, 27). In 1998 a poll by Earnscliffe found that over 86 percent of respondents agreed that "medicare embodies Canadian values" (ibid.). It had thus become near-impossible for any government or would-be government to question the merits of the Canada-wide pubic payment paradigm.

Many years after the enactment of the *Canada Health Act*, Monique Bégin, the former federal minister of health who had led the Liberals on this issue, acknowledged that medicare, as reflected in the *CHA*, had acquired a symbolic status. She also argued that it had become too narrow, too restrictive: "Legislation based solely on hospitals and doctors, as is the *CHA*, is not appropriate at all, and is even detrimental to good health policy" (Bégin 2002, 4). She argued that it could and should be reopened and proposed a list of reforms that included most of the issues that had been part of the First Ministers' Accord in 2000.

Bégin may not have been wrong that the issue should be reopened, but it has been more than 10 years since she delivered her message and not much has happened. For leaders to the right-of-centre, it appears that the overall popularity of medicare has entailed political risks vis-à-vis their electorates that they were just not willing to take. For leaders to the left-of-centre, the goal was to extend the services covered by the *CHA*. It appears, however, that they were unwilling to risk reopening the *CHA* without the certainty that the outcome would improve insurance coverage and that commensurate incremental financial resources would be made available for that purpose. Even during the years of fiscal plenty, this would have meant arguing for more money against other worthy causes. Implicit in this latter position was that there was nothing to be gained by attempting to improve the design of the *CHA* (using equity and efficiency criteria) within existing resources, even though it is difficult to find a leader, political or otherwise, who would design the medicare program as it exists now if she or he were starting from scratch. In evolving from a health insurance program to something politically sacred, the

CHA has seemingly narrowed the room for certain kinds of macro-health policy reform. Indeed, it has been argued that the values embedded in the *CHA* have become so entrenched in most provinces, both politically and in provincial health insurance legislation, that the narrowing affects reform prospects in individual provinces as it does at the pan-Canadian level (Gildiner 2006).

Relations between Provincial Governments and Provincial Medical Associations

When individual provinces first began implementing their publicly insured system of medical services, each decided to use the fee schedule of the existing not-for-profit insurance company that was owned or approved by the medical association in that province. This made it unnecessary for provincial governments to develop new fee schedules from scratch or to replace them entirely with alternative payment methods such as capitation or salary. Developing new fee schedules would have required governments to assess the value of primary care physicians relative to specialists and to take a stance as well on the relative value of different kinds of specialists and their procedures. The process would have been technically complex and politically very difficult. Introducing a method of payment other than fee-for-service would have been less technically complex but even more problematic to relations between governments and the medical associations and unions (Quebec only) that represented physicians. In contrast, adopting existing fee schedules was a simple approach. Adopting the schedule was also a way of assuring physicians that neither their livelihood nor manner of serving patients would be endangered by publicly financed medical services. The technical complexity could be avoided in the short run.

The short-run benefits of adopting existing fee schedules had long-run consequences. The adoption of these schedules established a pattern in the relationship between provincial governments and provincial medical associations that continues to this day. On the one side, provincial governments came to rely on medical associations for help in determining how to allocate periodic adjustments to physician fee schedules. On the other, provincial medical associations and unions came to value their insider role in allocating fees. Over time provincial governments recognized the medical associations in their provinces as the sole authorized bargaining agents on behalf of physicians. (Quebec had separate unions representing general practitioners and medical specialists.) Periodically, a newly elected provincial government would question and even challenge this recognition. But in each case the government backed off, apparently deciding that there was more to be lost than gained by challenging organizations representing physician interests.

Negotiating medical services budgets and their allocation was not the only role that provincial medical associations played relative to provincial governments, although it was the most publicized. By the 1990s, the provincial government–provincial medical association relationship had evolved stepwise into something greater (Lomas et al. 1992). Since fee negotiations alone did not provide a firm ceiling on the medical services budget, the fee negotiations were expanded to include items like physician supply and utilization intensity. Lomas et al. (1992) noted that items like the relative value of different services, alternative forms of payment like capitation and salary, and quality assurance also had the "potential" to be absorbed through this channel. They proved prescient. Tuohy (1999) subsequently described the relationship between provincial health ministries and provincial medical associations as one based on "mutual accommodation." Tuohy also observed a trend toward more formality in the way these bodies related to one another and confirmed that the agenda was becoming much broader.

Legislatures have given periodic approval to changes in physician remuneration, and provinces have acknowledged medical associations or unions as exclusive bargaining agents for physicians. But to our knowledge, the wider relationships referred to by Tuohy and Lomas have not been thoroughly debated in any of Canada's legislative bodies. They appear not to have been anticipated in the 1960s and 1970s when medical insurance was introduced. But they flowed logically out of the decisions taken then to continue with fee-for-service as the prime mode of physician payment. For more than a decade now, these arrangements have been governed by master agreements between the provinces and their medical associations. These agreements have, on the whole, become increasingly long, formal, and complex. They are also opaque. It is thus difficult for the outside observer to assess their impact.

Road Map

Chapter 2 elaborates on the methodology and theory that underpin our research. Chapters 3 to 7 analyze the six reform issues in Alberta, Saskatchewan, Ontario, Quebec, and Newfoundland and Labrador.

Chapter 8 analyzes the 30 cases to determine the kind of reform and extent of reform in each. It then accounts for the reform decisions, treating the five provinces as a single entity. Using cross-provincial and cross-issue analysis of the 30 cases, chapter 9 provides both a more comprehensive and yet fine-grained explanation of the reform decisions. Chapter 10 provides alternative ways of "measuring" reform. It also compares our findings to the existing literature.

Chapter 11 focuses on the period from 2004 to 2011. It analyzes the extent of reform and the evolution of the factors that shaped outcomes. Chapter

12, the final chapter, links the past to the future, asking what our studies suggest about the prospects for health policy reform going forward.

NOTES

1. These are observations often made by pollsters Nanos Research (2012) and Ipsos-Reid (2010), respectively.
2. The start date for Canada-wide hospital insurance was 1958 and for Canada-wide medical insurance 1966. However, the start date for the first provincial hospital insurance plans was 1 January 1947 and for medical insurance 1962.
3. The annex is based on reviews of these reports undertaken for this project by Kevin O'Fee. The reviews are available on the project website at http://www.queensu.ca/iigr/Res/crossprov.html.
4. Our focus in this book is on health-care *policy* reform, although in some places we refer simply to health-care reform for ease of reading. We acknowledge that much reform often occurs for reasons unrelated to policy change, for example, as a result of new breakthroughs in science and technology.
5. Mendelsohn's "review examined surveys from CROP, Decima, Earnscliffe, Ekos, Environics, Goldfarb, Ipsos-Reid, and POLLARA, as well as Canada Health Monitor/Berger Report, the Centre for Research and Information on Canada's annual 'Portraits of Canada,' and quantitative and qualitative data collected by the National Forum on Health (Government of Canada), the Saskatchewan Public Commission on the Future of Medicare, and a number of international studies" (Mendelsohn 2002, 1).
6. The 2009 OECD figure for total Canadian health expenditure as a share of GDP is slightly above the CIHI figure for the same year. The OECD adjusts national figures to ensure data comparability.
7. In addition to Canada, countries surveyed include Australia, France, Germany, Netherlands, New Zealand, Norway, Sweden, Switzerland, United Kingdom, and United States.
8. The *Medical Care Act, 1966* had no preamble that set out its lofty aims. The *Canada Health Act, 1984* has a preamble that spells out its overarching purposes.

CHAPTER 2

STUDYING HEALTH-CARE REFORMS

JOHN N. LAVIS

The basis of this book is a systematic study of health-care reforms in five Canadian provinces between 1990 and 2003. The beginning of the study period was a time when Canadians appeared to be outliers among high-income countries in considering their health system to "work pretty well" (almost 60 percent) and not need to be "completely rebuilt" (under 5 percent; Abelson et al. 2004). Over the ensuing decade these numbers shifted dramatically: in 1998 a larger proportion of Canadian respondents believed the system needed to be "completely rebuilt" than considered it to "work pretty well." The end of the study period coincided with the years in which the Romanow and Kirby reports were published (Commission on the Future of Health Care 2002; Standing Senate Committee 2002b) and two health accords were negotiated among federal, provincial, and territorial governments (Health Canada 2003, 2004). By then the proportion of Canadian respondents who considered the system needed to be "completely rebuilt" had dropped almost to 1988 levels, but the majority of Canadians believed (or continued since 1998 to believe) that the system still "needs fundamental changes" (Abelson et al. 2004; Health Council of Canada 2010).

As the research team was compiling the results of its analysis, there was a shift in Canadian politics. This shift saw the mainly centre and centre-left federal and provincial governments that were in office during the 1990–2003 period replaced by mainly centre-right governments. For this reason, it was decided to extend the analysis to include the period from 2004 to the end of 2011 to determine what effect this political shift might have had on health-care reforms. This addition to the research study is described in chapter 11. The sole point to note here is that the research for the later period rests on the base of the early (1990–2003) period. This chapter accordingly concentrates primarily on the methodology used for the 1990–2003 study period.

Health-care reform during the study period was something that all governments, a large proportion of the Canadian population, and most policy analysts appeared to believe should be undertaken in order to ensure timely access to high-quality health care for all Canadians and the country's health systems' financial and political sustainability. The rate at which reform took place seemed to be slower or less impactful than many thought desirable. However, health-care policy reform during this period did take place quite rapidly in some subsectors. For example, financial and delivery arrangements within the rehabilitation sector in Ontario changed dramatically over this period (Gildiner 2001). What appeared to move slowly was reform that touched significantly on the core "public payment/private delivery" bargains that underpinned much of the health system (Lavis 2004). The bargain with private practice physicians entailed care with first-dollar, one-tier public (fee-for-service) payment. It has proved remarkably enduring in every province, with reforms primarily taking the form of pilot or demonstration projects (Hutchison, Abelson, and Lavis 2001). The bargain with hospitals predates the bargain with physicians. It entailed private not-for-profit hospitals delivering care with first-dollar, one-tier public payment. Among the five provinces we studied, the hospital bargain was found in some provinces, for example, Ontario and Alberta, and not in others. In Quebec, hospitals became part of the formal public sector with regionalization in 1971, and in rural Newfoundland small cottage hospitals had been part of the public sector prior to its entry into Confederation.

Much of the existing literature on health policy in Canada has involved analysis at the sectorwide level (e.g., Maioni 1998; Tuohy 1999) or the specificities of certain subsectors (e.g., Gildiner 2001). There was a gap, however, between these two levels of study that needed to be bridged. The aim of the research has been to construct the bridge, or at least a large part of it, by focusing on reforms that touch significantly on the core public payment/private delivery bargains or seek to extend them beyond their parameters. By bridging the gap or a good part of it, the study team hoped to illuminate the particular challenges faced by those seeking to lead reform in this contested area as well as the factors that were conducive to reform when it happened. Specifically, the research was designed with four objectives in mind:

1. to describe the policy-making process for a purposively selected sample of six policy issues in each of five different provinces that differ in their affluence, population size, and urban-rural mix (Alberta, Saskatchewan, Ontario, Quebec, and Newfoundland and Labrador);
2. to determine how much reform had occurred as a result of these policy-making processes and identify the factors that explained the policy outcomes;

3. to determine if there were patterns in the factors that explained the policy outcomes across the six policy issues in each province and then across the five provinces; and
4. to draw on the factors identified in pursuing the second third objectives to derive policy implications for provincial/territorial and federal governments seeking to undertake health-care reform that touches significantly on the core "public payment/private delivery" bargains.

When we turned to the cross-provincial and cross-issue analyses and to deriving implications from these analyses, where our focus was much more on understanding why is it so difficult to reform health care in Canada, we addressed four questions:

1. What kind of health-care reform and how much occurred with respect to the six policy issues across five provinces during the 1990–2003 period?
2. Which factors facilitated reform and which factors impeded reform?
3. Was there a pattern in the distribution of factors within or (especially) across provinces and issues?
4. What can be done to create the conditions that make certain kinds of reform more probable and that is consistent with the effective functioning of the federation?

Questions 1 and 2 relate to objective 2, question 3 relates to objective 3, and question 4 relates to objective 4.

IDENTIFYING POLICY ISSUES FOR STUDY

The process of purposively sampling policy issues for study was fundamental to the study. This began by drawing on a sector-specific taxonomy of policy domains. The taxonomy distinguished among governance arrangements, financial arrangements, delivery arrangements, and program content (Lavis et al. 2002; and now fully elaborated at www. healthsystemsevidence.org and in Lavis et al. 2012). Governance arrangements can include who has what policy authority (e.g., centralization or decentralization), organizational authority (e.g., hospital accreditation), commercial authority (e.g., product licensing), and professional authority (e.g., scope of practice), as well as whether and how consumers and stakeholders are involved in decision-making. Financial arrangements can include how revenue is raised for health-care programs/services (i.e., financing), organizations are paid (i.e., funding), and professionals are paid (i.e., remuneration), as well as how products/services are purchased (e.g., prior approval requirements) and how consumers are incentivized (e.g., deductibles). Delivery arrangements can include decisions about how care is designed to meet consumers' needs (e.g., timely access to care), who provides care (e.g., substitution of one professional group for another), where (e.g., high-volume versus low-volume facilities), and with what supports (e.g., safety monitoring and quality-improvement systems). Program content can include which services, drugs, or devices are covered through publicly financed programs (or, while not the situation here, provided publicly through government-owned systems or reimbursed through private insurance systems).

Next the study team drew on the health-care policy literature and 10 key-informant interviews to identify six policy issues where reform had been attempted or undertaken in many if not all Canadian provinces, with at least one policy issue drawn from each of the aforementioned domains (Table 2.1). One of the policy issues—regionalization of health services delivery (a form of decentralization from provincial governments to subprovincial authorities)—was drawn from the domain of governance arrangements (Lomas, Wood, and Veenstra 1997). Two of the policy issues—needs-based funding for health regions/districts and alternative payment plans for physicians—were examples of changes to financial arrangements. Two of the policy issues—for-profit delivery of medically necessary services and waiting-list management—were examples of changes to the delivery arrangements domain. And one policy issue— establishing the terms of a prescription drug plan—was drawn from the program content domain.

Finally, for each issue the study team drew on the health-care policy literature, documentary analyses, and key-informant interviews to identify a "policy puzzle"—policy decisions and "non-decisions" or "no go" decisions that differed across provinces in ways that could not be easily explained without recourse to primary data collection (Table 2.1). Each provincial study coordinator then pursued a province-specific question about a policy decision for each policy issue, thereby contributing data to answering six cross-provincial policy puzzles. The policy puzzles related to governance and financial arrangements were and remain highly salient for health-care professionals in Canada. Practitioners care about whether they are accountable to themselves, hospital boards, regional health authorities, or provincial governments; whether resources will be allocated to their regions/districts based on historical factors or need; and how they will be paid, as shown by the activities of their professional associations and umbrella groups (e.g., Canadian Health Coalition). The governance and financial arrangements also have important implications for all Canadians, both as consumers and as the ultimate revenue source for health-care programs (whether as taxpayers, premium payers, or out-of-pocket fee payers), even if these arrangements are not as visible to them. Likewise, the policy puzzles related to delivery arrangements and program content were and remain highly salient for consumers and for health-care professionals in Canada. Consumers, for example, care about the privatization of medically necessary services (particularly hospital and physician services, which they treat differently from other types of services in this regard; Abelson et al. 2004), waiting lists, and access to prescription drugs for themselves and their families.

TABLE 2.1
Policy Issues under Study and Research Questions Asked

Policy Domain	Policy Issue	Research Question (i.e., policy puzzle to be explained)
Governance arrangements	Regionalization of health-services delivery	Why did some provinces establish health regions/ districts to assume responsibility for the management and delivery of a significant range of services, others for the coordination of the management and delivery of a significant range of services, and still others neither?
Financial arrangements	Needs-based funding for health regions/districts	Why did some provinces establish a needs-based funding formula that included health-related (not just demographic) measures of need to allocate funding to regions/districts, others a formula that included just demographic measures of need, and still others neither?
	Alternative payment plans for physicians	Why did some provinces establish an alternative payment plan based on capitation or salary for primary care physicians, others alternative payment plans based on minor modifications to fee-for-service remuneration, and still others neither?
Delivery arrangements	For-profit delivery of medically necessary services	Why did some provinces create a policy framework* that made possible the development of (parallel streams of) private, for-profit delivery of medically necessary services that had historically been delivered in private, not-for-profit hospitals, others framework(s) to constrain such developments, and still others neither?
	Waiting-list management	Why did some provinces establish a wait-list management system, others a wait-list tracking system, and still others neither?
Program content	Prescription drug plans	Why did some provinces establish a universal prescription drug plan in their efforts to cover previously uninsured persons, others a targeted plan, and still others neither?

Notes:
*Policy frameworks were considered to be those policy statements, statutes, and important regulatory decisions governing the delivery of diagnostic, surgical, and outpatient services historically affiliated with hospitals under the *Canada Health Act*; they do not address delisting of medical services or the contracting out of services like laundry.

SELECTING ANALYTICAL FRAMEWORKS TO EXAMINE AGENDAS AND DECISIONS

The research team followed the analytical convention of dividing the policy-making process into four stages was followed. Under this approach an issue makes it onto the governmental agenda (the list of subjects getting attention; Kingdon 2003); an issue makes it onto the decision agenda (the list of subjects that are up for active decision; Kingdon 2003); a choice is made to introduce or modify a policy to address an issue, or a choice is made to maintain the status quo; and (if applicable) a policy or modified policy is implemented. We recognize that such distinctions can be more heuristic than real (Table 2.2). Our focus was on the first three of these four stages. Through a review of the political science and public policy literature, we selected Kingdon's (2003) model of the agenda-setting process as the best suited to understanding the dynamics of governmental and decision agendas. According to this model, an issue comes onto the governmental agenda either because of events within the "problem stream" or events within the "politics stream." An issue comes onto the decision agenda because the problem, policy, and politics streams become coupled, thus creating a window of opportunity for policy choice (Kingdon 2003).

Through a separate comprehensive review of the literature, the study team identified four clusters of factors—institutions, interests, ideas, and external events—and a full array of subclusters that can explain policy choice (Bhatia 2002; Lavis et al. 2012). Institutions can include government structures (Immergut 1992; Pierson 1995), policy legacies (Pierson 1993), and policy networks (Coleman and Skogstad 1990). The core bargains with physicians and hospitals provide classic examples of policy legacies (Lavis 2004). Interests can include many types of actors, but for the purposes of the study distinctions were made among societal interest groups, elected officials, public servants, and researchers, as well as policy entrepreneurs (who can be drawn from any of the aforementioned types of actors; Kingdon 2003). Ideas can include knowledge or beliefs about "what is" (e.g., research knowledge), views about "what ought to be" (e.g., values), and combinations of these two factors (Lavis et al. 2002). External factors can include the release of major reports; political, economic, and technological changes; the emergence of new diseases; and media coverage.

The research team used both frameworks (which are referred to in this volume as the Kingdon and 3I frameworks, respectively) to guide the development of the interview schedule and to support the constant comparative analysis of data from the documentary analyses and interviews within each case study. The cross-provincial and cross-issue analyses drew primarily on the 3I—institutions, interests, and ideas—framework. We return to these issues below.

TABLE 2.2
Analytical Framework Used in the Study

Dependent Variables (and independent variables)	*Definitions (and examples)*
Governmental agenda	"The list of subjects or problems to which governmental officials, and people outside of government closely associated with those officials, are paying some serious attention at any given time" (Kingdon 2003, 3)
• Problems	Problems can come to light through focusing events, a change in an indicator, and feedback from the operation of a current policy or program
• Politics	Politics can include swings in provincial/national mood, changes in the balance of organized forces, and events within government (e.g., election)
Decision agenda	"The list of subjects within the governmental agenda that are [sic] up for active decision" (Kingdon 2003, 4)
• Problems	A problem can be defined as warranting governmental action by comparing current conditions with values concerning more ideal states of affairs, comparing performance with that of other jurisdictions, and putting the subject in one category or another (i.e., framing)
• Policy	A policy can come to policy attention through the diffusion of ideas, feedback from the operation of an existing policy or program, and communication or persuasion
	A policy can be deemed an appropriate solution if it is technically feasible, fits with dominant values and the current provincial/national mood, and is acceptable in terms of budget workability and likely political support or opposition
• Politics	Politics can be conducive to addressing a particular problem with a particular policy if the approach is congruent with the provincial/national mood, enjoys interest group support or lacks organized opposition, and fits the orientations of the current governing party or prevailing legislative coalitions
Policy choice	An explicit decision to change or to maintain the status quo
• Institutions	Institutions include three types of factors: • Government structures (e.g., federal versus unitary government) • Policy legacies (e.g., *Canada Health Act*) • Policy networks (e.g., executive council–appointed committees that involve key stakeholders)

... continued

TABLE 2.2
(Continued)

Dependent Variables (and independent variables)	Definitions (and examples)
• Interests	Interests include five types of actors: • Societal interest groups (e.g., medical associations) • Elected officials • Public servants • Researchers • Policy entrepreneurs (e.g., individuals who can couple a policy to a problem when a political window of opportunity opens)
• Ideas	Ideas include three types of factors: • Knowledge or beliefs about "what is" (e.g., research knowledge) • Views about "what ought to be" (e.g., values) • Knowledge and values combined
• External	External factors originate outside the immediate policy community under study, but they must in turn manifest themselves as institutions, interests, or ideas within the immediate policy community (e.g., societal interest groups may mobilize the media on a given issue). External factors include • release of major reports (e.g., commission reports) • political change (e.g., election or cabinet shuffle) • economic change (e.g., recession) • technological change (e.g., new imaging technology) • new diseases (e.g., severe acute respiratory syndrome) • media coverage (e.g., emergency room overcrowding)

COLLECTING AND ANALYZING DATA RELATED TO AGENDAS AND DECISIONS

For each policy decision under study, provincial study teams typically conducted a detailed documentary analysis, developed a timeline of key events related to the policy decision, conducted interviews with a purposive sample of public policy-makers and stakeholders who were familiar with the policy-making process, and analyzed the resulting data using the analytical frameworks described above.

For each documentary analysis, provincial study teams typically searched

- bibliographic databases to identify published descriptive or analytical research related to the policy issue or the broader policy area (all study teams except the one in Newfoundland and Labrador);

- media databases to identify coverage of events leading up to and including the policy decision (all study teams, although in Newfoundland and Labrador this was done primarily for the regionalization, wait-list management, and prescription drug case studies, and in Saskatchewan this involved a manual search of print media archives);
- Hansard to identify parliamentary debates related to the policy decision (all study teams); and
- websites and old telephone directories of relevant government departments to reconstruct the organizational chart for the periods when the policy decision was made and identify potential key informants (all study teams, although in Newfoundland and Labrador this was done primarily for the regionalization, alternative payment plan, and wait-list management case studies).

The provincial study teams developed a timeline of key events related to each policy decision, except for Newfoundland and Labrador where five decisions were "no go." The events include significant media coverage of related issues or actions, media releases or other public statements by government and stakeholder groups, releases of consultation documents or research reports, elections or cabinet shuffles, the policy decision itself as well as any related decisions, and any other events that appeared closely related to the policy decision. Each timeline typically consisted of the dates when each event occurred, a description of the event, the "institutions" (e.g., Ministry of Health) and key individuals involved in the event, historical references (e.g., media coverage), a brief comment on the "ideas" in play, a brief analysis of the significance of the event, and any more recent references (e.g., websites). The study teams that had constructed full timelines also developed a short version of the timeline for use in their interviews (the only exception being the prescription drug plan reform in Saskatchewan, which evolved so rapidly), which the provincial study coordinators modified as they gained additional insights into the temporal sequencing of key events.

Provincial study team members conducted interviews with a purposive sample of public policy-makers (i.e., public servants, politicians, and/or political staff in health and other departments) and stakeholders (e.g., heads of civil society groups and health professional associations) who were familiar with each policy-making process. The provincial study teams drew on the documentary analysis and timeline to identify each purposive sample, taking care to seek out a mix in the types of public policy-makers and stakeholders, as well as to seek out those who did not appear in either the documentary analysis or the preliminary timeline but who were identified by other study participants as playing an important role or having a unique perspective to offer about key events.

Typically one individual conducted all interviews in each province, but at least two individuals were involved in the analysis. Interviewees used a semi-structured interview guide coupled with (in most provinces) the short timeline that was provided as a prompt at the beginning of each interview. The interview guide dealt with each stage of the policy-making process in turn (i.e., governmental agenda, decision agenda, and policy choice) and within each stage dealt with the key individuals and groups, the perspectives they brought forward, and the actions they took. (In some provinces, such as Saskatchewan, the interviewees were not able to distinguish among these stages of policy-making, which may be attributable to the speed of decision-making for four of the six issues, and the analysis therefore focused on policy choice.) The interviews also explored hypotheses that had been developed during the documentary analysis and/or earlier interviews. The study team conducted a total of 238 interviews, with 67 in Alberta, 37 in Saskatchewan, 51 in Ontario, 53 in Quebec, and 30 in Newfoundland and Labrador. Each provincial study team employed a constant comparative method of analysis for each case study, drawing initially on the Kingdon and 3I frameworks described above, and proceeding iteratively to identify recurrent themes. The teams analyzed each stage of the policy-making process separately to the extent that documentation and interviews allowed. They also identified any discordance among interviews, or between interviews and publicly available documents. The provincial study teams did not engage in member checking. Each team wrote its case studies using a common methodology, but the style of presentation was decided by the provincial study coordinators. More details on methodology are provided on-line at http://www.queensu.ca/iigr/Res/crossprov.html.

CODING AND ANALYZING DATA ACROSS PROVINCES AND ISSUES

Drawing on 30 case studies (six policy issues, whether they involved decisions or "non-decisions," in each of five provinces), the central project coordinator identified a range of additional codes that facilitated cross-provincial and cross-issue analyses (chapters 8 and 9), applied the codes to each case study, sought feedback from the provincial study coordinators, and iteratively revised the codes based on this feedback and continued analyses.

Two sets of codes assist with describing the nature and extent of reform (i.e., our dependent variables):

1. The nature of reform is identified as being pro-reform, anti-reform, or counter-consensus relative to the grey literature. Factors that facilitate reform in the direction recommended by the grey literature are pro-reform. Both anti-reform influences and counter-consensus reforms

indicate opposition to the recommendations of the grey literature. However, anti-reform suggests attachment to the status quo, whereas counter-consensus reform indicates opposition to the status quo and movement in the opposite direction than that proposed in the grey literature (e.g., Saskatchewan reducing prescription drug coverage at a time when most calls were for expanded coverage).

2. The extent of reform is identified as being none, limited, moderate, significant, or comprehensive depending on the extent to which a provincial reform met the various elements that constituted the grey literature consensus in a given area (see annex 1 for details).

As noted in chapter 1, the grey literature refers to the major reports published during the study period and in the half-decade preceding it, particularly the systemwide reports that dealt with two or more of the six policy issues. These reports were often commissioned by provincial governments (four of the five provinces each published two reports during the period), less commonly by the federal government (with three reports published), and rarely by stakeholder groups (e.g., Canadian Medical Association). The first wave of such reports appeared in the mid-to-late 1980s and early-to-mid 1990s, a period of fiscal restraint (e.g., Commission d'enquête sur les services de santé et les services sociaux 1988; Health Canada 1997; Premier's Commission on Future Health Care for Albertans 1989a, 1989b). The second wave appeared in the late 1990s and early 2000s, by which time the fiscal situation had improved (e.g., Government of Newfoundland and Labrador 2002b; Commission on the Future of Health Care 2002; Ontario Health Services Restructuring Commission 2000). The same standard—whatever reform was advocated in relation to a given issue by all or a plurality of reports—was applied across all provinces regardless of the specifics of the report(s) from that province. The study team focused on the grey literature in order to avoid expressing normative preferences for what constituted "good" or "bad" reforms.

Having one set of codes and one categorization scheme for codes also assisted with describing the factors that influenced the nature and extent of reform in the 30 case studies. Note that the terms *factor, influence, independent variable,* and simply *variable* are used interchangeably in this volume. The categorization scheme indicated (a) whether a factor that influenced a policy decision was "major" or not; and (b) whether a factor could be considered endogenous or exogenous to the policy-making process that culminated in any given policy decision. As the case study findings were compiled and assessed in relation to research objective 3, an independent variable was occasionally relabelled (from the label used in Table 2.2) to make its meaning clearer or variables were grouped differently than initially anticipated to respond to patterns emerging in the data. For example, the original variable "political change (e.g., election or cabinet shuffle)" became "change in government/government leader that committed to reform through an election or leadership process and that acted expeditiously on the commitments upon taking office." Further, some interests were grouped as "insider interests."[1]

The advantage of coding the data in this way is that it allowed us to determine the frequency of association between independent variables and policy outcomes and, as a subset of that determination, the association between the independent variables that were most important (called "major" factors) and policy outcomes. These determinations were the basis for cross-provincial and cross-issue analyses. The downside is that it conveys a precision that qualitative data inherently lack. For example, it is a judgment call as to whether medical opposition to alternative payment plans should be coded as a policy legacy (i.e., the public payment/private delivery bargain) or as an insider interest. By being transparent about all aspects of the approach to coding (see annex 2 for details), we enable readers to assess the impacts of the coding approach on the conclusions.

EXTENDING THE ANALYSIS TO 2004–2011

As noted in the introduction to this chapter, the analysis was extended to include the period from 2004 to the end of 2011, which was a period of primarily centre-right governments. Our analysis of this recent period focused on three specific research questions.

The first question was whether the direction and magnitude of reform (i.e., the dependent variable in the analysis) had remained constant or had changed relative to the findings for the 1990–2003 study period. For this purpose, the study team took as the baseline the findings from each of the 30 case studies from 1990 to 2003 and analyzed the trajectory of policy reform in 2004–2011 relative to that earlier period. Three possibilities were examined in each of the 30 cases: (a) no change in the momentum of reform toward the grey literature consensus in the 2004–2011 period relative to the 1990–2003 period; (b) accelerated or new momentum toward the grey literature consensus in the 2004–2011 period relative to the 1990–2003 period; and (c) decelerated momentum toward the grey literature consensus or reversed direction with respect to the consensus in the 2004–2011 period relative to the 1990–2003 period.

The second question was whether the major independent variables from the 1990–2003 period remained important influences on the policy-making process in the 2004–2011 period. Unlike the first period, where independent variables were analyzed on a case-by-case basis and then aggregated in the cross-provincial and cross-issue analyses, in the second period we analyzed the independent variables in a more general way across all provinces and issues.

The third question was whether the major independent variables from the 1990–2003 period explained any of the three possibilities examined as part of the first question. The methodology is described further in chapter 11.

In the next five chapters, each of the five provincial reform experiences is described in turn. These chapters, and the case studies that underlie them, are the principal source for the coding for the 1990–2003 period described above.

NOTE

1. These adjustments are described fully in chapter 8. Moreover, the details about all factors are provided in annex 2 so that the reader can explore alternative categorizations of the independent variables.

Chapter 3

Health Reform in Alberta: Fiscal Crisis, Political Leadership, and Institutional Change within a Single-Party Democratic State

John Church and Neale Smith

Introduction

Like other Canadian provinces, Alberta undertook significant health-care reforms during the 1990s. The Alberta approach, while driven by fiscal pressures similar to those experienced by other provinces, was shaped by its own unique interplay of institutions, ideas, interests, technological change, and economic forces. A growing fiscal crisis, combined with a change in political leadership, but not in the governing party, led to aggressive reform in health care. Once economic growth returned, commitment to health-care reform waned. However, the enduring legacy of initial health reforms has been a shift away from the Ministry of Health and local health-care in decision-making institutions and interests (i.e., traditional forms of governance) to new decision-making institutions and interests (i.e., new forms of governance). Overall, this had a centralizing effect on decision-making.

The intent of this chapter is to discuss how Alberta addressed health policy reform around six key policy decisions: the regulation of health services delivery by private facility operators; the introduction of health regions; the introduction of a population-based funding model to support health regions; the introduction of a voluntary, centralized wait-times registry; the expansion of drug benefits to cover the children of parents moving off of social assistance to return to work, and palliative care patients; and the introduction of an alternative payment plan for physician remuneration aimed mainly at primary care. Although by the criteria employed in this volume, Alberta ranks second after Saskatchewan in terms of the extent of reforms achieved during the time period, only a modest degree of reform, overall, was realized. Significant institutional reform was achieved through regionalization and population-based funding. Privatization, although a priority of the premier, was only moderately achieved. Since the period studied, Alberta has abandoned most of the specific changes it made in favour of other policy options; however, the trend toward more centralized decision-making has continued.

After providing an overview of the political and policy-making context and the relevant sequence of events, the chapter details each of the six cases. The cases are analyzed within a framework that identifies the factors that explain the reform outcomes. The analysis is followed by a brief discussion of why more reform occurred in some cases than in others. The final section of the chapter recaps the major reforms and the roles played by ideas, institutions, interests, economics, and technology. The chapter concludes with a postscript that summarizes what has happened in Alberta in the several years beyond the period of study and why most reform, even that deemed significant, has not endured.

THE POLITICAL AND POLICY-MAKING CONTEXT

Politics in Alberta has several unique aspects that have shaped policy responses historically and during the time frame of the case studies. Among Canadian provinces, Alberta is unique in that it has operated virtually as a one-party state since the mid-1930s, the manifestation of a political culture with an unusual level of ideological cohesion (Bell 1992; Macpherson 1962). The Social Credit Party held power from 1935 until 1971, with Ernest Manning as premier for 25 uninterrupted years. Both Peter Lougheed and Ralph Klein were Progressive Conservative premiers for 14 years before retiring. These long periods of single-leader, single-party domination have reinforced the core political values of the province (Pal 1992, 16-22).

A major element of Alberta's political culture has been the idea that the role of the state is "residual." In this view, the individual is primarily responsible for his or her own well-being. Beyond the individual, the immediate and extended family, local community, and the private market are the sources of relief for personal hardship. Only as a last resort and on a temporary basis should the state become involved in the affairs of the individual (Guest 1997). A hallmark of long-term governments in Alberta has been a preference for private market solutions (Barr 1974; Dyck 1996, 505). Not surprisingly, the province has exhibited a marked tendency toward divestment and decentralization of responsibility for the provision of services to municipal and community levels (Hornick, Thomlison, and Nesbitt 1988, 52). In health care, Alberta has traditionally been reluctant to adopt a state-centred approach to health policy (Boase 1994; Church and Noseworthy 1999, 186-203).

Although private market solutions have been preferred, provincial wealth and intergovernmental pressures have acted as catalysts for state intervention. In this respect, Alberta, like other provinces, allowed progressive expansion in its health-care delivery system from the 1970s to the mid-1980s by financing incremental growth. After coming to power as premier in 1971, Peter Lougheed set about modernizing the province by developing key infrastructure (e.g., hospitals), expanding the health professional workforce, and granting substantial wage increases. Overall, two-thirds of Lougheed's tenure as premier occurred during a time when the province was experiencing unprecedented economic growth.

However, in a dramatic turn of fortune, oil and gas prices declined throughout the early 1980s, leading to a significant decline in resource revenue for government coffers. Although the rate of growth in provincial program expenditure gradually fell to below the inflation rate, the cost of servicing the debt increased significantly, from $22 million in 1981 to $880 million (i.e., 7.3 percent of provincial expenditures) by the 1989/90 fiscal year.[1] Don Getty succeeded Lougheed in 1985. During his years as premier, which ran to 1992, the province accumulated a net debt of $11 billion (Barrie 2004, 261). Limits to public sector wage increases were part of the resulting restraint efforts, which led to increased labour unrest (Tupper, Pratt, and Urquhart 1992, 49-50).[2] Faced with slipping political support in the successive elections of 1986 and 1989 (Pal 1992, 21-24), the Getty government began to consider alternative ways of financing and delivering health care (Alberta Health 1989; Church and Smith 2006; Philippon and Wasylyshyn 1996).

Two major reviews of the overall health system were initiated by the Getty government.[3] The Advisory Committee on the Utilization of Medical Services (i.e., the Watanabe Committee) was established in September 1987. Its mandate was to advise the Minister of Hospital and Medical Services on the "implementation of recommendations ... related to reducing or controlling increases in utilization of medical services" (Alberta Health 1989, 94). Three months later, the Premier's Commission on the Future of Health Care for Albertans was announced; its mandate was to conduct an inquiry on future health requirements for Albertans. The Watanabe Committee relied on expert advice, whereas the Premier's Commission consulted the public more broadly (Premier's Commission 1989a, 11-15). Reports from both processes were released in 1989. Both reports made recommendations on regionalization in health care. The Watanabe Committee recommended regional or local coordination among existing organizations. The Premier's Commission took a significantly different approach and recommended the creation of nine autonomous regional health authorities (1989b, 119). To paraphrase, it proposed a "serious redistribution" of "planning and power" away from Alberta Health to local communities, individuals, and newly created provincial entities. The commission also sounded the alarm on the implications of increasing expenditures in health care, indicating that total existing tax revenues would not be enough to cover the cost of health care (1989b, 107).

When the government's official response was released in November 1991, the vision was consistent with the directions and recommendations of the commission: a health-care system focused on community and individual-level responsibility, and on prevention and population health rather than illness treatment. Yet the government explicitly rejected the creation of autonomous health authorities in favour of a much weaker recommendation for "cooperative planning" at the regional level; that is, the Watanabe approach (Alberta Health 1991a, 39). With an election pending and a strong reaction against regional health authorities, especially in rural constituencies, the government backed away from the health governance issue. However, the Minister of Health foreshadowed what was to come when, in June 1992, she noted that the failure of a cooperative approach to reach solutions, prior to the 1994/95 fiscal year, might result in a more "prescriptive" approach by the provincial government (Alberta Health 1992, 2-3). The Minister of Health also reiterated the fiscal message from the commission that would become a government hallmark after the 1993 election (Alberta Health 1992, 4-5).

As the government moved closer to the 1993 provincial election, the campaign focused attention on a mounting provincial debt of $32 billion that had accumulated during the 1980s, due to deficit budgeting and the major plunge in oil revenues. The government had responded by cutting expenditures and raising taxes but remained unable to overcome the mounting financial problems. The net result was a loss of confidence in the strong state presence that had been initiated by Lougheed in an attempt to diversify the economy (Taras and Tupper 1994, 64).

Aside from these internal problems, the provincial Progressive Conservatives faced significant external challenges from the federal Reform Party, founded in 1987, and the federal Liberals. With a platform of fiscal austerity and smaller government, and its political base in Alberta, the Reform Party was an electoral threat to the provincial Progressive Conservatives. This set the stage for the emergence of a political agenda of radical expenditure reduction. Not surprisingly, political strategists of the provincial Progressive Conservative party argued that failure to address this issue could have serious electoral consequences. Replacement of the federal Progressive Conservatives, who had taken a soft approach to enforcement of the *Canada Health Act* while in power, by the Liberals meant renewed federal interest in health care (Tupper 2001, 465).[4]

The emerging political agenda on fiscal restraint was further solidified when Don Getty resigned as premier and as leader of the Progressive Conservative party and was replaced by Ralph Klein in late 1992. Klein had been quietly campaigning in rural Alberta for two years prior to Getty's resignation. The arrival of Klein signalled a shift in power, as the more moderate and affluent wing of the party, represented by Minister of Health Nancy Betkowski, was swept aside by the more right-wing constituency of the party that focused on fiscal austerity. While Lougheed had prided himself on prosperity through greater provincial develop- ment, one of the costs was bigger government. Klein reinvigorated the party in the 1990s by promising to downsize government and make Alberta prosperous again (Lisac 1995, 43). As such, he forged an alliance between the "conservative populists," concerned with big government, and the business lobby concerned with taxes, royalties, and privatization (Dickerson and Flanagan 1995, 11).

During his leadership campaign, Klein outlined what would become the blueprint for his first term as premier. As Martin (2003, 111) notes,

> [Klein] outlined five principles to restore integrity in government—realistic revenue predictions, a four year promise to eliminate the $2.2 billion deficit, a law prohibiting future deficits, a government retreat into core services and open arms to partnerships with the private sector.

Following the shift in party leadership from Getty to Klein, government embarked on an extensive public consultation process: the provincial roundtables. These roundtables were well-scripted exercises, arguably designed to sell Albertans on the new political agenda prior to a prov- incial election. The first in the series of roundtables on the provincial budget, held in the spring of 1993, was designed to convince Albertans that there was simply no alternative but to cut costs quickly or put the security of future generations in jeopardy (Lisac 1995, 85-90; Mansell 1997, 52). Given the significant anti-cutbacks coalitions that emerged in the late 1980s among school boards, municipalities, social service agen- cies, and public sector unions, reaching this consensus was no small feat (Tupper 2001, 465).

As part of its election strategy, the government passed the *Deficit Elimination Act* in the spring of 1993. The Act required government to eliminate the deficit within the next electoral mandate. Armed with this legislation and public confirmation of its political agenda through the roundtables, Klein called a provincial election and won a majority of seats in the provincial legislature.

Following closely on the heels of the election, government initiated a second series of roundtables solely focused on health care in August and September of 1993. The conclusions of these roundtables were consistent with the larger political agenda of fiscal restraint (Lisac 1995). Following the roundtables, the Health Planning Secretariat, a committee of the Legislative Assembly appointed by the premier to develop an implementation plan for health care, released a report entitled *Starting Points*. Based on the committee's interpretation of the roundtable discussions, the report recommended a "consumer-first" focus for service delivery, including maximum access and maximum choice; creation of a unified administrative and governance structure; integration of health services and institutions; a "wellness" focus to regional health services; greater opportunities for non-profit associations and the private sector to provide facilities; a funding formula for health regions; and a clear definition of roles for all major stakeholders (Alberta Health Planning Secretariat 1993).

Having legitimized the political agenda with an electoral mandate to cut costs and implement health-care reform, the government announced its Three-Year Business Plan for the Ministry of Health. This included planned expenditure reductions of $734 million (approximately 18 percent), from $4.2 billion in 1992/93 to $3.4 billion in 1996/97 (Alberta Health 1994). The major thrust of this reduction was directed at the acute care sector; for example, hospital beds were reduced from 4.5 beds to 2.4 beds per 1,000 people.

Two factors aided Klein in his early success as premier. The first was that although the provincial Liberal Party, under Laurence Decore, had presented Klein with a large opposition in 1993, and given him a good run for his money, once Decore departed from provincial politics the opposition became weaker in each succeeding election. That Decore had originally challenged Klein on a similar platform of fiscal restraint, but lost, meant that there was no alternative political agenda in the wake of the 1993 election.

Second, as the price of oil and gas recovered by 1996 and subsequently spiked by the end of the decade, government revenues rose to unsurpassed levels; thus, the government was able to balance its budget by early 1995, within the first Klein mandate, and run significant surpluses until late 2008 when oil and gas prices began to decline again. Within this context, the government was able to meet any political challenge with increased public expenditures (Barrie 2004, 267-69); however, the momentum for significant reforms in health dwindled once the larger fiscal crisis dissolved. By 1995, opposition to further expenditure cuts had begun to galvanize, and by 1996 government had started "reinvesting" in health care.

THE SIX CASES

Regionalization (1994)

Regionalizing Alberta's health services was seen as one way that the Alberta government could better manage its health expenditures.[5] The particular question examined in this first case study is, Why did the Government of Alberta establish regional health authorities (RHAs) to assume responsibility for the management and delivery of a significant range of health services?

In 1994, once fiscal targets were established at the provincial level, the government introduced Bill C-20 for the disestablishment of 200 local hospitals, public health boards, and continuing care boards, and the creation of 17 regional health authorities (RHAs) and two provincial health authorities, each with appointed governance boards and management infrastructures. The resulting legislation, the *Regional Health Authorities Act*, created RHAs responsible for the planning and delivery of a wide range of health services, within consolidated regional global budgets. This involved both the divestiture of programs and services previously planned or provided directly by the province, such as home care and communicable disease control, and the consolidation of existing acute care, home care, continuing care, and public health services under the new organizational structures. Mental health was to be phased into the responsibility of RHAs, while the Provincial Cancer Board would remain separate. Notable for their exclusion from the regional umbrella of service delivery responsibilities were ambulance services, which continued to be the responsibility of municipalities; physicians' services, which continued to be delivered by independent, fee-for-service physicians negotiating with the province through their provincial association; and services provided by non-hospital pharmacists.

Initial members of the regional health authority boards were appointed by the Minister of Health, in 1994 until July 1996, at which time a second wave of appointments occurred. In addition to governance by RHAs at the regional level, the legislation also mandated the creation of community health councils to act in an advisory capacity to RHAs.

What is most significant about this case is the impact it had on the local political power base specific to health care. Historically, the delivery of hospital services had been strictly a local concern. In most provincial jurisdictions, enabling legislation allowed local municipalities to raise revenues, through taxation, to build and fund hospitals. Legislation also enabled the establishment of local public health boards. Within the larger context of medical politics, physicians and locally elected or appointed hospital boards played a pivotal role in the development and operation of community hospitals. Subsequently, the entry of the provincial government into the health-care marketplace during the late 1950s shifted the source of funding for hospital services from the local to the provincial level; however, local hospital boards and local public health boards remained intact. In this context, the provincially elected member of the Legislative Assembly (MLA) assumed a key role as broker for local health-care interests within the provincial political arena (Lavis 2002; Taylor 2009). The shift to health regions disrupted this arrangement by eliminating local hospital and public health boards and diminishing the role of the MLA as broker for local health-care interests. As described below, the institutional changes precipitated by regionalization created new opportunities to address other fundamental health policy issues.

Population-Based Funding (1997)

Inherent in the introduction of a regionalized health system, with significant governance and service delivery integration, was the development of new funding mechanisms. [6] Prior to regionalization, Alberta had multiple funding formulas and processes for acute care, long-term care, public health, emergency, and home care programs and services. During the 1980s, various efforts were made to address weaknesses in these existing funding approaches (Smith and Church 2008). The introduction of RHAs motivated the government to develop a new formula for funding health regions that integrated historical, per capita, and population considerations. For this case, we asked the following question: Why did Alberta introduce a population-based funding model for regional health authorities?

The province's intent to regionalize the health system was stated in the *Starting Points* report, following the 1993 post-election Provincial Roundtables on Health. The document's comments about potential funding of the new RHAs foreshadowed many elements of the new model, including geographic and population indicators and the right of patients to access services anywhere in the province. After several years of studying the issue, including reviewing funding arrangements in Finland, Britain, and Saskatchewan, the government announced a new funding formula.

The population-based funding (PBF) model for RHAs was implemented for the 1997/98 fiscal year. Approximately 46 percent of the province's health expenditures were covered by the model; the balance was accounted for by provincewide services and other special allocations. Five key points are worth noting about the population-based funding model. First, it began with per capita allocations to the RHAs. Second, the per capita numbers were adjusted to account for certain measures of "need." Third, additional adjustments were made to account for the special circumstances of remote areas. Fourth, the model required that RHAs, whose residents received care outside their boundaries, reimburse the regions that provided such care for the cost of these treatments (i.e., an "import/export" adjustment). Fifth, a no-loss provision guaranteed that RHAs' funding would not be reduced from what would have been allocated under the previous system.

Under this model, funding levels for each RHA were determined first by calculating the total population, using data from the Alberta Health Care Insurance Plan registry. This was adjusted for age, gender, Aboriginal population (under 65 years of age), and low-income population (under 65 years of age). Other modifiers, such as standardized mortality rates, were considered but rejected, despite being recommended by a number of academics. There was also additional funding (i.e., "assured access"), outside population-based funding, for remote populations and a special allocation (i.e., the "cost of doing business") for the five northernmost RHAs.

Although the funding formula was reviewed and adjusted several times after its implementation, it continued to be the predominant means of funding services provided by RHAs throughout and beyond the period of our analysis.

Alternative Payment Plans (1998)

The Alberta Medical Association (AMA) negotiated several multiyear, master agreements with the Ministry of Health regarding physician reimbursement. Since the introduction of capped budgets,[7] the AMA has determined the distribution of the funding, within the collective agreement, across medical specialties. As a rule, master agreements did not specify clear deliverables on the part of individual physicians. After several years of negotiations, which were compelled by the fiscal crisis, the AMA and the government reached agreement introducing an alternative payment plan (APP) option as part of the 1998 Master Agreement. In this case, we examined why, in 1998, Alberta chose to introduce an APP (capitation) as an addition to existing payment mechanisms, and to develop a common set of principles to govern all physician remuneration models.

While a capped budget, with a 5.5 percent increase, had been negotiated between the Getty government and the AMA in 1992, the Klein government pressured physicians to accept new arrangements, including significant reductions in their compensation. Threatened by a potential cut of 40 percent (approximately $100 million) over three years, and the possible devolution of the physician service budget to RHAs, the AMA adopted a proactive response by suggesting APPs as a cost-saving measure. For government bureaucrats, APPs represented not only an opportunity for immediate savings but also a means to make physicians more responsible and accountable (AMA 1993).

In the 1995 negotiation, the AMA suggested a form of capitation payment, a fee-for-comprehensive-care model, as an additional means to fee-for-service by which physicians might be reimbursed (AMA, n.d.).

While negotiators on both sides of the table were in favour of the proposal, the deal was rejected by the cabinet and negotiations broke down; consequently, the AMA launched a public relations campaign (AMA 1996). The result, in late 1995, was a Letter of Understanding between the government and the AMA, which placed APPs on the government agenda. The agreement effectively ended the push by government to remove $100 million of funding from physicians, introduced APPs on a pilot project basis, introduced a joint management process, and enabled the RHAs as decision-making partners (Alberta Health, n.d.).

During the next round of negotiations, in 1998, APPs moved from their pilot status into a regular funding stream of the physician services budget, along with fee-for-service. The APP stream had several options including capitation, segregated fee-for-service, or contract. The move to embed APPs within the medical services budget reflected a growing level of trust between Alberta Health and the AMA. It also reflected a growing acceptance, among physicians, of a range of reimbursement methods.

In choosing to add APP (capitation) to a range of existing physician remuneration models, all governed by common guiding principles, Alberta decided to bridge organized medicine's desire to maintain fee-for-service with the political and bureaucratic desire to increase physicians' responsibility and accountability for expenditures within the medical services budget and across the broader system. In addition, the government reaffirmed the AMA's organizational status as the formally recognized, sole representative of physicians in Alberta.

Drug Benefits (1998–1999)

Although Alberta was once an innovator in pharmaceutical policy coverage (Grootendorst 2002), it pursued only incremental changes in drug benefit policies during the Klein "revolution." Illustrative of this approach were government decisions to extend publicly financed drug benefits for palliative care patients and to introduce a Child Health Benefit program for children of low-income families. The research question for this case study was: Why did Alberta expand its prescription drug plan to include palliative care patients and children of low-income families rather than adopt a universal plan?

Despite early government attention to the question of drug coverage—in *Palliative Care: A Policy Framework* (Alberta Health 1993) and the Publicly Funded Drugs in Community Settings Consultation in October 1997—no immediate policy change resulted from either initiative. However, in 1997 the government appointed MLA Dave Broda to head a Policy Advisory Committee on Long-Term Care (hereafter, the Broda Committee) to consult on key issues and recommendations for the future (Alberta Health and Wellness 1999b).

In its *Summary of Consultations with Public, November 1998 to March 1999*, the Broda Committee noted that "in-home intravenous therapy and palliative care drug programmes need to be provided" (Alberta Health and Wellness 1999a, 21). Coinciding with the release of the report was a $3 million commitment for a palliative care drug benefit program.

The second reform initiative, the 1998 Alberta Child Health Benefit Program, resulted from Alberta's commitment to the federal government's National Child Benefit (NCB). Under the NCB, the federal government increased the amount of money it provided to low-income families with children through the Canada Child Tax Benefit. Provinces had the opportunity to reduce their transfer payments to these families by an equivalent amount, as long as the savings were reinvested in other programs that provided benefits to the families. Each province could design specific programs in at least one of five areas: earned income supplements, child/daycare initiatives, early childhood services and services for children at risk, supplemental health benefits, and other initiatives (Government of Canada 2005).

Alberta extended coverage for optical and dental services, diabetic supplies, emergency ambulance transportation, and premium-free prescription drugs to the children of families leaving social assistance so that they could still access benefits that had previously been provided through the welfare system. This met the NCB objectives of addressing child poverty and "increas[ing] attachment to the workforce." It was initially estimated that 115,000 children would be eligible for these benefits (Government of Canada 1998); in 2002, the province reported that "approximately one-third [66,293] of eligible families enrolled" in the program (Alberta Human Resources and Employment 2002). In the 2003/04 fiscal year, Alberta Human Resources and Employment spent approximately $21 million on this program. This amount represented 2.7 percent of its spending on "People Investments" and about 1.9 percent of its total annual budget.

In summary, developments in public prescription drug coverage in Alberta during the 1990s were driven most strongly by ideological factors. Conservative governments were consistently opposed to universal programs and collective responsibility, as demonstrated by private coverage and copayments within public programs. Only select groups for which the public felt some sympathy and understood to be deserving became the beneficiaries of public programs. The lack of strong interest group voices meant that coverage expanded incrementally, as new services, based on existing models, were developed and as political attention temporarily shifted to focus on drugs.

Privatization (2000)

Technological change overshadowed many significant health reforms in Alberta.[8] The increasing capacity to perform complex interventions outside traditional health-care institutional settings led to the emergence of an increasing number of private clinics in Alberta (and elsewhere). In Alberta, where these activities were not regulated, significant growth occurred during the 1980s. The combination of unchecked market growth, shrinkage in the public sector, and pressure from citizens and the federal government to regulate this market led the Government of Alberta to pass legislation, in 2000, to regulate relationships between health regions and private contractors in providing certain "publicly funded" surgical services in private, for-profit facilities. The question that concerns us in this case is: Why did Alberta create policy frameworks that made possible private, for-profit delivery of medically necessary services that had historically been delivered in private, not-for-profit hospitals?

Given major budget reductions, the capacity of the health-care system since 1993 has been significantly reduced. In essence, the retreat of the Alberta government from the health-care marketplace created opportunities for medical entrepreneurs. As such, the government intended to encourage increased private-sector involvement in the delivery of services.

During the 1990s, the provincial government fought a running battle with local public interest groups and the federal government. While the province seemed willing to let private operators move in to occupy the market share vacated by the public sector, a local coalition of citizen and labour groups—Friends of Medicare—and the federal government became increasingly concerned that such activities directly violated the *Canada Health Act* and threatened the viability of the publicly funded health-care system. The ensuing debate was sustained by federal and provincial responses to the activities of local medical entrepreneurs and the Friends of Medicare.

In 1992, a private member's bill was introduced in the Legislative Assembly of Alberta to grant special charitable status to Howard Gimbel, a world-renowned ophthalmologist, to allow the proceeds from his private practice to be channelled into a private foundation to fund research activities; however, the legislation was withdrawn due to significant public and federal government outcry. Subsequently, an activist federal (Liberal) government became intent on enforcing the principles of the *Canada Health Act*. Alberta had developed a set of principles and was in discussion with the federal government about health-care privatization, but in 1995, Alberta, along with several other provinces, was penalized for violating the *Canada Health Act* by failing to enforce the extra-billing or facility fee aspects of the legislation.[9] Historically, Alberta had vehemently defended the right of physicians to extra-bill.

While the two orders of government were embroiled in a political battle, local entrepreneurs, mainly in Calgary, were busy developing new corporate ventures to increasingly deliver health-care services. In an environment of reduced public sector capacity, some regional health authorities

(RHAs) capitalized on private sector capacity by contracting out surgical services. In effect, the Calgary RHA sold "surplus" physical infrastructure to local medical entrepreneurs, and subsequently, these individuals performed a number of surgical procedures that would have normally been carried out in public hospitals. Starting with uncomplicated cataract surgeries, by the end of the 1990s the list had expanded to include major joint replacement surgeries; however, in all instances, private contractors were responsible only for uncomplicated cases. More complex patients or procedures continued to be handled by public facilities.

Although local entrepreneurs pressured the provincial government to approve these arrangements, RHAs, local health advocates, and the federal government pushed for a clear legislative framework to regulate these activities. In September 2000, the *Health Care Protection Act* was passed and regulations were drafted. The new legislation required all surgical facilities to be accredited by the College of Physicians and Surgeons of Alberta and approved by the Minister of Health. Insured surgical services could be provided by private health facilities only through contracts with health regions, in which facility fees were paid by the health regions to private contractors based on performance expectations and measures. In considering an application, the Minister was required to take into account the *Canada Health Act*, the public interest, and any possible adverse impacts on the publicly funded or administered system. The rationale for approving a contract was to be made public. The legislation contained provisions to protect patients from being forced to purchase "enhanced" services, at an additional direct cost, and also prohibited queue-jumping for insured surgeries.

The *Health Care Protection Act* allowed government to deal with a variety of issues but primarily regulated service delivery contracts between health regions and private health facilities. In essence, the legislation struck a balance among competing values of a stronger private sector role in health care, increased access and choice, regulation of increasing public expenditures pertaining to contracts, and quality assurance.

Wait Times (2003)

Expenditure reductions undermined the capacity of the public health-care system to meet increasing demands for services.[10] The most visible manifestation of this problem was the lengthy wait list for major surgical procedures. The research question for this case was: Why did Alberta establish a voluntary waiting-list tracking system rather than a centralized or decentralized waiting-list management system?

As Figure 3.1 illustrates, access to services appeared to be an increasing public concern, to which politicians were attuned, over the case study period.

FIGURE 3.1
Percentage of Albertans Reporting Access to Health Care as "Easy" or "Very Easy,"
1995–2004

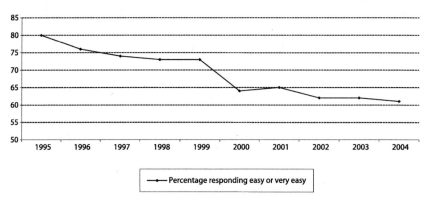

Source: Alberta Health and Wellness, *Public Surveys about Health and the Health System in Alberta*, 1995 through 2004.

In addition to the system's reduced capacity, the creation of regional governance and delivery systems provided local decision makers with a new perspective on the extent and nature of the problem. In short, once decision makers began addressing service delivery in more heavily populated areas and started dealing with resource allocation across multiple facilities, program wait lists moved from being a site-specific to a system-level problem.

The initial political response in 1996 was to devote additional public money to alleviate immediate demands for cardiac and joint replacement surgeries. In addition, the cabinet promoted private health care as a possible means of relieving pressure on the public system. As the decade progressed and long wait times persisted despite the infusion of additional resources, politicians and bureaucrats grew to better understand the complex relationship among surgeons, facilities, and other health providers, such as acute care surgical nurses. By the late 1990s, resources were targeted to address all three of these areas, as opposed to the earlier approach of targeting money to pay for more operating room time only. Stemming from the policy learning about the specific issue and a greater push by the Alberta government to implement a business planning model, a drive to develop performance indicators contributed significantly to the eventual government response to the issue.

To address the specific issue of wait times, Alberta introduced a voluntary, publicly accessible, Internet-based wait-list registry in 2003. The choice of a voluntary registry reflected the interplay of three factors: preference for minimal government intervention in social policy; preference for personal responsibility and choice; and recognition of the original bargain with organized medicine with its primary focus on professional autonomy. The underlying logic of the registry was to provide all stakeholders, including patients, with accurate and understandable information. In theory, patients and/or their physicians would be able to make appropriate choices about the best way to access necessary services. The voluntary aspect of the registry ensured that individual physicians were not coerced to surrender control over local information about wait times. It also recognized the disparity in the capacity of different regions to collect data on surgical and diagnostic procedures. Finally, in taking a voluntary approach, the government avoided a state-centred response. The boundaries within which a policy choice could be made necessitated an incremental approach to policy development and implementation.

Having provided an overview of the six cases, this chapter turns to examining the role played by ideas, interests, institutions, economics, and technology in shaping policy outcomes.

THE ROLE OF IDEAS, INTERESTS, INSTITUTIONS, AND EXTERNAL FACTORS

Role of Ideas

Health reform and policy in Alberta was driven by a number of over-arching value preferences. As discussed earlier, historically, Alberta had demonstrated a strong preference for limited government involvement in the lives of individuals. It preferred private market solutions to public policy problems. When national hospital insurance was originally being planned, Alberta advocated a non-compulsory, municipally decentralized approach, as opposed to the compulsory, centrally administered approached envisioned by the federal government (Taylor 2009, 169-70). Ernest Manning's Social Credit government led the opposition to the compulsory federal medical care insurance scheme (Barr 1974, 135). The Government of Alberta made its position perfectly clear in its submission to the federal Royal Commission on Health Services:

> We believe that only by maintaining a system in which private enterprise and individual initiative and personal responsibility combined with whatever financial subsidization is required from society collectively, can the best interests of our people in the field of health be successfully and adequately served (Alberta 1962, 4).

In fact, while the federal initiative was still under discussion, the AMA, in collaboration with the Alberta government and the insurance industry, launched a private, non-profit, contributory but non-compulsory plan to counter Saskatchewan's compulsory, universal plan (Saskatchewan's plan would become the blueprint for medicare). The Alberta initiative was designed primarily to subsidize coverage for low-income earners (Taylor 2009, 339).

Within the context of health reforms, in the 1980s and 1990s these sentiments were reiterated first by the Premier's Commission (1989b) and subsequently by the government (Alberta Health Planning Secretariat 1993). In the case of health-care regionalization, the Premier's Commission called for a redistribution of power away from the Department of Health and toward local communities to make them more responsible and accountable for managing health resources and for reflecting local priorities and needs. From the government's perspective, new ways to deliver services required increased private sector involvement, increased consumer choice, and increased direct payment for non-essential services (Alberta Health Planning Secretariat 1993).

During this time period, these traditional values merged with the values of New Public Management (NPM) and its emphasis on the devolution of responsibilities for direct service delivery away from line departments to existing or newly created structures and processes (Aucoin 2002, 37-52). This view was well supported by the position of the Premier's Commission that the role of government in health care should be long-term strategic planning, setting standards, allocating global funding, and ensuring coordination and communication.

The view of the commission on the appropriate role of government in health care reflected a broader concern about enhancing expenditure accountability to avoid reverting to simply throwing money back into the system. As an idea in good currency, accountability dovetailed with the political agenda of fiscal restraint. By 1991, accountability had been translated into needs-based planning, evaluation of outcomes, changes in provider behaviour, and increased consumer choice and responsibility (Alberta Health 1991c, 1).

In addition to these internal discussions about accountability, two other sets of popular ideas circulated in government and politics. The first set stemmed from the NPM ideas of Osborne and Gaebler (1992); these ideas were promoted by the new provincial treasurer, Jim Dinning,[11] who had come from the public service. The second set of ideas, which were more politically strategic in nature, emanated from Sir Roger Douglas's 1993 book, *Unfinished Business*. Douglas suggested that successful reform required moving fast and hard before effective opposition could be mobilized. While the second set was loosely linked to Premier Klein, he never confirmed that he had read the book (D. Martin 2003, 140.)

The end result of the cross-fertilization of these ideas in Alberta was the development of basic NPM components relating to business planning and performance measurement, within an environment focused on expenditure reduction, downsizing, and decentralization of decision-making away from line departments to other existing or newly created decision-making institutions. Within this context, government began to consider policy alternatives that would touch directly on all six cases.

As an idea, regionalization provided a convenient vehicle for the devolution of responsibilities, and to a lesser extent, authority for the delivery of an integrated and coordinated range of health services within fixed budgets and performance targets. Once the idea of health regions was accepted, some form of consolidated funding formula, at the regional population level, became essential.

Alternative payment plans (APPs) also fit into broader thinking because they were seen by the government and the Alberta Medical Association as a means of introducing greater accountability into the physician services' budget without removing individual physician or patient choice. In essence, the normalization of APPs allowed government to fund groups of physicians, with identifiable deliverables, within the context of a fixed budget. Recent Canadian Institute for Health Information data indicate that 14.4 percent of total physician payments (clinical) were allocated to APPs (CIHI 2008, 2011c).

The ideas of accountability and less direct state intervention also drove the policy choice in the case of wait times. The overall push to develop a business planning model with performance measures and the desire to maintain consumer and health provider choice led to the development of measurement tools to support the data requirements of a voluntary wait-times registry. The predominant thinking underpinning the drug case decisions was also residual.

Role of Interests

Politicians

Ralph Klein, sworn in as premier in late 1992, set the tone for a new policy style in which public servants, who had previously played more of a leadership role in policy development, took on a more supportive role to government MLA-led policy committees. In a loose sense, this was consistent with the NPM notion of moving decision-making away from line departments. Underpinning this shift in policy was an overriding sense among Conservative MLAs that "knowledge workers" had become too powerful and needed to be reined in by politicians, who, after all, had been elected to make decisions on behalf of the public (Taras and Tupper 1994, 61-83). Taking a page from Douglas's book, this scapegoating was extended to anyone who opposed the government's agenda (Lisac 1995, 53-54). The tendency of long-standing governments, of one-party-dominant political systems, to perceive their ideas as the only correct ones was evident here. In short, one was either for or against the government (Tupper, Pratt, and Urquhart 1992, 47, 59).

The overall shift in policy style and related expenditure cutbacks required building consensus within caucus and cabinet. To facilitate this, Klein[12] introduced sweeping changes to three major aspects of government: communications, ministerial staff, and committee structures. The first change centralized the communications apparatus of government into the Office of the Premier: "[Ministerial] communications officers were appointed by the executive director in the premier's office, and they reported to the director of communications in the Office of the Premier" (Brownsey 2005, 218).

The second change politicized the role of ministerial executive assistants (ibid., 219):

> All ministerial executive assistants were interviewed as to their perception of their role. In the course of the interview, if it was determined that the executive assistants did not see their role as political they were terminated. While ministers were free to hire their own executive assistants, Klein's chief of staff, Rod Love, ensured that they viewed their role as political operatives and not as neutral members of the bureaucracy.

The third major change involved replacing cabinet committees with standing policy committees (ibid.):

> In place of cabinet committees Love created what he described as Standing Policy Committees (SPCs). Comprised of both cabinet members and backbench MLAs, each standing policy committee is chaired by a private government member with the authority to hear public submissions. Ministers are appointed as vice-chairs of these committees. These chairpersons sit at the cabinet table to represent the views of their committee.

The new committee structure appeared to shift power back into the hands of the Tory caucus, especially rural MLAs, who had been alienated during the Getty era (White 2005, 118-23). For example, in the case of regionalization, the slight delay in introducing health regions and the large number of initial regions were a direct reflection of the influence of the rural caucus and the control of local hospitals (Hanrahan et al. 1992). The more substantial delay in regulating private providers reflected reluctance from the premier and from influential caucus members to intervene. The introduction of APPs was initially rejected by politicians because of the potential negative public perception of patient rostering.

While on the surface this created a more grassroots decision-making process, it also shifted power away from ministers and into the Premier's Office. In health care, this centralization of power allowed the premier to publicly contradict ministers and even reverse their decisions when he chose to do so.

Physicians

Physicians, collectively and individually, played an important role at the government agenda, decision agenda, and policy choice stages in the alternative payment plan (APP) and wait-times cases. In the privatization case, individual physician entrepreneurs played a significant role at the government agenda stage. They played a less important role in the regionalization case and appear to have played little or no role in the drug case. This variation reflected the extent to which each of these cases was integral to the core bargain between the Alberta Medical Association (AMA) and the government, with professional autonomy and method of payment being most central to the core bargain.

In the APP case, the AMA was key to bringing forward the issue and getting it onto the government's health reform agenda. Once on the table, the AMA, with its superior resources, controlled the decision and policy choice agendas. For wait times, the preferences of individual surgeons, shaped by the clinical autonomy aspect of the core physician bargain, heavily influenced the government's response. In the privatization case, physician entrepreneurs, concentrated in Calgary, forced and kept the issue on the government agenda. Individual physicians informed cabinet at the decision agenda stage. For regionalization, government deliberately excluded significant local physician input, fearing resistance that would slow the process. Such input was only reintegrated after regional structures were in place.

Bureaucrats

As previously mentioned, bureaucrats were challenged to manage a difficult policy environment during the 1990s; however, Alberta Health bureaucrats played an instrumental role in developing the thinking around accountability at the government agenda stage and in developing performance measures in the regionalization and wait-times cases. Provincial bureaucrats played a key role in the development and implementation of the new population-based funding formula. They were also influential in the development of policy options for the drug case. In the privatization, APP, wait-times, and regionalization cases, bureaucrats appear to have been less influential at the decision agenda and policy choice stages. The degree of influence that bureaucrats had at the different stages of policy-making for the different cases reflected the extent to which an issue was perceived as political as opposed to technical in nature.

Over time, the role of bureaucrats under Klein generally diminished for a number of reasons: centralization of decision-making in the Premier's Office, especially on the health file; general lack of trust in the bureaucracy; Klein's lack of trust in Alberta Health bureaucrats in particular because of his perception that health bureaucrats were resistant to proposed policy changes; downsizing; regionalization, which moved resources out of the line department; and the ascendance of government MLAs in the government decision-making process. Of the 16 ad hoc MLA committees initially created, 12 were linked to health-care reform (Church and Noseworthy 1999, 194). The shift to MLA committees represented a shift from decision-making through bureaucratic processes to decision-making through more politicized processes as well as a shift from more abstract and technical analysis to more practical (i.e., political) considerations (McArthur 2007, 245-60). The net result of the major changes to decision-making structures and significant expenditure cuts was a demoralized public service with a significantly reduced capacity to lead policy development or implementation.

Other Societal Interests

Other societal interests, such as citizens' groups, labour unions, and municipalities, appear to have been most prominent in the privatization, regionalization, and wait-times cases, which were more political in nature. The Friends of Medicare coalition of citizen and labour interests, in concert with the federal government, was instrumental in forcing the issue of privatization onto the government agenda and in heavily influencing the final policy choice. Local community and municipal interests were influential in delaying the legislation of health regions because of the implications for local control and the local economy. They were also influential in determining the relatively large number of regions that were originally established, although eventually this influence waned. The wait-times case was overshadowed by increasing citizen concerns with access to services. The policy response was designed to provide citizens with information that would continue to ensure they had choices about the services they received.

Role of Institutions

The policy legacies created by the *Canada Health Act* (*CHA*) and the implicit original bargains embedded in the legislation helped to shape the policy responses of the provincial government. In the privatization case, the requirements of the *CHA* forced Alberta to regulate the activities of private operators, despite the prevailing residual view of the state. The government response in the APP case was tempered by the recognition of the original bargain between the state and organized medicine. The "reasonable access" aspect of the *CHA* indirectly influenced government to address wait times. Devolution of RHAs' responsibilities occurred within a framework of continuing public accountability. In the drug case, federal resources were used to leverage policy change at the provincial level. Overall, the interprovincial process played an important role in achieving consensus on the general direction of reforms in the regionalization and APP cases. In wait times, federal-provincial relations were significant at the government agenda stage.

In addition to the more general changes to government structures and processes previously discussed, a number of institutional changes, specific to health care, were implemented to facilitate reforms. The provincial Ministry of Health, which had traditionally enjoyed a significant leadership role, was relegated to a support role for new health regions and other major stakeholders in implementing major health reform. With a significant reduction in human resources during the early stages of reform, Alberta Health effectively lost the capacity to take a leadership role (Church and Noseworthy 1999; Church and Smith 2006). Although the shift in the role of public administrators, within the context of New Public Management (NPM), was not unique to Alberta, the trend toward "hollowing out" the bureaucracy was vigorously pursued in Alberta compared to most provinces and territories (Gow 2004, 11; McArthur 2007, 247-48).

The replacement of close to 200 local hospital and public health boards, initially with 17 but eventually nine regional health authorities, effectively broke the link between local MLAs and hospital and public health boards. In essence, the pluralistic nature of local decision-making was replaced by more concentrated and centrally directed regional decision-making that involved fewer community representatives. This shift represented a direct assault on the core bargain with local communities about hospital governance. Klein, who had been mayor of Calgary, had personally dealt with the local empires built around hospitals and the salaries that hospital chief executive officers demanded.

While government successfully broke the traditional link between local physicians and local hospitals, new regional institutional mechanisms were eventually created to re-establish this linkage because it became apparent that attempting to move forward, without the support of local medical communities, would be problematic. Klein admitted, some years later, that leaving doctors out of the first round of reforms was a mistake (D. Martin 2003, 162). Overall, the government chose not to effect fundamental change to the core relationship with organized medicine. In the years following the introduction of health regions, new provincial-level institutional arrangements further entrenched the power of organized medicine. As the APP case demonstrated, the Alberta Medical Association was successful, in 2003, in officially representing all Alberta physicians in exchange for institutionalizing APPs. These same institutional mechanisms, however, introduced health regions as a third player at the system-level decision-making table. By bringing RHAs to the negotiating table, the province formalized a process for "tripartite" management of the health-care system, which enabled government to build sufficient consensus in order to discuss issues, beyond physician remuneration, related to primary care reform.

Role of External Factors

The Economy

The economic downturn of the mid-1980s set the stage for the change in political leadership and the subsequent agenda of fiscal restraint precipitating early health reform. Similarly, the rebound of the Alberta economy, in the mid-1990s, led to a significant reinvestment of resources in health care. This economic shift likely changed the nature of the reforms that occurred in the late 1990s. For example, the government rationale for an increased private role in the health sector was harder to justify once significant resources became available to support the publicly funded health-care system. Other reforms that required additional financial resources also became feasible.

Technology

In the privatization case, changes in medical technology made possible more medical procedures outside of the traditional hospital setting (Alberta Health 1991b, 1). The result of this was the unregulated growth of private health clinics in Alberta during the 1980s (Armstrong 2000). In short, an increasing number of physicians began to practice outside of publicly funded hospitals. The economic crisis in the late 1980s and early 1990s and the downsizing of the public health sector created a market opportunity for private, for-profit clinics. The return of resources to the public market in the mid-1990s may have curtailed the extent of the private market opportunity; however, population size and lack of sufficient population density (i.e., economies of scale) may also have limited the extent of the market opportunity (Church and Barker 1998).

   Technology played a role in the wait-times case because of the increased capacity to perform procedures outside of traditional acute care medical settings. Technology also enhanced the capacity to centralize and digitize information, particularly in the 1990s with the arrival and mainstreaming of the Internet.

WHY DID REFORM TAKE PLACE IN SOME CASES BUT NOT IN OTHERS?

The degree to which proposed reforms touched on one or more of the original core bargains, either independent physician contractors or publicly funded, locally controlled hospital services, determined the extent of reforms. Proximity to core bargains also affected which policy ideas were acceptable. Thus, in the APP and wait-times cases, government proceeded with the cooperation of organized medicine, because the chosen policy options either originated from doctors or were crafted to be acceptable to them. In both of these policy areas, proposed changes were voluntary.

In the APP case, the Alberta Medical Association largely determined the policy agenda and the policy response. Given the centrality of re-imbursement to the core bargain with doctors, physician interest in providing leadership on the development of APPs as a policy option is not surprising. In the wait-times case, the government had to balance the need to access local information controlled by individual physicians with the need to better coordinate service delivery at a regional and provincial level. In the population-based funding and drug cases, the core bargain with organized medicine was unaffected and government was able to implement policy change without significant opposition.

In the regionalization case, organized medicine was largely unaffected; in fact, government sought to make the changes without directly involving physicians. The devolution of the physician budget to health regions was not seriously contemplated because it lacked acceptability as a policy idea.

In the privatization case, the provincial government touched directly on the core bargain related to public funding and community control of hospitals, which angered community advocates, unions, and the federal Liberal government. The Liberal government characterized itself as the defender of the *Canada Health Act*, the institutional representation of the original core bargains.

A second important determinant of the extent of reform was the per-ceived fiscal crisis. Premier Klein's fiscal reform agenda and competency as a political communicator facilitated rapid expenditure reductions with little public opposition. Arguably, regionalization and population-based funding were initiated during the first Klein government mandate because a general fiscal crisis overshadowed other policy considerations. In fact, the overall agenda of deficit elimination allowed government to success-fully violate the second core bargain, relating to local community control of hospitals, by framing the decision as necessary to addressing the larger fiscal crisis. Once the price of oil had rebounded and the perceived crisis had passed, political will and public support to further significant policy changes in health care evaporated. By the time the privatization issue had fully matured, the rationale for increased private involvement was not supported by the fiscal environment. Beyond the first political mandate, there was no clear general policy direction; managing the embarrassment of wealth became the main preoccupation of government.

A third determinant of reform was the ideological lens through which government viewed policy. Although tempered by the amount of revenue generated through oil and gas, Alberta historically favoured a residual approach to social services, with a preference for private market solutions wherever possible. This preference was evident in the government's reluctance to regulate the private health-care market and its desire to allow choice for both providers and citizens in the alternative payment plan (APP) and wait-times cases. It also affected the rhetoric around the regionalization case and the number of regions originally created (local choice). This neoliberal ideological viewpoint dovetailed with emerging New Public Management (NPM) thinking from administrative and managerial sciences. The limited expansion of drug benefits reflected a belief that services should be targeted at those who are unable to compete in the private market and who are also deserving of societal support.

A fourth determinant, implicit in the first three, is political leadership. Undoubtedly, Klein's personal beliefs and political style were key to building and sustaining consensus, particularly during the preliminary years of fiscal reform when difficult decisions had to be made. Other politicians, such as Jim Dinning, were also important during this time period.

CONCLUSION

Health reform in Alberta has been shaped by a variety of exogenous and endogenous policy inputs. Declining government revenues resulting from a large unexpected drop in the price of oil and gas precipitated a fiscal crisis for government. Technological advancements during the 1980s made possible the delivery of an increasing range of health-care services outside traditional institutional settings. Moreover, the development of the Internet during the 1990s permitted centralization and digitization of the health-care system.

The inability of Getty's political leadership to address the fiscal crisis when it first broke in the mid-1980s, due to resistance from major policy actors (i.e., nurses, teachers, hospitals, doctors, municipalities, and public sector unions), instigated a successor government, under the leadership of Klein, that could work around existing elites and create new structures and processes (Laframboise 1986). A more nuanced interpretation of this idea is that when faced with significant resistance from powerful policy actors, government must alter existing institutional arrangements to facilitate the development of new patterns of interaction among these actors.

A change in political leadership also led to a change in ideation, and ultimately, to the style of government. To forge a new political consensus around deficit and debt elimination, the Klein government re-emphasized a major part of Alberta's political culture, the idea of the state as "residual," and married it with the emerging ideas of New Public Management. Although the same exogenous policy inputs were present during the late 1980s and early 1990s, it was only with the new aggressive political leadership and policy style of the Klein government that the existing institutional bias was overcome (Pierson 2000).

The messages emerging through the processes of policy development in Alberta indicated the cabinet's intentions to alter three sets of relationships underpinning the existing health-care system: the relationship of the provincial health ministry to other policy actors; the exchange relationship between individual members of the Legislative Assembly and local health-care constituencies; and the unmediated collective bargaining relationship between physicians and the province.

The government reinforced the new political consensus through institutional changes. Legislation, passed to mandate debt elimination and enhance accountability (i.e., business planning), facilitated a significant reduction in public expenditures. Legislative and expenditure changes rationalized the introduction of health regions, which were previously politically unfeasible. Creating a consensus was important because the introduction of health regions challenged the original bargain between local communities and the government over control of hospital services. The resistance of local municipalities and communities, especially Progressive Conservative constituencies, had formerly been a significant barrier to health reform. In essence, the traditional relationship between hospital administrators, hospital boards, and MLAs was replaced by a more centralized relationship between regional health boards, regional administrators, and government officials. These interactions were more removed from local communities than in the previous set of relationships.

Regionalization was a pivotal institutional change because it created a new institutional lens through which existing and emerging problems could be viewed. Policy ideas such as contracting out for delivery of surgical services, creating a centralized (although voluntary) wait-list registry, introducing a population-based funding formula, and introducing APPs became politically feasible because of the cascading impact of policy inputs and outputs on policy outcomes. By choosing to focus, initially, on larger institutional changes, the government created a new set of incentives to which major interests responded. Thus, regional health managers and appointed decision makers became responsive to a broader range of considerations about the health of local populations, as opposed to merely service catchment areas or the organizational survival of individual facilities. Over time, physicians became more supportive of a collaborative approach to practice and to different methods of remuneration.

The nature and extent of institutional change and interest response was tempered by institutional bias and political will. In formulating its overall response to health reform, Alberta was cognizant of the constraints of policy legacies. The presence of the *Canada Health Act* compelled the Alberta cabinet to address the issue of privatization far more aggressively than intended. The combination of local interest and federal government activism was essential to reinforcing the existing policy legacy. Previously, the legacy existed but had not forced Alberta to act due to a non-activist federal government.

Policy legacies relating to the original bargain between physicians and the state tempered the government's response in both the wait-times registry and APP cases. The government established buy-in from organized medicine to alter some aspects of the core bargain, namely, method of payment and sharing of patient information.

Viewed through a structural frame, health reforms in Alberta brought the values of corporate rationalists (challenging interests), concerned with improved system management (NPM), in conflict with the values of organized medicine (dominant interests), concerned with professional autonomy and control (Alford 1975). Regionalization was a favoured response of corporate rationalists because it aimed to address many of the shortcomings of the existing system (Weller 1977, 444-60). The introduction of regional health authorities, business planning, and institutions for the trilateral management of the health system suggests that the challenge was at least partially successful.

The concentration of administrative and decision-making authority at the regional level introduced a new source of power into the provincial health policy arena. Where government and organized medicine had previously negotiated the nature of the health-care system, health regions evolved into a third substantive partner—a potential counterbalance to the other two parties—at the provincial decision-making table. As a result, the Alberta Medical Association positioned itself to protect its members' interests by agreeing to partner with the government and the regions in order to "manage" the health system. In exchange, the interests of organized medicine were accommodated by reaffirming the AMA as the sole representative for all physicians. Essentially, health reforms impacted physicians by creating incremental change and, in turn, by reinforcing feedback.

Overall, the Alberta government was successful at redirecting resources to create new incentives at the individual provider and organizational levels. In the process, opportunities emerged for new partnerships and patterns of interaction between the major interests in health care, for example, between RHAs and organized medicine. By their nature, these partnerships are slowly altering medical practice and health-care service delivery.

Postscript

In the wake of this study, a number of significant changes have occurred. These changes have largely replaced the major reforms that occurred during the 1990s and early 2000s. The first change was the replacement of Ralph Klein by Ed Stelmach as premier in early 2006. Whereas Klein was populist, media savvy, outspoken, and combative, Stelmach's leadership style was more laissez-faire and bland; however, in the same way that Klein sought to distinguish himself from the previous premier by significantly deviating from prior health policies, Stelmach also sought to distinguish himself from Klein by embarking on his own policy priorities.

 During the latter part of his premiership, Klein relied more heavily on the advice of Jack Davis, CEO of the Calgary Health Region (1999–2008), who had also been deputy minister of health (1996–1997) and senior deputy for the government (1997–1999). That Davis continued to make his authoritative voice on health policy heard, in public forums, after Klein's departure became an increasing irritant (as did other local voices) to the Stelmach administration. What made this even more aggravating for Stelmach was that the increasing expenditures in health care, resulting from the cacophony of local voices, failed to yield more efficient and effective service delivery. Because the Klein government had sought to weaken the local health-care power base by eliminating hospital and public health boards, the re-emergence of local voices had already become a burning political issue prior to the change in provincial political leadership.

After Stelmach was elected as premier in early 2008, the government moved swiftly to dissolve the existing regional health authorities. The nine regional health authority boards were replaced by a single provincial health authority—Alberta Health Services—with a government-appointed board responsible for the delivery of health services across the whole province. In effect, the nine remaining local authoritative voices, with 127 provincially appointed regional board members who might have opposed government actions, were eliminated. They were replaced by 15 provincially appointed decision makers, a far cry from the approximately 3,000 local decision makers involved under the old local hospital and public health boards. In addition, the government centralized other services, such as emergency response (i.e., ambulance), that had traditionally been under the control of local municipalities and were, in fact, a matter of local option. Several previous efforts to integrate the delivery of these services had failed. In essence, the government created the equivalent of a health maintenance organization, albeit with a separation between purchaser and provider (Ruttan 2009).[13] After pilot testing home care in 2010, Alberta continues to move toward activity-based (i.e., fee-for-service) funding for hospitals and emergency services as a way to create more efficiency through financial incentives (a market-like discipline). Interestingly, this is where Alberta was headed prior to the introduction of health regions and population-based funding (Derworiz 2010).

The privatization aspirations of the Klein government appear to have faltered. A recent competition to award contracts for eye and joint surgery for the province left several of the previous contractors out in the cold. At least one contractor, HRC, which had been the source of controversy around the contracting out of acute care services to private providers during the late 1990s, declared bankruptcy after being taken over by another private corporation. The government stepped in to financially support the beleaguered company (Howell 2010). While discussions about various options for increased private involvement in health care occasionally occur, there does not appear to be the same overt push for increased privatization as there was during the Klein era. A more subtle approach, such as unbundling services in long-term and continuing care, appears to be the current direction. The idea that private market solutions are the best way to go in Alberta's health-care system has taken a significant body blow.

Most other reforms discussed in this chapter have evolved without changing as much as regionalization or the population-based funding model. While alternative payment plans have continued to develop incrementally, the government appears to have shifted its emphasis to other aspects of its relationship with physicians. Primary care networks are designed to coordinate physicians together with each other and with regional services, such as public health, to ensure continuity of care and access. Changing the method of payment is not a requirement of these networks. At least one insider reports that the government's interest in APPs has waned because of their failure to produce cost savings. From the physician point of view, the increasingly cumbersome bureaucracy associated with establishing and maintaining APPs has made them less attractive. In essence, as government has moved to standardize the processes and increase accountability with respect to APPs, physicians have backed away from the idea.

The Internet-based, voluntary wait-times registry was shut down after the establishment of Alberta Health Services. Having said this, aspects of a wait-times registry have reappeared on the Alberta Health and Wellness website that links to Alberta Health Services. This relates to a continuing emphasis on public accountability and performance management. The current configuration of data shows wait times for major joint replacement surgery (knee and hip), coronary artery bypass, and emergency room treatment (complicated and uncomplicated) for individual hospital sites. Alberta Health Services has also set performance targets in all of these areas. Overall, while the specific nature of health reforms in Alberta has evolved, corporate rationalist managerial tools for performance management have persisted and been refined. The trend toward standardization of delivery and centralization of decision-making has also increased. The days of local control of health-care decision-making appear to be a thing of the past in Alberta.

Notes

1. A string of failed attempts to support economic diversification through low-interest business loans made a significant contribution to the growing provincial debt.
2. Having said this, social services expenditures increased by 53 percent and health by 34 percent between 1981 and 1989. Other departments such as environment, transportation, and utilities experienced major cuts during the same time period—92 percent and 77 percent, respectively.
3. Don Getty succeeded Peter Lougheed as leader of the Progressive Conservative Party of Alberta and was premier from 1985 to 1992.
4. Tupper (2001) notes that during the Mulroney era in federal politics, Alberta and the federal government worked collaboratively on a variety of issues including free trade. Alberta was politically well represented in the federal Cabinet.
5. For a full discussion of this case, see Church and Smith (2008).
6. For a full discussion of this case, see Smith and Church (2008).
7. Since the early 1990s, the Alberta government and the AMA have negotiated a fixed amount of money for physician services.
8. For a full discussion of this case, see Church and Smith (2006).
9. A grace period to allow the provinces to come into compliance with the legislation had expired in 1987, but compliance had never been pursued by a federal Progressive Conservative government.
10. For a full discussion of this case, see Church and Smith (2009).
11. Dinning also served as a link to the more moderate urban wing of the party.
12. It was well known in government circles that Klein relied heavily on Rod Love for advice on these matters.
13. The structures and processes for decision-making around the allocation of research investments in health and other policy areas have also been centralized with a major focus on demonstrable impact (measurable performance outcomes).

CHAPTER 4

SASKATCHEWAN'S HEALTH-CARE POLICY REFORM IN THE ROMANOW ERA: FROM RESTRAINT TO RESTRUCTURING

TOM MCINTOSH AND MICHAEL DUCIE

INTRODUCTION

This chapter examines the nature and extent of health reform decision-making in the province of Saskatchewan during the premiership of Roy Romanow, who led the province from 1991 until his resignation a decade later. The early 1990s saw the beginning of the greatest period of health-care reform since the adoption of publicly funded medical insurance by Saskatchewan in 1962. Like the other four provinces covered in this volume, however, Saskatchewan also chose to impose stringent restraints on public spending in response to growing levels of debt. As is discussed more fully below, the budget restraints had a significant impact on the province's health reform plans. The reforms began in 1991 with the election of Roy Romanow's left-of-centre New Democratic Party (NDP) government and were, for the most part, introduced within the first three years of his administration; however, developments continued throughout his time in office, as aspects of the reform program were refined and the social and economic situation within province improved.

Six specific health policy reform decisions are examined in this study. These decisions begin with Romanow's first provincial budget and carry on throughout his tenure and into that of his successor, Lorne Calvert. The first decision, to cut access to the once generous provincial drug plan, came about because of specific economic circumstances in the province. The next three decisions—the creation of a regionalized governance structure, the attempt to move to population needs-based funding for health services, and the attempt to move physicians away from fee-for-service payments—were part of an explicitly articulated vision of health reform that eventually became known as the "wellness agenda." The passage of the 1996 *Health Facilities Licensing Act*, which limits the ability of entrepreneurs to open private for-profit health facilities, was a response to events outside the province. It also allowed the government to shore up its standing as a "defender of medicare" in the aftermath of controversial decisions to close or convert over 50 small rural hospitals. The final decision examined here, the creation of a centralized, mandatory wait-list registry, emerged as the result of growing public concern over wait times within the system and the failure of the government's initial attempts to spend its way out of the problem. None of these decisions fundamentally altered the basic structures of publicly provided health insurance, but that was not the intention. If anything, these decisions were an attempt to extend and reconfigure medicare in the directions first proposed by Tommy Douglas in the 1940s and by Emmett Hall in the 1960s.

The Saskatchewan reform process displays the importance of the interplay of ideas between elected officials and the civil service. At the same time, the difficult economic conditions in the province, the inability of the political opposition to mount an effective counterattack to the proposed reforms, and the complicated relationship between the government and key health-care stakeholders were important determining factors for the changes that took place from 1991 to 2003. It is comforting, however overly simplistic, to consider the Romanow government's health reform agenda as a triumph of "ideas" that were generated by independent, forward-looking research and implemented by strong "institutions," that is, a professional civil service working closely with a strong political executive, that either sidelined or co-opted opposing "interests" (the health professions, unions, legislative opposition, etc.).

The spending restraints of the early to mid-1990s certainly helped facilitate the health-care decisions examined below and, to some extent, emboldened the government to act despite opposition from important health-care interests. Rather than add money to the system to propose new incentives for change, the government was, in effect, forced to shift spending within the system in a way that drove cuts to the public drug insurance program. Those interviewed for this study defended these decisions but not in a prideful way. On the more positive side, the closure and conversion of small rural hospitals facilitated the process of regionalization and the decisions that stemmed directly from it. The closures and conversions were key to attempts to reorganize the governance of the system and shift the system's focus away from doctor and hospital services. As is explored more fully below, the fiscal challenges faced by the Romanow government proved, in some ways, to be a necessary but insufficient condition for the reforms and also undercut public support for the reform agenda.

The changes to health care in Saskatchewan during the Romanow years were significant and, for the most part, lasting. But they did not fundamentally alter the key elements of medicare, as it was created in the late 1960s and early 1970s. This chapter demonstrates how Saskatchewan has gone further than the other four provinces analyzed in this volume, and arguably, further than most other Canadian provinces, in achieving its health reform goals. However, economics, politics, and the self-preservation instincts of key actors in the system necessitated compromises that slowed, diverted, and blunted some of the more ambitious elements of the agenda.

THE POLITICAL AND POLICY-MAKING CONTEXT IN SASKATCHEWAN

The early years of the Romanow government were marked by fiscal restraint and the contraction of publicly provided health and social services, as the province teetered near bankruptcy brought about by years of overspending by Grant Devine and his Conservative administration. As the province began to achieve a greater level of fiscal security, the Romanow government fundamentally reformed the governance and financing of the provincial health-care system according to a "wellness agenda." The NDP's election platform had promised to shift health care away from its preoccupation with doctor and hospital services and toward preventative and population health services. This was to be accomplished by integrating the range of health-care services, with a greater focus on primary care to be delivered by interdisciplinary teams of health-care providers, and a governance structure aimed at articulating the health needs of local populations.

Successful implementation of the reforms planned by the Romanow government was consistently undercut by the political fallout of the restraint measures. The reduced access to the provincial prescription drug plan, discussed in detail below, and the closure and conversion of 50 small rural hospitals as part of the province's rationalization of acute care delivery, gave rise to a public perception that the "wellness agenda" was, in fact, merely a code for neoliberal fiscal restraint and the undermining of Tommy Douglas's vision of accessible and publicly funded care. It was a politically difficult position for a social democratic government in a province that valued, and continues to value, a national medicare system.

The Romanow government had the advantage of facing a weak and divided opposition in the provincial legislature throughout much of its tenure, especially during its first term in office. The Progressive Conservative Party won only 10 of the province's 66 seats in 1991, and the Liberals won only one seat. Revelations of improprieties while in office led to a further decline in Tory fortunes in 1995 when the party won only five seats, whereas the Liberals captured 11. The NDP was left with a reduced but still overwhelming majority in a smaller 58 seat legislature. In 1997, four Tory and four Liberal members of the Legislative Assembly (MLAs) jumped their respective ships and formed the Saskatchewan Party under the leadership of former Progressive Conservative, Elwin Hermanson.

The attempt to create a single, unified opposition was undercut by the refusal of both opposition parties to formally disband. In 1997, the Progressive Conservative Party did decide to withdraw from provincial politics for 10 years but not to terminate itself permanently. In 1999, the Liberals managed to elect only four members (later reduced to three in a by-election loss to the Saskatchewan Party), the Saskatchewan Party 25 members, and the NDP 29 members. With half the seats in the Legislative Assembly, the Romanow NDP government negotiated a coalition agreement with the Liberals that saw two of the Liberals appointed to cabinet and the third to the Speaker's chair. The coalition agreement split the Liberals internally. Leader Jim Melanchuk was defeated in a leadership convention and refused, along with Speaker Ron Osika, to leave the coalition government. He identified as an Independent until eventually joining the NDP. The Liberals failed to win a seat in either the 2003 or 2007 elections.

From 1991 until 1999, Romanow, much like the federal Liberal leader Jean Chrétien, had a comfortable majority in the legislature, which was coupled with a weak, divided opposition that was unable to mount effective campaigns against the NPD-proposed changes. Even after winning a minority government in 1999, Romanow's successful negotiation of the NDP-Liberal coalition agreement allowed the government to operate as a de facto majority government, especially after the expulsion of the Liberal MLAs from their own party.

The government's relations with key stakeholders in the health-care system are also important for understanding how and why specific decisions were made. Because of the scope of the reforms, the precarious economic situation, and the challenges of recruiting and retaining health-care workers, Saskatchewan government–stakeholder relations in the health sector were a complicated balancing act of interest promotion, turf protection, and a recognition that open warfare between parties would be ultimately damaging to all those concerned. Whatever desire there might have been, for example, for the government to "take on" doctors in a fight to reorganize their role in the system, the government was cognizant that policy shifts that might cause doctors to leave the province were best avoided. In turn, the Saskatchewan Medical Association (SMA) could not be openly hostile toward government out of fear of both undermining public confidence in the system and alienating its own membership. As for the Saskatchewan Union of Nurses, which represents registered nurses across the province, it had traditionally staked out positions much in line with the goals of the Romanow reforms and, like other labour organizations, had been an official supporter of the provincial NDP. At the same time, the series of health worker strikes in the mid-to-late

1990s, mostly over wages and staffing levels driven by fiscal restraint, significantly damaged the government's relationships with health-care unions throughout the latter half of Romanow's time in office and during the Calvert administration.

As important as these factors are, there is also a prevailing culture within stakeholder organizations that further mitigates open conflict with the government. The legacy of Saskatchewan as the "birthplace of medicare" looms large in the province. It is a point of pride for its residents. The Saskatchewan Medical Association, in the aftermath of the 1960 doctors' strike, took on the mantle of one of medicare's chief architects and has been a consistent defender of its principles and its preservation inside the province and within the medical community nationally. Similarly, most of the major players within the system see themselves, to some degree, as participating in the project initiated by Tommy Douglas and the Co-operative Commonwealth Federation (CCF) in the 1940s. Though this does not eliminate the traditional sources of tension between the government and stakeholders, or among stakeholders themselves, it does serve to deflect these sources of tension toward negotiation, consultation, and compromise rather than the more adversarial relationships one sometimes sees in other Canadian jurisdictions.

THE SIX CASE STUDIES

As indicated in chapter 1, the intent of this study was not to examine the Romanow government's approach to health reform in and of itself. Rather, as part of a larger multi-province study involving researchers from across the country, the goal was to examine a series of decisions in specific health-care sectors and subsectors in order to understand the forces that drove particular issues onto the health reform agenda and the factors that shaped their outcome. The larger study was also motivated by a desire to understand whether and why different provinces chose different solutions to similar health problems and whether there was any evidence that provinces learned much from the reform experiences of other provinces.

That the health reform decisions considered here track the period of Romanow's time in office is coincidental but also provides an important narrative thread to the analysis of how those reforms happened in Saskatchewan. The reforms move chronologically from those motivated by the fiscal imperatives of a near-bankrupt province to the articulation of a new vision of publicly funded health care. This vision was rooted in an appreciation of the limited ability of a physician- and hospital-centred model to create healthy populations. Interestingly, the attempt of the Romanow government to embark on its "wellness agenda" in the mid-1990s owed as much to the original vision of medicare proposed by people like Tommy Douglas and Justice Emmett Hall as it did to contemporary understandings of the determinants of population health (Labonte et al. 2005; McIntosh, Jeffery, and Muhajarinel 2010).

The study examines reform decisions in respect of six issues in Saskatchewan from 1990 to 2003: prescription drug policy, the regionalization of the health system's governance structures, the move to needs-based funding mechanisms within the provincial system, the creation of alternative payment plans for primary care physicians, for-profit delivery of health services, and wait-list management. On each of these issues, we examine specific decisions:

- Why did Saskatchewan restrict access to the province's prescription drug plan in 1992 and 1993?
- Why did Saskatchewan choose to regionalize the governance of the provincial health system by creating 32 health districts?
- Why did Saskatchewan implement a needs-based funding formula for health districts as part of its process of regionalization?
- Why did Saskatchewan choose to negotiate modified fee-for-service remuneration plans for primary care physicians rather than more comprehensive capitation or salary arrangements?
- Why did Saskatchewan choose to create a legislative framework that would make private, for-profit facilities legal but unlikely to succeed?
- Why did Saskatchewan create a mandatory wait-list management system to prioritize access to surgical services in 2002?

This study is based on a series of interviews with key informants conducted over the course of approximately a year, between 2003 and 2004. A total of 27 individuals were interviewed: past and present public servants, politicians directly involved in the decisions, and representatives of health-care stakeholder organizations (unions, regulatory bodies, professional associations, and others). The interview subjects were chosen through a snowball sampling method. The initial group of candidates suggested further candidates to be interviewed. A number of subjects were interviewed about more than one of the six policy decisions under investigation, which resulted in 37 separate interviews. At least five and as many as eight individuals were interviewed for each case. Only two individuals refused to be interviewed (for unstated reasons). In all instances, the interviews were recorded, transcribed, and coded using NVivo software, using a coding framework developed by the research team.

In addition, as described in chapter 2, for each policy decision we conducted a detailed documentary analysis and developed a timeline of key events related to the policy decision.[1] For documentary analysis we searched both PubMed and the Social Sciences and Humanities Research Index databases for material relevant to the issues under study (though there was little on the actual decisions made in Saskatchewan) as well as government, stakeholder, and research organizations' websites. This was supplemented by searches of legislative debates in Hansard and the archives of the Regina *Leader-Post* and the Saskatoon *Star-Phoenix* newspapers. The resulting data (including the interviews) were analyzed using the Kingdon and 3I frameworks (see Table 2.2 in chapter 2).

The decisions on regionalization, needs-based funding, and alternative physician payment schemes were, in fact, the heart of the Romanow government's wellness agenda. The latter two issues were, to a great extent, subsets of the first: the decision to regionalize the governance of the health-care system. These were the structural reforms that led to greater coordination of health services across geographic areas, greater integration of services across the continuum of care, and a shift from institutional and physician-focused care toward an emphasis on interdisciplinary, primary health-care teams. The other three decisions were, in some respects, more isolated ones. The cuts to the provincial drug plan came very early in Romanow's first mandate at a time when the province was in a serious fiscal crisis. The legal framework for private for-profit facilities came in response to a series of pressures to fill a policy gap in the regulatory framework governing the provincial health system. The creation of the Saskatchewan Surgical Care Network was a response to the growth of wait times for some services. These six reforms, combined, illustrate the nature of health-care reform during the Romanow and Calvert administrations in Saskatchewan.

Limiting Access to Prescription Drugs

Saskatchewan's drug plan, immediately upon its inception in 1974, was one of the most generous plans in the country in terms of universal coverage. The *Prescription Drug Act* of 1974 laid the foundation for the program, which included a fixed copayment system: all patients were charged a dispensing fee of $3.95 per prescription. Over time, the plan grew to what was seen as unsustainable cost levels, and in 1987, changes were made in an attempt to offset increasing costs. Between 1987 and 1993, a number of incremental changes were made with the same goal. In 1992 and 1993, the government drastically increased both the deductible and copayments under the plan. The exact numbers are outlined in Table 4.1.

Most of the participants in this study, who had fairly diverse backgrounds, indicated fiscal imperatives as the main factor for such fundamental change in the drug plan. One participant explained that "every year, of course, the drug plan escalated at a rate beyond what they thought it should, as a percentage, and then all of a sudden, they just started toying with ... deductibles to the point now ... there basically is no deductible." Another participant acknowledged that drug plan costs would escalate

TABLE 4.1
Changes to the Saskatchewan Provincial Drug Plan, 1987–1993

Year	Deductible ($)			Copayment (%)		
	Regular Family	Senior Family	Single Senior	Regular Family	Senior Family	Single Senior
1987	125 (annual)	75 (annual)	50 (annual)	20	20	20
1991	125 (annual)	75 (annual)	50 (annual)	25	25	25
1992	190 (semi-annual)	75 (semi-annual)	50 (semi-annual)	35 to $375 maximum, then 10	35 to $375 maximum, then 10	35 to $375 maximum, then 10
1993*	850 (semi-annual	850 (semi-annual)	850 (semi-annual)	35	35	35

Note: *In 1993, the drug plan changed so that anyone who did not qualify for special assistance was required to pay the above deductible and copayment.
Source: Saskatchewan Health (2010, 9).

if government did not take action or employ some sort of "cost containment or cost management."

A dilemma for the government was how to create significant savings through cuts to the drug plan, while making sure that the poor and medically indigent were still covered through the provincial plan. As one senior government official described it, "First of all, we needed to realize savings for deficit reduction. Secondly, if we were going to do that, we had to protect low-income families and we had to protect people who suffered catastrophic situations." In addition, many respondents noted that most unionized workers and white-collar public sector workers were already covered under private insurance plans as part of their collective agreements. This mitigated the potential political fallout from key elements of the government's electoral base.

The process of reforming the drug plan began with budget analysts and was driven by the Treasury Board and Department of Finance rather than the Department of Health, according to one government official. To the extent that the changes were driven by central agencies inside government, they were also done as part of a very traditional budget-making process whereby few, if any, outside bodies were given an opportunity to weigh in on the issue. In retrospect, however, none of the stakeholder groups interviewed noted any particular objections to the changes that were made. It appears that stakeholders recognized the fiscal limitations of the government.

Political actors involved in the decision regarded this action as one of the low points of the NDP's term in office. They expressed regret and frustration that the financial situation in the province had effectively forced their hand. Indeed, one person interviewed said that she had not supported the decision at the time, though others noted that the decision was taken with the full support of the cabinet. Given that the purpose of these policy changes was to save money, it must be noted that there was no consensus among our participants as to whether this goal was achieved, especially over the medium to long term. A study by Marchildon and O'Fee (2007, 118-19) found that initial savings brought about by the transformation of the program from universal to catastrophic coverage were short-lived and that drug expenditures began to rise again in the mid-1990s. The choice of the drug plan for immediate funding cuts was due, in part, to the manner in which prescription drugs were integrated into the overall health-care system. It was one of the few areas that were either self-funded or funded through a private insurance program (Commission on the Future of Health Care 2002, 189-210). This allowed the government some degree of freedom to make the cuts without unduly impacting middle-class residents of the province.

The Road to Wellness: Regionalization

In light of what was to follow in the area of health reform, the decision to cut access to prescription drugs was of relatively minor importance. Between 1992 and 1994, the Romanow government embarked on an ambitious package of reforms aimed, first, at restructuring the governance of the whole provincial health system and second, at reorienting the organization, funding, coordination, and delivery of primary and acute health-care services. Restructuring was undertaken with the intent of integrating and rationalizing the delivery of health services in an effort to place the delivery of primary health care, much of it outside traditional health-care institutions, at the core of the system. Along with the changes came a new driving philosophy for health care: health promotion and disease prevention, or "wellness."

The reorganization of the health system in Saskatchewan involved a sequential two-step approach: restructuring the system into health districts and shifting the focus to primary health care. The rationale for this two-stage approach was relatively simple. Working on the assumption that the existing governance structures were in fact a barrier to primary health-care reform and the better integration of services, the government believed that it needed first to "wipe the slate clean" by removing those elements of the system that it felt would be resistant to change. Individual boards of hospitals and other institutions could be expected to resist changes that had the potential to alter fundamentally their mandates, affect their budgets, and threaten their existence. By replacing these boards with district boards that had clear mandates to integrate and coordinate services across a broader geographic region, the government believed it would be able to move forward on implementing a more fundamental reorientation of the system.

Interviewees consistently named three people who were key drivers in the process and served as "champions" of the proposed changes: health minister Louise Simard, deputy minister of health Duane Adams, and assistant deputy minister of health Lorraine Hill. They were responsible for "making sure timelines were met and agendas were met and policy was being developed." According to the interviewees, these three worked in concert to drive the process of reform forward and win support from both political and bureaucratic leaders in the province. This situation illustrates the symbiotic relationship between the elected and bureaucratic levels of government that is often needed for the successful implementation of major policy changes. For example, Adams had been a long-time provincial public servant during the Blakeney government, who decamped to Health Canada during the Devine administration. He returned to the provincial civil service as deputy minister of health following the election of the Romanow government. Elected officials and public servants shared a common vision as to the type of reforms required for the health-care system.

But, as became apparent, the second part of the plan, the wide-scale implementation of new primary health-care "wellness" models and the heightened emphasis on prevention and health promotion, secured limited implementation. Few new primary health teams were established, and investments in prevention and health promotion remained relatively small. A series of decisions—some related to the restructuring of the health system and some to the financial crisis in the province—created a widespread public perception that the government's commitment to wellness was, in fact, code for government cutbacks and retrenchment of services. This perception limited the extent of the second phase of reform.

In *A Saskatchewan Vision for Health* (Saskatchewan Health 1992), the roles of the newly created health districts within the health system were set out as follows:

- conduct health needs assessments and develop district health plans;
- integrate and coordinate health services within the district;
- manage all health services within the district;
- develop community health centres (e.g., health and social centres, cooperative health centres, community clinics or wellness centres);
- ensure that all health services within the district meet specific provincial guidelines and standards; and
- be governed by a single health board. (17)

The health boards were to be two-thirds composed of locally elected members with the others appointed. The belief was that the health boards would reflect local control and responsibility which, in turn, would enable services to be tailored to meet specific regional needs.

One of the reasons for the initial success of the reform initiatives may have been the willingness of stakeholders to participate in the consultations that were promised by the government. There was real support from health leaders, who recognized the need for change and supported the general philosophical thrust of the government's plan. The broad objectives of reform, namely, to reorient the system toward prevention and primary health care, were consistent with a consensus of policy analysis dating at least as far back as the Lalonde report (Lalonde 1974). Agreement with the goals of the reform plan, however, did not always translate into support for specific changes or initiatives that had the potential to reorganize the distribution of power and authority throughout the system.

This was particularly true of the response of health professionals, for example, doctors and nurses. One participant described physicians as staying outside the process, not expecting government to actually go through with such large-scale reforms. Physician indifference may also have been due to the fact that medical services budgets were not to be regionalized, leaving intact the negotiations over the fee-for-service schedule between the Saskatchewan Medical Association (SMA) and the provincial government. It was not until after the reforms were introduced that physicians weighed in on the changes and expressed their displeasure. Any initial SMA support for reform evaporated once the type and extent of reform was unveiled, especially the decision to close or convert 52 small rural hospitals. Opposition also came from Saskatchewan Union of Nurses, who believed that the strategy would result in a significant layoff of nurses. The opposition to the reforms from these stakeholders, whose authority within the system was bolstered by high levels of public trust and confidence, put the government somewhat on the defensive. Reform became increasingly identified as a means to disguise cutbacks and retrenchment of the system. This view painted the health professions as the defenders of medicare against a government obsessed with cost-savings.

The government defended the closure of a small number of hospitals and the conversion of a much larger number to community "wellness centres" on the basis that these facilities were unable to provide quality acute and emergency care. These protestations failed to persuade the opposition and, in the view of some respondents, may well have hindered the government's ability to implement some of the subsequent decisions that were part and parcel of the reform agenda. Indeed, Adams admitted that the closures and conversions were as much about efficiency and cost-savings as they were about the quality of care; it was the black horse of health-care reform, with regionalization being the white horse (Adams 2001c). In the public's view, health reform and hospital closures had been rolled into one entity.

Politically, it seems the government failed to recognize the symbolic importance of the hospital in a small rural community. Along with schools, a post office, and a bank (all of which were also disappearing from small towns), a hospital was a signifier of a community's existence. The "H" on the highway said to all who passed, "There's a community here." Economically, hospitals provided jobs that helped maintain struggling family farms in those communities. Losing the hospital, whatever quality or extent of services it could provide, was akin to saying, "that community no longer exists." But as a number of respondents pointed out, it was well recognized that residents would often forego their local hospital in favour of a larger one nearby.

In and of itself, the concept of regionalization was never about cuts to the health-care system; rather, it was a way to make the system more efficient and to improve the delivery of services through better integration and coordination. The problem was that regionalization coincided with the hospital closures and conversions in communities that were, in many cases, already struggling to sustain their own existence. Opposition to the changes from some quarters within the health professions effectively linked the two outcomes and undercut public support. The creation of health districts already meant the loss of separate institutional boards for local hospitals and other institutions in favour of district boards to govern larger geographic areas. When this was coupled with the actual closing or conversion of small rural hospitals, the government opened itself up to charges that regionalization was just a smokescreen for cost-saving at the expense of rural residents of the province.

The Road to Wellness: Needs-Based Funding and Alternative Payment Plans for Physicians

A key component of restructuring the way health services were delivered was how those services were to be funded. The government's goal was to replace the historical funding formula, based on the past use of services within each institution, with one that allocated funding in accordance with some measure of the health needs and health status of the population served by the new health districts. This new formula was intimately tied to the goals of both regionalization and the wellness initiative, in that it aimed to link the allocation of funds to the population being served and not to the institutions within the districts. If one of the goals of regionalization was to focus attention on the population's health needs within each district, then it only made sense that the allocation of funds to the district be accorded through some measure of that population's health needs and be driven by the services needed to meet those needs. The institutions within those districts would be funded to provide services that met those needs and not simply on the basis of the level and type of services provided in the past. As discussed more fully below, the creation of the population needs-based funding (PNBF) formula in 1994 was driven from inside the civil service, which saw it as a logical extension of regionalization.

Prior to the changes, "individual health facilities were line item funded.... Funding was based mainly on approved volumes of service, derived largely from past levels of use" (McKillop, Pink, and Johnson 2001, 230). Using historical usage patterns to project expenses was a generally accepted method of budgeting, but proved less effective as individual institutions jockeyed for their budget allocation. Even in an era where there was no growth in the overall health budget, individual institutions would lobby for a greater budget, if only to keep up with inflation, at the expense of other institutions that consequently would face budget reductions. One senior public servant familiar with the development of PNBF offered that with former methods of budgeting, there tended to be institutions that were constant winners and losers.

The PNBF formula was implemented in two stages in Saskatchewan. In 1994, it was applied to the funding of non-primary acute care and, a year later, expanded to include both non-primary and primary acute care. Primary acute care refers to the provision of primary care services in an acute care setting, like a hospital emergency room. Primary acute care is not the same as emergency care; it is the delivery of non-emergency care in an emergency room environment. Of the five provinces considered in this volume, Saskatchewan and Alberta were the two that went the furthest in the move to implement PNBF as a key component of their regionalization projects (McIntosh, Ducie, et al. 2010).

The creation of the PNBF formula in Saskatchewan was a technocratic exercise driven by officials within the Department of Health and a small group of outside experts brought in to design the actual allocation formula. Since the changes involved complex technical measurements of need (based on population demographics and health status within each district) and did not affect either the fee-for-service schedule that determined the pay of individual doctors or the wages paid to nurses, the changes attracted little media attention and, perhaps more importantly, little public or stakeholder opposition. Indeed, the key opponents of such a move would likely have been the governing boards of the institutions themselves, but they had ceased to exist upon the creation of the districts. As a number of those involved in the development of the formula noted during interviews, the PNBF formula was, despite its technical complexity, relatively easy to implement insofar as the process was entirely internal to the civil service and the experts charged with its creation.

The model adopted in Saskatchewan was based on the work of McMaster University health economist, Stephen Birch, and his collaborators (Birch and Chambers 1993; Eyles, Birch, et al. 1991). One participant, a public servant responsible for much of the work leading up to the funding change, stated:

> We found [Birch and Chambers'] model and found that they were available to us out of Ontario and got them and others to come and sit on the technical advisory committee.... And we got another economist out of Alberta.... We kind of went across ... who are some of the experts in funding allocation and brought them together at the table with us.

It was these experts who provided the formula that government used to determine funding for the new districts. Because a population-needs-based formula is necessarily complex, the civil service deferred to a technical advisory committee to create the actual formula.

Although some of the stakeholder organizations within the system did express mild concerns about the application of the formula after its implementation, mostly to do with how the reallocation of funds might affect some jobs in some institutions, there was little noticeable opposition to the move. Instead, according to both government officials and the stakeholder groups themselves, the stakeholder groups focused on other aspects of the reform package that had a more direct impact on their members, such as layoffs due to regionalization and hospital closures. Although many of the primary care initiatives were never implemented, the needs-based funding formula became, at least for a while, the principal form for allocating health-care spending in Saskatchewan.

The success of the implementation of the PNBF formula in Saskatchewan seems to rest on its technical complexity, which made it easier to exclude political or non-expert opinions from the discussion, and the fact that it did not directly impact the financial situation of either physicians or nurses. Insofar as payments to physicians continued to be governed by the fee schedule negotiated directly between the SMA and the government, and nurses continued to bargain collectively over their remuneration, they seem to have paid little attention to how the rest of the system's funding was being changed. However, subsequent modifications to the PNBF have restored some of the more traditional forms of historical usage patterns to the allocation formula (Marchildon and O'Fee 2007, 59; McIntosh, Ducie, et al. 2010).

Distinct from the funding of health districts, but still a key component of the wellness agenda articulated by Romanow, was the desire to shift a larger number of physicians from traditional fee-for-service arrangements to different capitation and salary payments. But, unlike the PNBF formula decision, the government encountered significant resistance from the Saskatchewan Medical Association. The SMA took the view that changing the mode of payment would alter one of the more fundamental aspects of the bargain that had been struck between the government and the organization representing the Saskatchewan physicians in 1962, the year when public medical insurance was first implemented in Saskatchewan. That bargain had been designed to ensure the independence of physician decision-making. Despite considerable literature documenting the successes of alternative payments in other parts of the world, support for alternative payments on the part of government, and a willingness by individual physicians to take a look at alternative forms of payment, there was not significant movement away from the fee-for-service payment system in the province during the Romanow and Calvert governments.

In 1992, the Saskatchewan government set up the Alternative Payments Unit as a branch of Saskatchewan Health and began a number of pilot projects in various communities across the province. The physicians in the pilots, who were part of diverse primary health-care teams, were paid using a capitated payment plan. This plan included a service delivery component and focused on team performance expectations rather than individual results. According to those interviewed from the department and the Saskatchewan Medical Association, the pilots were not viewed as having achieved either significant health improvements for patients or satisfaction for physician participants. As such, the attractiveness of alternative payment schemes among physicians remained low. The 2001 Commission on Medicare, chaired by Ken Fyke, re-emphasized the desirability of interdisciplinary health-care teams.The government's *Action Plan for Saskatchewan Health Care* (Saskatchewan Health 2002) reflected its response to the Fyke report's recommendations.

Interestingly, Saskatchewan has had a relatively long experience with the provision of medical services through alternative payment arrangements. Following the introduction of medicare, there were numerous experiments with community clinics in both rural and urban centres. Ranging from single physician practices in small towns to larger multi-professional teams in urban centres, these clinics have long been held up as a model for a different way of providing integrated, coordinated care, but there is no evidence to suggest that they have been widely influential in the struggle over physician payment. Although alternative payment plans for primary care physicians have been around since the 1990s, there was no widespread shift toward them during the years covered here. In fact, in 2003, fee-for-service still accounted for 98 percent of the payments made to primary care physicians by the Medical Services Branch of Saskatchewan Health (Saskatchewan Health 2004, 7-8). The Primary Care Network teams, set up under the *Action Plan* after 2002, remain the predominant, voluntary, alternative payment program.

At this point, it should be noted that a discussion of alternative payment invariably includes a discussion of primary health care. In the words of one government official, "the issue of APPs [alternative payment plans] came forward as a means of having physicians work more with other providers without losing income and the desire to have physicians be within the overall responsibility structure of the RHAs [Regional Health Authorities]." Alternative payments were a mechanism to get physicians working with other health practitioners in a collaborative way. The framework for this was the Primary Care Network teams, which placed a physician with a diverse group of health-care professionals, including nurses, nutritionists, physiotherapists, social workers, and psychologists. The goal was to promote cooperative relationships among practitioners in order to provide comprehensive health care, prevention, and maintenance (Saskatchewan Health 2002, 11). This could only be done by getting physicians away from fee-for-service and onto a more patient-centred system.

The desire to divert physicians away from fee-for-service was strongly promoted from within the health bureaucracy. The Alternative Payments Unit was responsible for setting up various pilot projects across the province that consisted of primary care teams wherein physicians were paid on a non-fee-for-service basis. Members of this particular unit were enthusiastic about new models of remuneration as a means of bolstering quality of care over quantity of care. But at the same time, there were also those within the government who argued that a change in remuneration mechanisms would be just "too much change all at once and … not enough work had been done with the physicians in terms of physician buy-in." In light of the number of dramatic, systemic changes that had already been introduced, other members of the government and civil service were insistent that any changes to fee-for-service would have to be done on a voluntary basis. To do otherwise would invite conflict with the Saskatchewan Medical Association.

The government's decision to try to move doctors off fee-for-service was strongly informed by the work of Morris Barer and Greg Stoddart (1991, 1999), who argued for a population-focused physician funding plan. In an attempt to encourage participation in alternative payment mechanisms, the government brought in physicians from other jurisdictions, including those from Ontario's health service organizations, to speak to Saskatchewan's physicians about their experiences with alternative methods of payment. Despite the evidence of the effectiveness of alternative payment plans, the physician culture of Saskatchewan remained strongly in favour of fee-for-service methods of payment such that little movement occurred.

There is some evidence, however, that physician pay schemes are being reformed within the medical community. Younger physicians consistently decry the lack of work/life balance they observe in their older colleagues and express concern about the "business" side of running a medical practice. The growing number of women in the profession poses new challenges of working while raising a child. Younger doctors are more likely to have spouses who also have important professional obligations outside the home, which must be taken into account in the physician's work life (Canadian Labour and Business Centre and the Canadian Policy Research Networks 2005). Alternative payments fit with this change as physicians would no longer feel obligated to push many patients through to guarantee a certain level of income. As some participants suggested, it may prove that a generational shift will provide a more appropriate landscape for an alternative payment program.

Limiting Access to Private For-profit Care

The ambitious nature of the "wellness agenda" reforms put forward by Romanow took a significant toll on the government and its political support. Regionalization of the system, which the public associated with hospital closures and conversions and fiscal restraint, came at a significant price in terms of the province's credibility as a defender of medicare. Although defending medicare should not be equated with a defence of the status quo, the creation of health districts and the attempts to push the system away from hospital-based, physician-centric acute care clearly created significant anxiety for the public and other community stakeholders. That the anxiety may have been misplaced or misunderstood was neither here nor there; it was real and it was damaging to the government's ability to move forward with the agenda. However, a decision in 1996, driven by politics and these particular circumstances, reasserted the government's position that it was defender of a universal, accessible, and publicly administered health-care system.

In 1996 the government of Saskatchewan passed the *Health Facilities Licensing Act*, which was designed to clarify the legal status of any privately operated facility that might be opened in the province. The legislation did not make it illegal to operate private for-profit clinics in the province but rather clarified a process for their accreditation and regulation (McIntosh and Ducie 2009). In effect, the legislation allows clinics to operate if they meet the regulatory standards set by the Saskatchewan College of Physicians and Surgeons and rely entirely on private payment for the services they provide. In other words, clinics cannot have a dual revenue stream combining monies from the private and public systems. As with individual physicians, a facility was required to choose either public or private payment as its sole source of revenue. The legislation prevents facilities from charging extra fees for "Cadillac services"— services deemed superior to those offered in publicly funded facilities. Furthermore, before a license is issued there must be a determination by the Minister of Health that there is a demonstrated need for such a facility in the proposed location. The legislation permits private, for-profit facilities, but the stipulation that there must be complete reliance on private revenue renders it highly unlikely that any such clinic would be able to make a profit in a small market like Saskatchewan. As of 2010, no such facility has been approved in the province.

Physician representatives interviewed for this study commented that the power given to the Minister to make decisions about private facilities was excessive. In the words of one interviewee, "It was absolute power.... It basically allowed the Minister to determine, based on a very broad set of criteria, whether or not there would be [a private facility] and some of it was smudgy enough like *need*, that it allowed the Minister to essentially say no to any and all requests for private clinics." The Saskatchewan Medical Association (SMA), although it was unhappy with the legislation, chose not to make its displeasure public. At the same time, knowing that at least some elements within the SMA would be opposed to the legislation, the government and the SMA "had several meetings and discussions, and in the end, they [the government] made it clear they were going to introduce the legislation, but [the SMA] did get some changes to it that [it] could live with."

The *Health Facilities Licensing Act* (*HFLA*) was the product of a relatively short policy process. According to one informant, "compared to many legislative agendas, this moved forward relatively quickly." However, while the actual policy did not undergo a lengthy policy-making process, "the government had a sense that this was the road they would like to go down ... much before the actual tabling of the Act.... At least for a year or more, we [the SMA and government] were in discussions. There was some length of time during which the government contemplated this before they moved forward." However, according to most respondents, the time between the decision made and the actual tabling of the legislation was relatively short. Once tabled in the legislature, the *HFLA* was passed without much determined opposition. Most participants close to the process argued that the ideas behind the legislation came straight from the level of cabinet, if not directly from the Premier's Office (McIntosh and Ducie 2009).

As such, it appears that the key rationale for the *HFLA* was philosophical. Private payment for publicly insured services was antithetical to the government's worldview and certainly ran counter to its traditional defence of medicare. Moreover, the legislation filled a regulatory void that even critics admitted needed to be filled. According to most respondents, they just wished for a slightly less stringent regulatory framework. At the same time, a number of those interviewed noted that developments outside the province may have sped up the decision-making process. Private cataract clinics were opening in Alberta at this time and there were rumours of similar clinics being proposed in Saskatoon. The recent adoption of the North American Free Trade Agreement (NAFTA) had also sparked significant concern, especially by the political left, that free trade would threaten Canada's social safety net if it allowed private enterprise to gain traction in the Canadian health-care sector. In this view, then, the

HFLA served to close the door to such operations by making them legal but unlikely to be profitable.

Within the context of the Romanow government's overall health reform agenda—that is, regionalization, the wellness agenda, and the restructuring of public facilities—the *Health Facilities Licensing Act* was consistent with the government's objectives of modernizing medicare. While critics would argue that the *HFLA* froze an outdated vision of health-care delivery, one that needed to be amended to support private payment, the legislation served to fill a regulatory gap that had been unanticipated decades earlier.

One cannot forget that the *HFLA* came at a time when the government had already made a number of controversial health policy decisions, including cutting the drug plan and closing of rural hospitals in an effort to save costs and restructure acute care in the province. The closure and conversion of rural hospitals did significant political damage to the NDP's support in rural Saskatchewan and was seen by many as antithetical to the Douglas vision of medicare that the NDP was expected to protect. For those who viewed the changes wrought by regionalization (and its related reforms) either as disconcerting or as a disguise for fiscal restraint, the strict terms of the *HFLA*'s approach to private facilities in the province reiterated the government's overall commitment to the public oversight of the delivery of health care.

Crisis of Confidence: Waiting for Care in Saskatchewan

The late 1990s brought a new issue to the fore that threatened to permanently undermine the public's confidence in the model of universal, needs-based access to medical care. The issue of waiting times for elective surgery and advanced diagnostic testing had incrementally moved from the margins to the centre of the health-care debate in virtually every Canadian jurisdiction. Ultimately, the Romanow and Calvert governments would respond with the creation of a centralized, mandatory surgical registry, which would employ standardized assessment tools to consolidate and manage access to surgical and diagnostic services across the province. But this did not happen without some false starts along the way.

Two reports released in 1998 were important in focusing public and government attention on the issue of wait times: the Fraser Institute report, and the Health Canada report *Waiting Lists and Waiting Times for Health Care in Canada: More Management, More Money?* (McDonald et al. 1998). The Fraser report singled out Saskatchewan for having the longest wait times and wait lists in the country (Ramsay and Walker 1998). Despite widespread criticism from policy-makers and academics about the think tank's methodology, several respondents indicated that the Fraser report was particularly damaging to the Government of Saskatchewan. On the other hand, the Health Canada report, according to one interviewee, was useful in that it "basically set the foundations of the work that followed, which showed that wait lists were poorly managed."

According to one government official, immediately following the Health Canada report the Saskatchewan government made two crucial moves in the evolution of waiting-list policy in the province. First, it commissioned the Task Team on Surgical Waiting Lists to "describe a fair and transparent system for scheduling elective surgical procedures" and to "recommend the steps necessary to implement the waiting list system across the province." Second, Saskatchewan joined the Western Canada Waiting List Project, which "designed tools for the purpose ... [of creating] an objective measurement of urgency which can be compared between patients with fairly similar conditions."

The Task Team submitted its report on 17 March 1999. The government's initial answer to the recommendations was to announce on 26 March 1999 a $12 million wait-list initiative in the 1999/2000 health budget. Several interviewees, including physicians, viewed the creation of this fund as an attempt by the government to spend its way out of the wait-list problem. The fund essentially transferred one-time monies to the health districts in Regina and Saskatoon (and later, Prince Albert and Moose Jaw) with the idea that such a cash flow would increase capacity and thus decrease surgical waiting lists. However, both government officials and physician representatives noted that the money poured into districts to buy more surgical capacity was not necessarily being used for that purpose.

A subsequent provincewide study, *Surgical Wait List Management: A Strategy for Saskatchewan* (Glynn, Taylor, and Hudson 2002), was released in January 2002. Among the nine recommendations was the call for an electronic surgical registry in Saskatchewan, the development of priority criteria tools, and the designation of a surgical services coordinator to allow for communication between the district, the patient, and the physician. These ideas were eventually moulded into the Saskatchewan Surgical Care Network (SSCN), which was launched in 2003 and has continued to evolve ever since.

The government created the SSCN in an attempt to achieve data consistency across communities and institutions and transparency to the public about how long people might be expected to wait for surgery in their community. The SSCN was an advisory committee to Saskatchewan Health responsible for providing advice on three points: first, planning and managing surgical services in Saskatchewan; second, developing standards and monitoring performance; and finally, communicating with the public and health providers on issues pertaining to surgical access. Consistency and transparency were expected to create a fairer allocation of services and bolster the public's confidence in the system.

Interview subjects noted that the Acute and Emergency Services Branch of Saskatchewan Health, with the help of some physician champions outside the leadership of the SMA, convinced the government that the SSCN was the most viable option to the wait-list problems facing the province. In short, individuals within Saskatchewan Health, armed with independent analysis by outside researchers and supported by physicians willing to make the case to their colleagues, argued that the "wait-list problem" stemmed from the way in which the system allowed lists to be managed by individual doctors, hospitals, and health authorities, rather than from a mere lack of resources.

It is interesting to note that although some actors within the health system were unenthusiastic about the Saskatchewan Surgical Care Network, there was little in the way of organized opposition from stakeholders, especially physicians. Despite the prospect that the SSCN would have some impact on how physicians and surgeons practised medicine, the Saskatchewan Medical Association, according to those interviewed, remained officially neutral on the appropriateness, design, and implementation of the SSCN. At the same time, interview subjects noted the key role played by a small number of physician champions who used their positions of authority within major hospitals to push for acceptance of the SSCN by the medical community. Since inception, a number of validity studies have been conducted, which may have alleviated some of the initial concerns. Support for its further refinement and development appears unswerving. It is apparent that the SSCN has had some success in reducing wait times, but it has since been superseded by other efforts undertaken by the Saskatchewan Party government of Brad Wall (first elected in 2007), which built on the foundation laid by the SSCN. Wait times remain, though, a key issue for the public despite the incremental progress made by the SSCN and its successor initiatives.

CONCLUSIONS: DECISION-MAKING PROCESSES AND THE EXTENT OF REFORM

This chapter has examined six very different issues in the Saskatchewan health-care system—from fiscal restraint to the restructuring of governance and from drug policy to the "bargain" with physicians. Although our analysis does not yield any simple, overarching observations about how or why particular decisions were made, we can draw some general conclusions about how health care decision-making unfolded during the Romanow era.

First, as has been noted throughout the study, there was a privileged place for ideas, research, and policy analysis inside the provincial civil service. This is evident from the ways in which the Romanow government approached the development of the wellness agenda and made subsequent decisions on regionalization, population needs-based funding of health districts, and moving physicians away from fee-for-service payments.

Second, the important role of ideas was fostered by the close working relationship between the civil service and the political executive in the province. The interviewees repeatedly made clear that the close institutional relationship between key civil service actors and key political actors allowed the government to respond to issues as they arose, by implementing the *Health Facilities Licensing Act*, for instance. This working relationship also enabled the government to push forward complicated responses, for example, the "wellness agenda" and the Surgical Care Network, to complicated issues.

These responses were abetted by the lack of a significant political opposition in the province during the first half, at least, of Romanow's decade in power. This changed somewhat in the late 1990s, when the opposition was stronger. Indeed, the government's initial attempt to spend its way out of the wait-list issue may well have reflected its desire to show people, including the opposition and the media, that it was doing "something" about wait times.

Third, there was, and continues to be, a curious dynamic between the government and the various interest groups within the health-care system. In a small jurisdiction like Saskatchewan, access to policy and decision-making is relatively easy for stakeholders to achieve. Coupled with a culture in the province that makes support for medicare the default position for virtually all politicians and stakeholders, this surely helped ease the ability of the civil service and the political executive to engage with stakeholders in a way that undercut the impetus to launch public opposition to the proposed reforms.

Finally, there were those occasions when the government felt forced to take decisions it would not have taken otherwise. The cut to the drug program unveiled in Romanow's very first budget was, no pun intended, a "difficult pill to swallow" for all those concerned. In office for only a few months after a decade of Progressive Conservative rule, the NDP government experienced pressure to make a decision that some involved would later express regret about or attempt to distance themselves from. It was also the only decision of the six led by actors outside the Department of Health. Interestingly, the *HFLA* reflects a different response to external pressures: a quick, publicly accepted introduction of legislation to cut off potential developments before they happened and in such a way that did not create conflict with the pro-NAFTA federal government.

More difficult is an assessment of how much reform the Romanow and Calvert governments achieved during their time in power. The kind of macro reform enunciated by the National Forum on Health (1997a) and later by the Commission on the Future of Health Care in Canada (2002) headed by Romanow himself, has still yet to be achieved in Saskatchewan.

Yet, judged differently, one can say that considerable progress was achieved. Saskatchewan's own blueprints for reform in the form of, first, the Murray report (Saskatchewan Commission on Directions in Health Care 1990) and later, the Commission on Medicare (2001), headed by Ken Fyke, may provide a more appropriate standard by which to judge the progress made. The "wellness agenda" reforms were clearly built on the work of the Murray Commission, despite its having been appointed by the previous Progressive Conservative government, but were also part of the inherent political structure of the NDP. Douglas himself spoke of policy aimed at avoiding ill-health as the "next phase" of medicare. The Lalonde report in the 1970s had laid out the importance of healthy lifestyle choices, and researchers increasingly focused on the social and economic determinants of healthy populations. All of this would have resonated with key actors inside the NDP government and the Saskatchewan civil service. The election of the Romanow government opened a window of opportunity for policy change at a moment when the problem, the solution, and the politics were aligned in a manner that allowed for policy innovation (Kingdon 2003, 2006).

Two of the decisions illustrate the distance between policy-making, decision-making, and policy implementation in a world of competing interests and agendas. The move to a population needs-based funding formula was successfully implemented, but over time was increasingly modified in response to institutional interests and pressures from within the system to preserve funding. In this case, it seems that a significant reform was eroded by the need to keep peace within a system that had already seen significant levels of upheaval over the previous few years.

Second, there was simply a lack of will to engage in a sustained battle with physicians to make alternative payment plans mandatory. Had fee-for-service been the only desired type of reform, the government might have been more forceful with the physician lobby. But in the context of systematic changes, reform fatigue set in. For both the government and the public, the issue proved to be just "a bridge too far." There was neither the capacity nor the political will to take on another contentious and divisive battle.

It is apparent that the wellness agenda got sidetracked but not completely derailed by fiscal restraints. The Fyke report clearly built on the reforms achieved, however imperfectly, to provide a new blueprint for regionalization, primary health care, and integration of services (Commission on Medicare 2001). That the Calvert government's response to Fyke, in the form of its *Action Plan for Saskatchewan Health Care* (Saskatchewan Health 2002), remained the touchstone for reform in the post-Romanow era, speaks to the continuity of the health-care reform project in the province despite whatever zigs and zags have been necessitated by the circumstances of the day.

NOTE

1. The one exception was the decision to cut the drug benefits for budgetary reasons. The interviews make it clear that the decision was taken quickly and with little consultation or "back and forth" between actors involved.

CHAPTER 5

HEALTH-CARE REFORM IN ONTARIO: MORE TORTOISE THAN HARE?

JOHN N. LAVIS, DIANNA PASIC, AND
MICHAEL G. WILSON

If the province of Ontario were one of the two characters in the fable about the tortoise and the hare and the race were health-care reform, Ontario would more closely resemble the tortoise during the 1990–2003 period. Whereas other provinces acted almost spritely when they regionalized health services delivery, Ontario held back, acting as the "control group" for such ambitious reforms. Ontario did occasionally pick up a bit of speed in its efforts to ensure timely access to high-quality health care for all citizens or the system's financial and political sustainability. The province established both a wait-list tracking system (the Cardiac Care Network) and a new prescription drug plan (the Trillium Drug Program). But it is in the domain of the core "public payment/private delivery" bargains where Ontario's slow and steady approach might yet win the race for most significant reforms (Lavis 2004). The province prepared the groundwork for the private for-profit delivery of medically necessary services (although this yielded fairly small impacts) and, more notably, established an alternative payment plan for primary care physicians that has attracted ever more physicians away from the traditional fee-for-service payment plan (Hutchison et al. 2011; Kralj and Kantarevic 2012).

While it is far from clear that changing the core bargains with hospitals and physicians in Ontario will translate into timely access to high-quality health care, better health outcomes, or greater financial and political sustainability for the system, structural reforms were the holy grail of the period and were being called for by many commissions and task forces, both provincially and nationally (National Forum on Health 1997a; Ontario Health Services Restructuring Commission 1999). Ontario's reforms were not comprehensive, however, even though their effect over time could be. The province prepared for a fundamental change to the core bargain with hospitals—private not-for-profit hospitals delivering care with first-dollar, one-tier public payment—but a privatization-inclined governing party would have had to be in office for several consecutive terms to accomplish the change, which turned out not to be the case. The province also prepared for a fundamental change to the core bargain with physicians—private practice physicians delivering care with first-dollar, one-tier public (fee-for-service) payment—but here consecutive governing parties have continued to support the change.

The policy decisions under study in Ontario differ in their nature, timing, and significance (Table 5.1). One decision—the decision not to regionalize health-services delivery—was a "non-decision" during the study period whereas the other five were decisions to do something differently even if the "somethings" differed dramatically in scale. The timing of the decisions ranged from 1990 with the establishment of the Cardiac Care Network through to 2002 with the second of two policy decisions that created a policy framework that made possible the private for-profit delivery of medically necessary services.[1] The significance of the policy decisions ranged from a reinforcement of the status quo (with the decisions not to regionalize and not to redistribute resources to regions with the greatest need) to the establishment of a major new entitlement for catastrophic drug coverage (through the Trillium Drug Program) and the beginning of a change—and what could become a dramatic transformation—in the core bargain with physicians (through the establishment of an alternative payment plan).

The intention of the research in Ontario was to answer the six following questions:

1. Why did Ontario choose not to establish regional health authorities or health districts to assume responsibility for the management and delivery of a significant range of health services?
2. Why did Ontario establish a needs-based funding formula that included only demographic measures of need to allocate funding to hospitals?
3. Why did Ontario establish an alternative payment plan for primary care physicians based on a blend of capitation and fee-for-service (FFS)?
4. Why did Ontario create a policy framework that made possible the development of private for-profit delivery of medically necessary services that had historically been delivered in private not-for-profit hospitals?
5. Why did Ontario establish a voluntary, centralized, wait-list tracking system with a strong potential for management and not another type of tracking system or a management system?

TABLE 5.1
Research Questions Asked and Policy Decisions under Study and Their Significance

Policy Issue	Research Question	Policy Decision under Study	Significance of the Policy Decision in the Context of the Challenges Faced in the Policy Domain
Regionalization of health services delivery	Why did Ontario choose not to establish regional health authorities or health districts to assume responsibility for the management and delivery of a significant range of health services?	Decision not to regionalize (or a "non-decision" about regionalization) in the period between 1991 and 1994	Policy decision reinforced the status quo (i.e., provincial government–driven, rather than a more locally driven, health-care system)
Needs-based funding for health regions/districts	Why did Ontario establish a needs-based funding formula that included only demographic measures of need to allocate funding to hospitals?	Decision in 1992 to allocate hospitals beds on the basis of population size, with the target being the district with the lowest number of hospital beds, and not allocate funding on the basis of health-related measures of need	Policy decision reinforced the status quo (i.e., hospital funding that did not redistribute resources to regions with greater need, which are typically also regions of lower socioeconomic status)
Alternative payment plans for physicians	Why did Ontario establish an alternative payment plan for primary care physicians based on a blend of capitation and fee-for-service (FFS)?	Establishment of Family Health Networks in 2001 that provided a choice of blended payment (capitation based on age and sex profile of patients with some FFS and bonus elements) or reformed FFS	Policy decision began a dramatic transformation of the core bargain with physicians
For-profit delivery of medically necessary services	Why did Ontario create a policy framework that made possible the development of private for-profit delivery of medically necessary services that had historically been delivered in private not-for-profit hospitals?	Series of decisions amending the *Independent Health Facilities Act, 1989*, to allow the development of private for-profit delivery of medically necessary, high-tech diagnostic services (1996), and parallel (i.e., public payment and private payment) tiers of access to these services (2002)	Policy decision surreptitiously prepared the groundwork for a privatization agenda that could have been pursued by a privatization-inclined governing party over several consecutive terms in office
Wait-list management	Why did Ontario establish a voluntary, centralized, wait-list tracking system with a strong potential for management and not another type of tracking system or a management system?	Establishment of the Cardiac Care Network in 1990 for cardiac surgery	Policy decision established a wait-list model that failed to gain traction in many less technical and visible domains
Prescription drug plans	Why did Ontario establish a targeted prescription drug plan and not a universal plan or no new plan?	Establishment of the Trillium Drug Program in 1995 to extend publicly funded prescription drug benefits to anyone paying an income-related sliding-scale deductible	Policy decision established a major new entitlement for catastrophic drug coverage, which left many citizens (with significant but not catastrophic drug expenditures) uninsured

6. Why did Ontario establish a targeted prescription drug plan and not a universal plan (that would reach everyone regardless of whether they chose to pay an income-related sliding-scale deductible) or no new plan?

We begin this chapter by highlighting key features of the policy-making context in Ontario, describing the policy decisions under study, and providing an overview of key events such as major changes to or within the governing party. Next we briefly describe the methods we used to study the six policy decisions, focusing in particular on methodological features unique to this provincial case study. Then we move on to describe the policy-making process for each of the six policy decisions in turn, for which we draw on both a brief timeline of key events and a description of the factors that explain the policy outcome arising from each process.[2] Our analysis identifies patterns in the explanatory factors across the six policy domains. We conclude by highlighting key messages from this provincial analysis.

CONTEXT FOR HEALTH-CARE REFORMS

Two shifts in the Ontario policy-making context between 1990 and 2003 appear as germane as the period's constants. The first shift was the transition in governing party from the centre-left Liberals to the left-leaning New Democrats and then to the right-leaning Progressive Conservatives, and then (just after the end of the study period) back again to the centrist Liberals. These changes in political orientation were all the more remarkable for having followed decades of one-party (Conservative) rule. The second shift was the emergence, during the New Democrats' tenure in office, of a recession and significant government deficits—which was a departure from the province's long-term trajectory of relatively healthy public finances.

The relative constants in the Ontario policy-making context during this period were far more numerous:

- a deeply entrenched public payment/private delivery bargain with hospitals and physicians
- a relatively tightly defined boundary around the health-care sector with medically necessary hospital and physician care at its core
- a joint management committee that involved physicians in the policy-making process for medically necessary care
- a well-organized and resourced provincial medical association but typically poorly organized and resourced groups representing other health-care professionals and "consumers"

- a largely independent and hierarchical public service with frequent turnover of the deputy minister (and health minister)
- a moderately well-established health services and policy research community that was often not effectively engaged by the Ministry of Health and Long-Term Care
- relatively little value accorded to system innovation
- generally positive federal/provincial relations (during the early years of the study period) and interprovincial relations
- pressures arising from technological change (e.g., ambulatory surgery, outpatient diagnostic procedures, new prescription drugs, and home-care services) and new diseases (e.g., HIV/AIDS)
- occasional, proactive, in-depth media coverage of particular policy issues

Many but not all of these constants are shared with other provinces. The first of these constants—the public payment/private delivery bargain—proved to be the most salient in our research.

The election of Liberal majorities in 1987 and 2003 provide metaphorical bookends for the period under study, with the NDP and Progressive Conservatives forming majority governments through most of the study period (Table 5.2). Only the NDP election was widely perceived as an "upset" that brought to power a political party that was not fully prepared for the transition from opposition party to governing party (Rae 1996). The policy decisions were made under the watch of four premiers (David Peterson from the Liberals, 1987–1990; Bob Rae from the NDP, 1990–1995, and Mike Harris and Ernie Eves from the Progressive Conservatives, 1995–2002 and 2002–2003, respectively) and seven health ministers (Elinor Caplan from the Liberals; Evelyn Gigantes, Frances Lankin, and Ruth Grier from the NDP; and Jim Wilson, Elizabeth Witmer, and Tony Clement from the Progressive Conservatives). The establishment of the Cardiac Care Network took place under the Liberals; the decision not to regionalize, the decision to allocate hospital beds on the basis of population size, and the establishment of the Trillium Drug Program took place under the NDP; and the creation of a policy framework that made possible the development of private for-profit delivery of medically necessary services and the establishment of an alternative payment plan for primary care physicians took place under the Progressive Conservatives.

METHODS USED TO STUDY THE CASES

As described in chapter 2, for each policy decision we conducted a detailed documentary analysis, developed a timeline of key events related to the policy decision, interviewed a purposive sample of public policy-makers and stakeholders who were familiar with the policy-making process, and

TABLE 5.2
Timeline of Major Changes to or within the Governing Party and the Policy Decisions under Study in Ontario

Year	Changes to or within the Governing Party	Policy Decisions
1987	• Liberal majority elected with David Peterson as premier and Elinor Caplan appointed as health minister (after decades of Conservative party rule)	
1990	• NDP majority elected with Bob Rae as premier and Evelyn Gigantes as health minister	• Establishment of the Cardiac Care Network (case 5)
1991	• Frances Lankin replaces Evelyn Gigantes as health minister	• Decision not to regionalize in the period between 1991 and 1994 (case 1)
1992		• Decision to allocate hospitals beds on the basis of population size (case 2)
1993	• Ruth Grier replaces Frances Lankin as health minister	
1995	• Progressive Conservative majority elected with Mike Harris as premier and Jim Wilson appointed as health minister	• Establishment of the Trillium Drug Program (case 6)
1996		• Decision to amend the *Independent Health Facilities Act, 1989,* to allow the development of private for-profit delivery of medically necessary, high-tech diagnostic services (1996) (case 4)
1997	• Elizabeth Witmer replaces Jim Wilson as health minister	
1999	• Progressive Conservative majority re-elected with Mike Harris as premier	
2001	• Tony Clement replaces Elizabeth Witmer as health minister	• Establishment of Family Health Networks in 2001 (case 3)
2002	• Ernie Eves replaces Mike Harris as premier	• Decision to amend the *Independent Health Facilities Act, 1989,* to allow the development of parallel (i.e., public payment and private payment) tiers of access to medically necessary, high-tech diagnostic services (case 4)
2003	• Liberal majority elected with Dalton McGuinty as premier and George Smitherman appointed as health minister	

analyzed the resulting data using the Kingdon and 3I frameworks (see Table 2.2 in chapter 2; Bhatia 2002; Kingdon 2003; Lavis et al. 2002; Lavis et al. 2012). For each documentary analysis we searched seven bibliographic databases (Canadian Research Index, CBCA, EconLit, MedLine, Political Science Abstracts, Social Sciences Index, and Sociological Abstracts) and one media database (Lexis Nexis). For the documentary analyses related to the establishment of the Cardiac Care Network and Trillium Drug Plan, we also hand-searched the *Ontario Medical Review* and the *Canadian Medical Association Journal* for the years 1986–1990 and 1990–1995, respectively.

We conducted 51 interviews with public policy-makers and stakeholders in Ontario, with a range of seven to ten interviews for each policy decision. We encountered only 15 individuals whose contact information could not be located, who declined to be interviewed because they were not knowledgeable about the policy decision or they could identify others who were more knowledgeable, or who could not be scheduled despite repeated efforts. Eight individuals never responded to our requests for an interview for the two related policy decisions that reinforced the status quo (i.e., deciding not to regionalize and deciding not to redistribute resources to regions with the greatest need), although some of these were the same people. Ten individuals declined to be interviewed about creating a policy framework that made possible the development of private for-profit delivery of medically necessary services. Consequently, for this case we may have heard only part of the story; we cannot be certain whether some key individuals felt constrained in what they could say or were not heard at all.

FINDINGS – SIX STUDIES IN HEALTH-CARE REFORM

Case Study 1: Deciding Not to Regionalize

The visible elements of the public policy-making process associated with considering whether to regionalize—that is, whether to establish health regions/districts in Ontario to assume responsibility for the management and delivery of a significant range of health-care services—took place over a three-year period between 1991 and 1994. The Premier's Council on Health Strategy, a creation of Ontario Liberal premier David Peterson, released a report on devolution in the spring of 1991, which was not long after the election of NDP leader Bob Rae (Ontario. Premier's Council on Health Strategy 1991). Three years later the council's successor, the Premier's Council on Health, Well-Being and Social Justice, released two reports on devolution, one of which described a framework for evaluating pilot projects in the devolution of the management and delivery of a significant range of health-care services (Ontario. Premier's Council on Health, Well-Being and Social Justice 1994a, 1994b). None of these reports contributed to or coincided with regionalization being on the government's decision agenda: the champions of the first report were no longer in office when the report was released, and the champions of the next two reports, most of whom came from outside government, appear not to have been successful in creating the political will to act on their recommendations.

Ontario had experimented in the past (and would experiment again beyond our study period) with various forms of regionalization, but often with little actual transfer of decision-making authority. In 1973 the Ontario government established District Health Councils to assist in health planning for 16 districts (and specifically in advising about the allocation of any new funding); however, they were given no decision-making authority, and not even an advisory role about base budgets. The Rae-led NDP government introduced regional offices for the Ministry, although the transfer of decision-making authority from the "central" Ministry of Health (i.e., deconcentration) was minimal. The Harris-led Progressive Conservative government, which replaced the NDP government, established Community Care Access Centres as regional access points for long-term care services and the Health Services Restructuring Commission as a mechanism to plan hospital mergers on a region-by-region basis, both of which meant some form of concentration in decision-making authority at the regional (as opposed to local) level (Ontario Health Services Restructuring Commission 2000). This government also devolved some authority over public health services, and health and social services, to the municipal level. It was only in 2004 and 2005 that a McGuinty-led Liberal government revisited the idea of regionalization, which had first been introduced by the Peterson-led Liberals 15 years earlier, and established Local Health Integration Networks (Ministry of Health and Long-Term Care 2004).

The issue of regionalization appeared on the governmental agenda through the work of the Premier's Council on Health Strategy. The council's Integration and Coordination Committee had identified what they perceived to be a lack of locally sensitive planning in the health-care system and a lack of involvement of local communities in decision-making about their health-care system. However, the issue of regionalization never really moved to the decision agenda despite it moving to and remaining on the agenda of the Premier's Council on Health, Well-Being and Social Justice, the successor to the Premier's Council on Health Strategy. Both Premier's Councils framed the problem and the policy proposal in the same way, albeit with the refinement by the second Premier's Council that devolution be piloted and evaluated before widespread implementation. Nevertheless, political forces both inside government (such as the premier and the hospital branch of the Ministry) and outside government (such as the Ontario Hospital Association and the Ontario Medical

Association) were either unsupportive or actively opposed to the change. As we describe in the next case study, the lack of support and / or the opposition was in small part related to empirical research that had found that needs-based funding, which was seen as an obvious policy to accompany regionalization, would have resulted in substantial reallocations across regions, and this in an era with large deficits and a troubled economy.

Case Study 2: Deciding to Allocate Hospitals Beds (Not Dollars) on the Basis of Population Size (Not Need)

The public policy-making process associated with considering whether to introduce needs-based funding—whether to fund districts, or hospitals, on the basis of need rather than funding hospitals within each district on the basis of a mixed global budget / case-based method—took place over a very brief period in 1991 and 1992. As described in the previous section, both Premier's Councils had been toying with the idea of devolution. A northern District Health Council had commissioned McMaster University professor Stephen Birch to explore what a needs-based "virtual" district budget would look like.[3] The Ministry of Health, inspired by the District Health Council's experience, commissioned Birch to produce a report on how hospital budgets would change if needs-based funding were implemented in Ontario; the report was later turned into a peer-reviewed journal article (Birch and Chambers 1993). Meanwhile, two events drew attention away from districts and needs-based funding and toward hospitals and cost containment. A provincial auditor's report that highlighted "questionable practices by hospitals" and "loose procedures" by the Ministry of Health drew the health minister's attention toward hospital accountability (Archer 1991; "Getting a Handle on Hospital Costs" 1991). And an economic downturn drew the treasurer's attention towards cost containment, which meant that any reallocations on the basis of need became a zero-sum game.

The issue of needs-based funding had been on the governmental agenda for some time as District Health Council members repeatedly pointed out the lack of financial framework (even virtual district budgets) within which they could provide advice to the Ministry of Health. This problem was given new visibility within the Ministry of Health through the work of a northern District Health Council. But as with regionalization, the issue of needs-based funding never really moved to the decision agenda. The one needs-based funding proposal on the table (which had been outlined in Birch's report) would have resulted in substantial reallocations across districts. The same political forces in the devolution debate were at play here, with the added complication that an auditor's report and an economic downturn had given the minister of health reason to focus on hospital accountability and cost containment, not virtual or real district-level budgets or zero-sum reallocations across districts.[4]

Case Study 3: Deciding to Establish an Alternative Payment Plan for Primary Care Physicians

The public policy-making process associated with considering whether to establish an alternative payment plan for primary care physicians in Ontario based on a blend of capitation and fee-for-service (FFS) began within a year of the Progress Conservative party taking power in June 1995. Health Minister Jim Wilson announced in the summer of 1996 an implementation committee to guide the establishment of pilot projects that would enable the Ministry of Health to evaluate both a capitation and a reformed FFS model. Two years later, in May 1998, his successor, Elizabeth Witmer, and Ontario Medical Association (OMA) president William Orovan announced the launch of five pilot projects to evaluate the effectiveness of what were then called Primary Care Networks. In March 2001, which was four months before the release of the evaluation report and still well in advance of funds beginning to flow to Ontario from the federal government's Primary Health Care Transition Fund (Barnes 2006), Elizabeth Witmer's successor, Tony Clement, and Premier Mike Harris announced the establishment of the Ontario Family Health Network, an arm's-length agency tasked with facilitating the rollout of what were by then called Family Health Networks.

The build-up to reform had taken six years, and yet it was not the first time that alternative payment plans had been announced as the future of primary care. The governments of the day had launched Health Service Organizations in 1973 and Community Health Centres in 1982, and a government-appointed committee had called for Comprehensive Health Organizations in 1987 (J.R. Evans 1987; Gillet, Hutchison, and Birch 2001; Hutchison, Abelson, and Lavis 2001). What was different this time was the sustained effort that followed the announcement to offer significant financial returns to physicians who enrolled in Family Health Networks (and later in Family Health Groups).

As this brief historical summary would suggest, the issue of an alternative payment plan for physicians had been on the governmental agenda for decades. There had been a long-standing perception that FFS remuneration (compared to alternative remuneration methods) created the wrong incentives for primary care (such as a focus on services, not value for money). This perception had been reinforced by many reports over the years (J.R. Evans 1987; Hastings 1972; Kilshaw 1995). As a new governing party took office, there were additional concerns about shortages of primary care physicians and a declining interest among physicians in a comprehensive model of primary care, as well as strained relations between the provincial government and the Ontario Medical Association (which arose, in large part, due to claw-backs imposed on physicians' billings above defined levels in order to reduce the government's deficit).

The issue of an alternative payment plan for physicians moved to the decision agenda as a result of the confluence of a problem (in this case perceived problems with FFS remuneration) brought into focus yet again through a report, a viable policy option, and a political desire to lay the groundwork for four years of peace with the OMA. The report was issued by the Health Services Restructuring Commission (1999) and endorsed by the Ontario College of Family Physicians and the new Coalition for Primary Health Care. The viable policy option was the widespread implementation of the five pilot Primary Care Networks, which involved a choice of two remuneration methods (reformed FFS with thresholds based on the number and characteristics of enrolled patients, and capitation with payments based on the number and gender of patients served). The political desire emerged from the re-election of the Progressive Conservative party who faced as one of their first orders of business in the health sector the need to negotiate a new four-year agreement with the OMA.

The final policy chosen in 2001 was the establishment of Family Health Networks that (a) provided a choice of blended payment (capitation based on age and sex profile of patients with some FFS and bonus elements) or reformed FFS; (b) required rostering for blended payment; (c) provided incentives for providing preventive services; (d) provided indirect incentives to hire nurses, nurse practitioners, and others; (e) required 24/7 coverage through on-call arrangements involving the group or network; (f) provided an incentive for computer purchases to make possible the use of electronic health records; (g) provided an incentive for continuing medical education; (h) provided a centrally administered telephone advisory service; and (i) placed few limits on patient choice. Patients were not required to join a Family Health Network and were allowed to change physicians up to twice a year; they were required only to notify their physician if seeking care elsewhere (Lee 2003; Ontario Family Health Network 2005).

This policy choice appears to have arisen from the confluence of many institutional, interest-based, ideas-based, and external factors. Six policy legacies were in play. Two of the policy legacies diminished the prospects for a change to the prevailing physician-remuneration method: the core bargain's focus on physicians instead of the services they have historically provided; and the Ontario Health Insurance Plan's focus on paying individuals instead of groups. The remaining four policy legacies were conducive to a change: (a) policies that had led to some negative connotations for fee-for-service remuneration among primary care physicians;

(b) a policy that allowed nurse practitioners to join primary care teams; (c) a set of pilot projects that had been endorsed by the OMA; and (d) a prototype for the widespread adoption of an alternative payment plan by physicians. The combination of a well-established policy network that privileged physicians in policy-making about primary care and a desire among some members of the OMA for change provided the opportunity for a breakthrough. A report by the Health Services Restructuring Commission (1999) had proposed a relatively significant reform that made the aforementioned pilot projects seem almost incremental in nature and hence a reform that could be more readily embraced. Moreover, the combination of concerns about shortages in primary care physicians, a declining interest among physicians in a comprehensive model of primary care, and the long-standing perception that FFS remuneration creates the wrong incentives for primary care meant that any governing party would have been open to the possibility of a breakthrough. The re-election of a Progressive Conservative party that was in a relatively strong bargaining position for the next four-year agreement with the OMA, the willingness of the OMA to allow money to be reallocated from the FFS pool of funds to alternative remuneration methods, and the relatively healthy public finances that made it possible to offer significant financial returns to physicians who joined a Family Health Network, all created the conditions necessary to achieve a breakthrough.

Case Study 4: Making Possible the For-Profit Delivery of Medically Necessary Services

The public policy-making processes associated with making possible the for-profit delivery of medically necessary services, which we have called a counter-consensus reform—were not very visible to the public because the processes were often embedded within much bigger legislative changes or announcements. The documentary trail for the processes is almost non-existent, and the bigger legislative changes were sufficiently highly charged that (as mentioned previously) some participants were not willing to be interviewed about the smaller-scale changes related to this case. The first decision involved amending the *Independent Health Facilities Act* (*IHFA*), originally introduced in 1989 under the Liberals, to allow the development of private for-profit delivery of medically necessary "high tech" diagnostic services. The 1996 amendments, undertaken as part of Bill 26, the *Savings and Restructuring Act*, eliminated the preference in the *IHFA* for Canadian-owned, not-for-profit independent health facilities (IHF). The amendments, while later called "sleeper legislation" (Gilmour 2003), had little short-term impact because the cap on the price of an IHF license meant that there was little incentive to make the large capital expenditures needed to provide these services.

The series of decisions that made possible a parallel stream of private payment for medically necessary services began in June 2002 with a statement embedded in a budget announcement (Government of Ontario 2002) and ended five months later (in November 2002) with the Ministry of Health and Long-Term Care issuing a request for proposals for five new CT scanners and five new MRI scanners (with another 15 to come later; Boyle 2002). The budget announcement outlined plans to allow the operation of CT and MRI scanners in private for-profit clinics, and made clear that these clinics would be able to provide both medically necessary (i.e., publicly insured) and non-medically necessary (i.e., un-insured or privately insured) streams of these services. Amendments to the *IHFA* regulations allowed the provision of CT and MRI scans outside of private not-for-profit hospitals. Additional amendments to the *IHFA* regulations, which were made as part of Bill 179, the *Government Efficiency Act*, removed the cap on the price of an IHF license. This policy decision gave IHF operators the opportunity to sell their facilities to the highest bidder (and thus to recoup capital expenditures before the expenditures had been amortized); it also gave them the incentive to call "medically necessary" services "unnecessary" because the higher revenue from the latter would help to offset their investments in a license. Shortly thereafter, Health Minister Tony Clement announced plans to provide up to 20 new MRI machines and five new CT scanners (Rachlis 2002), which would be allowed to operate through existing independent health facilities, and the Ministry issued the request for proposals.

Challenges in the delivery of medically necessary diagnostic services had appeared on the governmental agenda in 1999 and 2000, largely as a result of a report by the Fraser Institute (about the number of CT and MRI scanners per capita in Canada compared to other OECD countries; Wilson and Zelder 2000), a report by the Ontario Association of Radiologists (2002) about Ontario hospitals' waiting times for a number of diagnostic procedures, and statements by both the Canadian and Ontario Associations of Radiologists that there were shortfalls in machines and technologists). The Ontario Health Coalition, a network of grassroots organizations, viewed the issue as a widespread problem of access. The Commission on the Future of Health Care in Canada later legitimized these concerns in its November 2002 report.

When the issue moved to the decision agenda in 2002, however, it had come to be framed more as one about a shortage in machines, rather than as a shortage in both machines and technologists or as a more widespread access problem. The viable policy option was identified as making possible the for-profit delivery of these services (rather than hospitals being allocated a share of the federal government transfers that were provided to purchase such machines, and training more technologists). The "politics stream" within this agenda-setting dynamic appeared particularly influential here with a new party leader taking over as premier and a new health minister being appointed, both of whom shared the type of "free market" values that would lead them to see more potential for change among for-profit facilities than not-for-profit hospitals.[5]

While the proximal factors at play at the time of policy choice in 2002 included a broad array of institutions, interests, and ideas, a premier and a health minister with strongly held values carried the day for this counter-consensus reform. The institutional factors included two policy legacies. First, the *Canada Health Act* covers only hospital-based and physician-provided services, which means that services provided outside of hospitals (and with no or partial involvement of physicians) are not bound by the Act's first-dollar, one-tier coverage requirement. In the absence of additional legislation covering private health-care facilities, patients would have had to pay for health care that had historically been provided in hospitals and considered "medically necessary," or they could have chosen to pay to receive faster access or higher-quality care. Second, the *Independent Health Facility Act* filled this gap by making provisions for private health-care facilities to receive both facility fees (to cover their capital and operating costs) and physician fees from the government (instead of from patients) in return for providing "medically necessary" services. The interests at play included societal interest groups, specifically the Ontario Association of Radiologists advocating for more machines and technologists but not at the expense of hospitals; the Ontario Health Coalition and its partners advocating for improved access but not for-profit delivery; and the Ontario Hospital Association highlighting concerns about staff poaching, queue jumping, and spillover effects if a parallel stream of services were provided in private for-profit clinics. The interests also included elected officials and specifically the premier and health minister, who were interested in pursuing more for-profit delivery. The ideas in play included views about what "ought to be," specifically, "free market" values. It was the combination of the latter two factors—an engaged premier and health minister who both placed great emphasis on a particular set of values—that appears to have carried the day. (Two more distal factors also played a role: a political change in the form of a new premier and health minister coming to power, and a technological change in the form of many new indications being identified for CT and MRI scans.)

Case Study 5: Establishing a Wait-List Tracking System for Cardiac Surgery

The public policy-making process associated with the establishment of the Cardiac Care Network in 1990 took place over a 26-month period between May 1988 and July 1990 (Wilson 2004). In May 1988 media coverage began about patient deaths on wait lists. In July 1990 the Provincial

Adult Cardiac Care Network (later renamed the Cardiac Care Network) was established and given authority for overseeing a voluntary, centralized wait-list tracking system for cardiac surgery. The network had the potential to become a management system: it had a central database for tracking patients' clinical severity and hospitals' throughput, regional coordinators tasked with data submissions and local coordination, and an independent governance mechanism that gave voice to cardiologists and cardiac surgeons. But it was quite clearly established as a tracking system only, albeit one that was well ahead of its time and one that set the benchmark against which other provincial systems (both inside and outside Ontario) were compared for many years (Davies 1999; Moralis 1996; Monaghan et al. 2001; Trypuc 2001).

The issue of wait lists for cardiac surgery appeared on the governmental agenda in May 1988 because of intense media coverage about patient deaths on wait lists (e.g., Tyler and Maycheck 1989). A lack of resources was argued by many to be the immediate cause of the problem; however, others argued that the root causes included the lack of a systems approach (e.g., surgeons with wait lists in their pockets rather than a central registry with patients tracked using agreed-upon risk scores) and competition among hospitals. Regardless of how the problem was framed, the consequences were the same: a decline in public confidence in the health-care system.

The issue of wait lists for cardiac surgery moved to the decision agenda in 1990. Research suggested that wait lists for cardiac surgery were a large and growing problem but, more importantly, feedback from hospitals suggested that more money had not had a significant effect (Naylor 1991; Naylor et al. 1993). The lack of effect was attributed to care not being allocated on the basis of need (i.e., a lack of equity) and low hospital throughput (i.e., a lack of efficiency). Political forces were also at play with the health minister facing growing public concerns about the ability of the system to meet patients' needs. Meanwhile the Provincial Working Group on Cardiovascular Services had reviewed the wait-list tracking system in Toronto (called the Metropolitan Toronto Triage System; Kaminski, Sibbald, and Davis 1989), which had attributes that they felt were key to a well-functioning system: it was voluntary, centralized, focused on cardiac surgery, and independent of the provincial Ministry of Health (Keon 1991). A confluence of a continued problem that had not been solved simply with more resources, a health minister "under the gun," and a workable policy option in a constituent jurisdiction were coupled in a way that brought the issue to the decision agenda.

Like the alternative payment plan case study, this policy choice appears to have arisen from the confluence of many factors. The institutional factors included (a) the policy legacy of the Metropolitan Toronto Triage System, a system endorsed by the St. Michael's Hospital review panel, which had looked into several patient deaths at that hospital (Kaminski,

Sibbald, and Davis 1989); and (b) the policy network that had been created first through the Metropolitan Toronto Triage System and then through the Provincial Working Group on Cardiovascular Services (Keon 1991). The interests at play included societal interest groups—specifically cardiologists and cardiac surgeons—and elected officials. In particular, the health minister was seeking to reduce the political harms arising from media coverage of deaths on the wait lists and, in the longer run, restore public confidence in the health-care system. The ideas in play included knowledge or beliefs about "what is" and views about "what ought to be." Research on risk scores, for example, informed "what is." Views about "what ought to be" reflected a desire for efficiency and equity: efficiency in hospitals' meeting target volumes in throughput, and equity in allocating surgery (specifically cardiac surgery) on the basis of need and not the "squeakiness of the wheel." A more distal factor that also played a role was the intense media coverage of deaths on wait lists.

Case Study 6: Establishing a New Publicly Funded Prescription Drug Benefit

The public policy-making process associated with the establishment of the Trillium Drug Program in 1995, which extended publicly funded prescription drug benefits to anyone paying an income-related sliding-scale deductible, took place over a 33-month period between February 1992 and November 1994 (Wilson 2004). In February 1992 the provincial government established the Drug Programs Reform Secretariat to reform provincial drug programs to make them accessible to more Ontario residents, to improve the quality of prescribing, and to make the programs more affordable. On 30 November 1994, on the eve of World AIDS Day—the day that AIDS Action Now! (a societal interest group) planned to hold a fifth high-profile demonstration to demand a catastrophic drug plan for individuals with life-threatening illnesses—Ontario premier Bob Rae announced that the provincial government had decided to extend the Ontario Drug Benefits (ODB) plan (with as yet unspecified cost-sharing arrangements) to include patients not already covered under the ODB plan or by private insurance (Walkom 1994, 1995). A process that began as an initiative led by public servants within the Ministry of Health ended with a highly visible political decision made by the premier. The Trillium Drug Program officially began in April 1995, just over four months after the premier's announcement.

While anyone not already covered under the ODB plan or by private insurance is eligible to apply for the Trillium Drug Program, the income-related sliding-scale deductible means that the program disproportionately benefits those with low incomes and high drug costs. People with high incomes typically do not benefit from the program unless their drug costs are very high. For example, at the time the program was introduced an individual with an income of $100,000 per year would have had to pay $4,100 of their prescription drug costs before receiving any assistance through the program (Wright 1995). People living with HIV/AIDS, cancer, cystic fibrosis, and rare diseases like Gaucher's disease would be among those who often faced catastrophic drug costs. For example, the drug costs for the 15,000 HIV/AIDS patients in Ontario in 1994 were estimated to be between $40 and $50 million (Papp 1994).

The issue of making changes to prescription drug plans in an effort to cover previously uninsured or underinsured persons appeared on the governmental agenda in the lead up to the provincial government's establishment of the Drug Programs Reform Secretariat. Public servants had identified that drug program expenditures were growing exponentially, which was driven in part by the emergence of "breakthrough" drugs and the open-ended nature of the Special Drugs Program (a program that covered the costs of specific, very expensive prescription drugs, such as some experimental HIV/AIDS treatments).

The issue moved to the decision agenda late in 1994. Rapidly escalating drug expenditures continued to be seen as a problem, but the consultation led by the Drug Secretariat had also identified a new problem—the unmet needs of those aged 55–64 who had no job or had lost their drug benefits when the economy was in rough straits. Political forces were also at play as the premier faced an emotionally charged campaign by AIDS Action Now!, which included a press conference with a plea from a dying AIDS patient and a threat to burn in effigy a mock-up of Premier Bob Rae. Meanwhile, public servants had been working on the design of a new drug program that (a) extended the ODB plan to anyone paying an income-related sliding-scale deductible (although the scale was contested at this time); (b) had no eligibility requirement linked to a particular illness (like AIDS), health status (like end-of-life care), or drug class (like the drugs covered by the Special Drugs Program); and (c) provided full-family access to the full Ontario Drug Benefits formulary (thereby removing any incentive to leave a job in order to gain access to this plan, which would have run counter to the governing party's desire to move people from "welfare to work"). A confluence of two problems, politics, and a workable policy option were coupled in a way that brought these issues to the decision agenda.

Like both the alternative payment plan and the wait-list management case studies, this policy choice appears to have arisen from the confluence of many factors, and not just the highly visible political pressure brought to bear on the government of the day. The institutional factors included two policy legacies: the ODB plan, with a formulary and fully operational administrative process, and HealthNet, which provided an online submission and adjudication process for the ODB plan. The interests at play included societal interest groups (specifically AIDS Action

Now! and less visibly a group led by a Toronto lawyer with Gaucher's disease), elected officials (specifically the premier who was facing a pending election, which he lost within seven months of the decision to establish the Trillium Drug Program), and public servants (specifically officials who had identified an unmet need among those aged 55–64, and officials who had managed a program that they felt worked—the ODB plan). The ideas in play included knowledge or beliefs about "what is" (the exponential growth of drug program expenditures and the unmet needs of those aged 55–64) and views about what "ought to be" (equity across income groups, disease groups, and age groups). Four more distal factors also played a role: AIDS had appeared as a significant new disease, "breakthrough" drugs had begun to appear for diseases like AIDS (and Gaucher's disease), the media provided extensive coverage of the life-and-death consequences of patients having access to these drugs, and tough economic times made it difficult to propose a free plan or even a plan with a small deductible.

Cross-Case Analysis

A health-care reform that did not touch significantly on the core "public payment/private delivery" bargains that underpin the Canadian health-care system went forward, much as others have done in the past. The Ontario government established a targeted prescription drug plan (the Trillium Drug Program) in its effort to cover previously uninsured persons and, in so doing, went some way toward extending the public payment element of the core bargain into a new sphere. But the bargain was not nearly as generous as the bargains struck with hospitals and physicians more than three decades earlier. Public payment for prescription drugs was far from being first-dollar or one-tier in the Trillium Drug Program. Nevertheless, a problem (rapidly escalating prescription drug expenditures) brought the issue to the governmental agenda. The coupling of this problem and a newly identified problem (an unmet need among those aged 55–64), politics (a highly visible interest-group campaign), and a workable policy option brought the issue to the decision agenda. A confluence of many factors appears to explain the final policy choice.

On the other hand, two health-care reforms that had the potential to touch significantly on the core public payment/private delivery bargain with hospitals floundered. Both regionalization and needs-based funding constitute an incursion into the community autonomy that was to have been safeguarded by the "private not-for-profit hospitals" part of the public payment/private delivery bargain with hospitals. In both cases, a perceived problem brought the issue to the governmental agenda: a lack of locally sensitive planning and community involvement in decision-making (regionalization), and a lack of a financial framework for District Health Councils (needs-based funding). But no policy entrepreneurs rose to the fore to couple these problems with a viable policy proposal and the politics of the day. Two successive Premier's Councils endorsed a move toward regionalization yet, unlike every other Canadian province, the Ontario government did not fully embrace the idea, at least during the period of study (1990–2003). Select District Health Council members endorsed a move toward needs-based funding, but a new focus on hospital accountability and cost containment meant that the Ontario government never fully embraced this idea either. In both cases a prominent interest group opposed the idea, but no major campaign was required to send the idea to the back burner, where needs-based funding largely remained (until 2010 with the gradual phasing-in of the Health-Based Allocation Model, which has both needs-based and activity-based elements) and where regionalization remained for over a decade (until the formal creation of Local Health Integration Networks in 2006).

A health-care reform that had the potential to touch significantly on the core public payment/private delivery bargain with physicians but that preserved key elements of the bargain went forward. A wait-list management system would have constituted an incursion into the professional autonomy that was to have been safeguarded by the "private practice" part of the public payment/private delivery bargain with physicians. In this case, the alternative that was adopted left largely intact the professional autonomy of cardiologists and cardiac surgeons. All that the Cardiac Care Network asked of them was that they used an agreed-upon risk score to assess their patients' clinical severity and that the hospitals in which they worked added these data to the central registry and met particular throughput targets. A problem—deaths on the wait lists—brought the issue to the governmental agenda. With the recognition that the problem could not be solved with more resources alone, the coupling of this problem with the politics (a health minister trying to retain public confidence in the health-care system) and a workable policy option (the Metropolitan Toronto Triage System model) brought the issue to the decision agenda. As with the Trillium Drug Program, a confluence of many factors appears to explain the final policy choice made in establishing the Cardiac Care Network.

Similarly, a health-care reform that touched on the core public payment/private delivery bargain with hospitals but that took place over time, in the shadows of larger legislative changes and announcements and with limited negative near-term consequences, also went forward. For-profit hospitals (or more accurately for-profit clinics providing services that have been historically provided in hospitals) constitute an incursion into the community ownership that was to have been safeguarded by the "private not-for-profit hospitals" part of the public payment/private delivery bargain with hospitals. Moreover, a parallel stream of private payment for medically necessary services constitutes an incursion into the equity principle that was to have been safeguarded by the "one-tier public payment" part of the bargain. In this case the Ontario government over two successive terms in office created a policy framework that made possible the development of private for-profit delivery of medically necessary services that had historically been delivered in private not-for-profit hospitals. But the services were primarily restricted to CT and MRI scans, two services for which patients had long been receiving care in nearby US cities, and even then only in the small number of independent health facilities that were granted licenses for new CT and MRI scanners. A problem (challenges in the delivery of medically necessary diagnostic services) brought the issue to the governmental agenda. The coupling of this problem and more general concerns about access, politics (a new premier and health minister), and a workable policy option brought the issue to the decision agenda. But at the stage of policy choice we see a different pattern: it appears to be the combination of two factors—an engaged premier and health minister who both placed great emphasis on a particular set of values—not a broad constellation of factors that carried the day.

Most surprisingly, a health-care reform that touched significantly on the core public payment/private delivery bargain with physicians but that took place over time and with significant positive near-term financial and non-financial advantages to "early adopters" also went forward, but this time after years of failure. Alternative payment plans constitute an incursion into the entrepreneurialism and professional autonomy that was to have been safeguarded by the public payment/private delivery bargain with physicians. In this case a perceived problem (the long-standing perception that FFS remuneration created the wrong incentives for primary care) brought the issue of an alternative payment plan for physicians to the governmental agenda and kept it there for several decades. The confluence of this problem—brought into focus through yet another report, a viable policy option, and a political desire to lay the groundwork for four years of peace with the OMA and for a financial basis for reallocating funds from the fee-for-service "pool" to alternative payment plans—brought the issue to the decision agenda. And as with the establishment of the Trillium Drug Program and the Cardiac Care Network, a confluence of many factors appears to explain the final policy choice. As more and more physicians leave a purely private practice for the new models supported by alternative payment plans, the reform now appears to have been the beginning of a change, and possibly a dramatic transformation, in the core bargain with physicians.

CONCLUSION

Strong policy legacies, particularly those arising from the core bargains with hospitals and physicians, do appear amenable to influence, albeit not with the "big bang" that advocates of comprehensive structural reform typically advocate. Notwithstanding the core bargain with hospitals, the Harris-led Progressive Conservatives were able to create a framework that made possible the development of private for-profit delivery of medically necessary services that had historically been provided in hospitals. But their counter-consensus reform took place over an extended period of time and in the shadows of larger legislative changes and announcements. Moreover, their reform had limited to no near-term consequences and would have required them (or a like-minded government) to pursue the reform over successive terms in order to have a vibrant for-profit delivery sector competing with the well-established not-for-profit sector. Notwithstanding the core bargain with physicians, the same governing party was able to establish an alternative payment plan for physicians. This reform also took place over time and with significant financial and non-financial incentives to the "early adopters." As we discuss in chapter 11, the reform gathered steam over the subsequent decade (Hutchison et al. 2011; Kralj and Kantarevic 2012), raising the prospects for an eventual larger role for government (through contracts) in the fiercely guarded professional terrain of physicians.

And this brings us back to the fable of the tortoise and the hare. Two of the reforms we studied—making possible the for-profit delivery of select medically necessary services and establishing a new publicly funded prescription drug benefit—turned out not to be the start of any sweeping changes in the health sector. On the other hand, one of the reforms—establishing a wait-list tracking system for cardiac surgery—influenced the development of other wait-list systems in the province, such as those for cataract surgery, hip replacement and knee replacement, as well as for CT and MRI scans. Moreover, one "no go" decision and one "near no go" decision—deciding not to regionalize and deciding to allocate hospitals beds (not dollars) on the basis of population size (not need)—were followed within a decade by bold decisions. In 2006, Ontario regionalized its health-care system with the creation of Local Health Integration Networks, and in 2010 began the move toward needs-funding with the gradual phasing-in of the Health-Based Allocation Model. Most interestingly, the decision to establish an alternative payment plan for primary care physicians has been systematically followed up by a steady stream of decisions that have translated into significant numbers of physicians now practicing under the terms of formal contracts with the Ministry of Health and Long-Term Care and under a blended payment mechanism, which has altered the traditional, public fee-for-service payment mechanism in use for more than three decades. The contracts hold the potential for having public imperatives compete with the professional autonomy that has long been associated with the private practice part of the core bargain. At least with this issue, the province of Ontario more closely resembles the tortoise that eventually outpaces the hare.

As with any research study, readers may take issue with our interpretations of the case studies, particularly in terms of the factors that influenced whether and how decisions were made. However, we believe that our provincial study has two main strengths that reduce the likelihood of differences in interpretation. First, we combined two complementary data-collection methods—interviews with a purposive sample of 51 public policy-makers and stakeholders who were familiar with each policy-making process, and a detailed documentary analysis. From the documentary analysis, we developed a timeline of key events as a prompt to those being interviewed. Second, we used a constant comparative method to analyze the data using two analytical frameworks—the Kingdon and 3I frameworks—that are well grounded in the theoretical and empirical literature (Bhatia 2002; Kingdon 2003; Lavis et al. 2002; Lavis et al. 2012).

That said, the study did have one general weakness: the potential for recall bias among those interviewed, particularly in the few instances where there was no document trail against which we could compare their recollections. The privatization case study had its own unique weakness. As mentioned previously, 10 individuals declined to be interviewed about the creation of a policy framework that made possible the development of private for-profit delivery of medically necessary services. In the case of privatization, then, we cannot be certain whether we have heard the full story; even those who agreed to be interviewed may have felt constrained in speaking about such a politically contentious issue. However, our systematic approach to collecting and analyzing data, and our transparent reporting of the findings, allow those who might disagree with our interpretations to re-examine our data and reach their own conclusions about why health-care reform in Ontario happens and, more frequently, why it does not.

NOTES

1.   We chose the Cardiac Care Network case, even though it was at the boundary of our time range for case selection, because it was a landmark decision that informed how best to approach waiting lists in Ontario and in some other parts of Canada.
2.   Tables providing a timeline of key events related to each case and a summary of the factors that influenced agendas/decisions in each case are available at http://www.queensu.ca/iigr/Res/crossprov.html.

3. District Health Councils provided advice to the Ministry of Health about any new funding made available to their respective districts, but they had no overall financial framework within which they operated.
4. But Birch's report did exert a significant influence in the Saskatchewan government's decision to implement a needs-based funding system, as reported by McIntosh and Ducie in chapter 4.
5. Some of those interviewed linked the position of the health minister to the leadership race; however, this sequencing conflicts with the documentary analysis.

CHAPTER 6

QUEBEC REFORMS FROM ROCHON TO COUILLARD: THE LONG AND WINDING ROAD

MARIE-PASCALE POMEY, ELISABETH MARTIN, AND
PIERRE-GERLIER FOREST

INTRODUCTION

Quebec's health and social services system has been under tremendous pressure since the beginning of the 1990s. The manner in which the Quebec governments in the period under study, 1990 to 2003, responded to these pressures was at once similar to and yet different from the way in which other provinces responded. The similarity reflected the common exposure to new realities such as the information technology revolution (with implications both for management of health services and clinical practice), the availability of effective but expensive new breakthrough drugs, the stress on public finances, and the aging of the population.

The difference was in part due to history. The growth of the welfare state in Canada (especially from 1963 to 1968, the Pearson years), including health services, coincided with the flowering of Quebec's Quiet Revolution. Where other provinces looked to Ottawa for leadership, Quebec blazed its own trail. As the one jurisdiction in North America with a French-speaking majority, Quebec's situation was unique. The determination to preserve and enhance this uniqueness was shared by most French-speaking Quebecers. Accordingly, francophone Quebecers relied on the Quebec state, the key institution that they controlled, to promote modernity and solidarity. One area of difference between Quebec and other provinces that affected health services was in public administration. By the beginning of the 1990s, Quebec's health system had been regionalized for two decades. Its regional infrastructure thus had deeper roots than elsewhere in Canada. A second was in the role of labour. Where

unions elsewhere in Canada looked to the federal government on matters of health-care policy, Quebec unions focused on the Quebec state to
which they had a close attachment.

During the study period, there was more dissatisfaction in Quebec with
the health system than in most other provinces (Mendelsohn 2002, 39,
47-48). Demands for structural and political change to Quebec's health
system were ongoing. In response, governments commissioned reports
to assess needs and in most cases to provide recommendations. Yet, with
one important exception relating to prescription drugs, little reform was
achieved on the six issues that we studied.

In some sense, this chapter seeks to account for a paradox. Quebecers
studied more intensively their health system than was the case in other
provinces. Like other Canadians they approved of the health "model,"
but they were less approving of performance. They had well-researched
reports on the various issues and a substantial policy research community to assess the reports and debate the issues. Both political parties that
formed governments appointed, at least for a few years, ministers of
health who were not only well-respected in political and governmental
circles but also medical doctors with strong credentials in the medical
community. How can we explain the reform record?

With a view to illustrating health reform policy decisions undertaken
in Quebec during the turbulent period from 1990 to 2003, we examined
reforms on six significant issues: prescription drug insurance coverage,
the for-profit delivery of health-care services, wait-list management, the
creation of family medicine groups/introduction of alternative physician
payment plans, the regionalization of health services governance structures, and the effort to move to needs-based funding. The last reform,
needs-based funding, occurred in 2004, after our predefined period of
study, but we include it here because of its long gestation period. For each
of these issues, we studied a specific policy decision or non-decision and
framed the research question accordingly:

1. Why did Quebec adopt a universal pharmaceutical insurance plan?
2. Why did Quebec ignore the Arpin report, which advocated a greater
   role for private for-profit services?
3. Why did Quebec establish a decentralized wait-list management
   system?
4. Why, when Quebec implemented family medicine groups, did it make
   only minor changes to the fee-for-service payment system?
5. Why did Quebec choose to transform the regional health and social
   services boards established in 1992 into regional health and social
   services agencies instead of transferring regional powers to the local
   level?
6. Why did Quebec take so long to implement a population-based approach to the allocation of resources for medical and social services?

To answer these questions, we conducted in-depth face-to-face interviews with individuals who had either participated in the political process at the time or belonged to an organization impacted by that policy. We also reviewed the entire body of scientific and grey literature published on each case. We conducted our interviews between May 2004 and December 2005 and spoke to 51 individuals: current and former public servants, politicians involved with the policies in question, and representatives of health-care stakeholder organizations (unions, regulatory bodies, professional associations, and others). As described in chapter 2, interviewees were chosen through a purposive sampling method: we identified a list of likely candidates and then, drawing on their input, we identified additional candidates who met our sampling criteria. Some interviewees were asked about more than one of the policy decisions. In all, we conducted 53 distinct interviews, all of which were recorded, transcribed, and coded using NVivo software and an initial coding framework developed by the research team.

This chapter begins with an overview of the policy context in Quebec, describing the principal recommendations of the Commission of Inquiry on Health Services and Social Services and identifying key events (including changes in the governing parties) during our period of study. Next we describe the policy-making process for each of the six policy decisions studied, organizing our analysis around Kingdon's (1995) three phases of the policy-making process: the governmental agenda, the decision agenda, and the choice of a policy. The key factors behind each policy decision or non-decision are then discussed in order to determine whether these factors form a pattern.

QUEBEC'S POLITICAL AND POLICY-MAKING CONTEXT

To describe the context in which Quebec made the policy decisions studied here, we begin by discussing the Rochon report, a seminal analysis of the situation in Quebec that helped to frame issues during the 1990s. We then set out Quebec's political context during our study period.

The Rochon Report

The reforms proposed by the Rochon report, published in 1988, can be traced back at least two decades to the work of the Castonguay-Nepveu Commission, a commission of inquiry into health and social services created in 1966. In 1970, the work of this commission led the government to adhere to a federal-provincial program for medical services, the *Health Insurance Act* (Loi sur l'assurance maladie; Québec 1970). In 1971, the government adopted the *Act Respecting Health Services and Social Services*

(Loi sur la santé et les services sociaux; Québec 1971), which established 12 regional health and social services councils to advise the Ministry of Health on regional policy.

In 1985, a government led by the Parti Québécois appointed Dr. Jean Rochon to head a newly formed commission (Commission d'enquête sur les services de santé et les services sociaux) charged with evaluating and proposing improvements to the system that had been in place since 1971. Generously funded,[1] the Rochon Commission had the wide-ranging mandate to study the functioning, financing, and development of Quebec's health and social services structures. The Rochon report had far-reaching results: with the exception of prescription drug insurance, each of the policies studied by our team would eventually be impacted by its recommendations (Commission d'enquête sur les services de santé et les services sociaux 1988). In the more immediate term, however, the report prompted Minister Thérèse Lavoie-Roux and then Minister Marc-Yvan Coté of the newly elected Liberal government to publish ministerial orientation papers proposing various reforms (Ministère de la Santé et des Services sociaux 1989, 1990). While these papers did not lead to substantive change, they nonetheless paved the way for new health and social services legislation in the province (Québec 1991).

One of the most important reforms suggested by the Rochon report related to governance. Criticizing the operations of the regional system, Rochon suggested transforming the councils into regional health and social services boards invested with true management authority, tax-generating powers, and mechanisms for genuine public participation. Rochon also proposed that government resources be decentralized toward regional authorities governed by boards of directors elected by and accountable to the regional population. Cognizant that the government was being held ransom by interest groups, Rochon advocated a fundamental redistribution of power among the various organizational structures and levels of administration of Quebec's health-care system.

Rochon made his recommendations from the position that Quebec had a strong public health and social services system that should be maintained and reinforced and whose viability should be ensured. He based these convictions on three arguments. First, he contended that the public system had proved its capacity to provide adequate quality of care at reasonable cost. Second, he felt that systems such as Quebec's had the merit of ensuring that all residents had more or less equal access to health and social services. Third, he esteemed it vital that the state remain receptive to the demands and the needs of vulnerable populations in order to constantly improve its responsiveness. With this latter point in mind, he suggested that the province adopt a formal health and social welfare policy (la politique de la santé et du bien-être). The province did so in 1992.

In addition to articulating a new vision of health care for Quebec, the Rochon report recommended practical measures designed to increase accessibility to care within the public system. First, the report declared that fee-for-service payments did nothing to enhance monitoring for vulnerable populations or for patients with chronic diseases and suggested introducing elements of capitation funding and investing in primary care. Second, the report suggested implementing a regional budget allocation system based on adjusted per capita calculations that would take health and social services programs into account. The report also backed a population health approach that would allow communities to develop programs adapted to their environment, their social profile, their residents' lifestyles, and their population's ability to take charge of its welfare.

The Political Context between 1990 and 2003

One of Canada's 10 provinces, Quebec is unique in several respects: its official language (French as opposed to English or both English and French), its legal system (civil law, not common law), its immigration policy (Quebec has negotiated the responsibility to select immigrants), and its generous social policies (parental leave programs, public daycare, and more). Quebec is also characterized by a reluctance to collaborate too closely with the federal government on health-care issues, preferring an interpretation of the Constitution in which health is treated as an exclusively provincial responsibility. Quebec has accordingly tended to adopt an empty-chair policy in Ottawa over past years, declining to participate in a number of joint provincial-federal health-care initiatives (Forest 2007) even while managing a health system that cannot but be impacted by events elsewhere in the country.

To a large extent, the history of Quebec's health-care policies can be captured in buzzwords. During the 1990s, the most popular buzzword in Quebec (as in most provinces) was "rationalization." At that time, the economic context was difficult across Canada leading to a severe deterioration in public finances in all provinces. Other chapters in this volume detail the way in which Ontario, Alberta, Saskatchewan, and Newfoundland and Labrador coped. In Quebec, the government's determination to balance the budget led to unprecedented financial cutbacks (Normand 1996). As a result, between 1993 and 1997, some 300 health-care establishments were closed or merged. The number of health-care workers in the province fell from 240,000 in 1990/91 to 235,000 in 1995/96 and 216,000 in 1997/98, as thousands of workers left the health-care system to take advantage of an early retirement program. Nursing staff alone went from 100,000 in 1995/96 to 93,000 in 1997/98. The number of beds for general and specialized care was slashed from 28,800 in 1990 to 20,500 in 2001. The number of hospital beds dropped 26 percent between 1996 and 2001 (St-Pierre 2001). In 1995 alone, several community hospitals were closed and nine Montreal hospitals shut their doors or changed the nature of their operations. Long-term care was also affected: the system went from being able to accommodate 52,500 long-term-care patients (including those who needed housing) in 1990 to 48,600 such patients in 2001 (St-Pierre 2001). Meanwhile, with much of the health-care system being reorganized to promote the shift toward outpatient care, day surgeries grew 20 percent between 1993/94 and 1997/98 (Bergeron and Gagnon 2003; Bernier and Dallaire 2000). The spending cuts were planned by the Quebec Liberal Party, which was in office when the recession began, but were implemented by the Parti Québécois (PQ) after it won the September 1994 general election. The PQ's goal in instituting such massive cuts was to reach a zero deficit.

The legacy of the cutback policies implemented in the 1990s was not long in making itself known. What began as problems of access to health care soon led to emergency room overcrowding of crisis proportions. The change in situation led to a change in buzzword: "accessibility" was the new mantra, and attention focused on the need for the health-care system to find ways to fill the population's needs. The early 2000s saw new investments in health care, but by this time new management techniques and governance principles had gained visibility and policy-makers had become increasingly preoccupied by the idea of accountability. With the goal of improving accessibility and coordination of care, the reforms of those years pursued objectives of accountability, efficiency- and effectiveness, all principles of New Public Management theory (Aucoin 1990; Denis 1997; Farrell and Morris 2003). But problems of accessibility continued and public dissatisfaction remained high.[2]

In addition to economic factors in the 1990s, the 1995 referendum called by the Parti Québécois was another important force behind the policies implemented during this period. Only a few thousand votes decided that Quebec would not pursue negotiations to separate from Canada (Venne 1995). The closeness of the vote affected virtually everyone in the province and greatly influenced the Parti Québécois, which before leaving office in 2003 undertook a number of innovative health-care policy decisions designed to demonstrate its uniqueness among Canadian political parties. In 2003, the Quebec Liberal Party under Jean Charest won a majority of seats pursuant to a campaign centred on problems of accessibility to health care (Parti libéral du Québec 2002). These parties, the Parti Québécois and the Quebec Liberals, were the two main political forces during the 1990–2003 period although the third party, the populist right-of-centre Action démocratique du Québec, was not without some influence.

The two largest policy differences between the Parti Québécois and the Liberals related to the status of Quebec within Canada and the role of the state. The Parti Québécois purported to promote economic development while respecting principles of social progress, territorial sovereignty, the common good, equity, solidarity, social justice, and sustainable development (Parti Québécois 2008). The Liberals favoured a reduced role for the state and a greater role for individual rights, espousing liberal economic policies and a strong role for Quebec within the Canadian federation (Parti libéral du Québec 2008). Four of the reforms studied here took place under the Parti Québécois: prescription drug insurance, for-profit delivery (the Arpin report), waiting lists, and alternative payment plans. Two of the reforms took place under the Liberals: regionalization (which, as we shall see, was closer to decentralization than to regionalization) and needs-based funding. During the period of study, only one minister of health and social services held office under the Liberal party: Dr. Philippe Couillard.

THE POLICY-MAKING PROCESS: SIX CASE STUDIES

In this section, we present the results for our six cases in chronological order.

The Prescription Drug Insurance Plan: A Public-Private Partnership (1996)

Our first case—and the only one of the six that resulted in major reform—consists of Quebec's 1996 decision to adopt a universal public-private prescription drug insurance program. Twenty-five years of public health care with only limited prescription drug coverage had produced growing inequity and an increasing public outcry. Quebec's policy response was to create an innovative new program founded on collaboration between public and private insurers (Pomey et al. 2007).

Since the establishment of the public hospital insurance system in Quebec on 1 January 1961, medication had been provided to all hospital patients free of charge. Unemployment insurance recipients were also qualified for free drugs. In 1973, the Quebec government published its Outpatient Circular, which granted free drug coverage to patients with certain serious illnesses when treated outside of a hospital (Reinharz, Rousseau, and Rheault 1999). In 1975, the benefit was extended to seniors and adults between ages 60 and 64 who received the federal income-tested guaranteed income supplement or spousal allowance. Prior to 1997, some 4.5 million Quebecers subscribed to private group insurance plans, mainly through work, but some 1.1 million Quebecers had neither private insurance nor public coverage of their medication costs (Gratton 1996).

Quebec's new prescription drug program (Régime général d'assurance médicaments) took effect 1 January 1997. Under this program, private sector companies collaborate with a public insurer to ensure that all provincial residents are covered for the same range of prescription drugs at a cost largely adjusted to income. The law (Québec 1996) requires all

Quebecers to belong either to a private plan offered by their employer or professional association or to the public plan administered by Quebec's Health Insurance Board, the Régie de l'assurance maladie du Québec (RAMQ 2006). In 2006, 4.4 million residents were covered by private policies and 3.2 million were members of the public plan (RAMQ 2006). Coverage in the private sector varies from plan to plan, but the law limits beneficiaries' out-of-pocket costs and determines certain coverage conditions, such as which drugs the plans must cover (RAMQ 2004).

Our study participants identified a number of factors that led Quebec to adopt this drug insurance legislation. In the governmental agenda phase of the policy decision, discontent with the Outpatient Circular was an important institutional and interest-related element. Under this Circular, the government provided free medication to victims of six specific diseases;[3] at the same time, victims of other diseases, for which prescription drugs were just as expensive, had no subsidies at all. Growing numbers of people criticized the system as discrimination on the basis of disease, and the media ran stories of people dying for want of drugs they could not afford. Non-covered patients were increasingly demanding coverage for their treatment, and covered patients clamoured for access to the latest medication. After successive provincial governments commissioned a series of reports on the question (Comité d'experts sur l'assurance médicaments 1996; Comité de révision de la circulaire 1994; Ministère de la Santé et des Services sociaux 1995a), it became increasingly clear that the Outpatient Circular should be replaced with a fairer regime.

Another institutional factor that helped put a new drug insurance program onto the government agenda was the shift to ambulatory care. Advances in technology, especially new drugs, meant that it was increasingly possible for certain illnesses to be treated and for patients to convalesce outside of hospital, thus reducing health-care costs. As long as drugs remained free in hospital but charged out of hospital, however, the shift to ambulatory care would be compromised.

Under the influence of Jean Rochon, idea-related factors helped to move the issue from the governmental agenda to the decision-making agenda. Prior to his appointment as minister of health and social services in 1994, Rochon, a medical doctor, had worked in public health at the World Health Organization. He believed strongly in the merits of universal, free drug coverage and succeeded in moving the prescription drug policy reform to the electoral platform of the Parti Québécois for the 1994 campaign (Parti Québécois 1993). When the party gained power, it was already convinced that implementing a universal prescription drug program was consistent with its progressive social image.

Once on the decision-making agenda, however, the choice of a policy was largely determined by financial and interest-related factors. Jean Rochon commissioned Claude Castonguay, former minister of health and social affairs under the Quebec Liberals and ex-insurance industry executive, to determine the options (Comité d'experts sur l'assurance médicaments 1996). The first scenario elaborated by Castonguay consisted of a universal public regime with or without user contributions. This strictly public regime was to be funded by global taxes and some user fees and had the support of large segments of the public. Rochon and various health professionals including hospital pharmacists also supported a universal public regime, believing that the best way to ensure equity was to have a state-run program. Nonetheless, three principal factors made it all but impossible politically. First, private insurance companies opposed it on the grounds that they would lose clients. Private insurers were (and still are) significant employers in Quebec and represent an important interest group. Many are small, home-grown companies, and loss of this client base threatened their existence. Second, private pharmacists complained that a public regime threatened the two-tiered system whereby they charged higher prices for medication and higher dispensing fees to private plan beneficiaries than they did to beneficiaries with public coverage. It also jeopardized sales in the sense that pharmacists sold drugs to the privately insured that the public system refused to purchase. Because pharmacists were in direct contact with the public, and the government counted on them to explain the new coverage system to their clients, antagonizing the pharmacists would not have been good strategy. Third, a purely publicly financed system would have meant transferring the payment of $895 million in premiums from companies on to individuals, a move that would have alienated the public.

The second scenario elaborated by Castonguay consisted of a universal private regime. Private insurers would be called upon to insure all Quebecers, including seniors and the socially assisted. This scenario was also dismissed by the insurers, who were unwilling to cover the insolvent and those with high medication costs.

The third scenario was a regime that would protect the public against the risk of incurring catastrophic costs. The government would cover the cost of medication for people whose health problems generated expenses that greatly exceeded their capacity to pay. This regime was comparable to that which already existed under the Outpatient Circular, but coverage would be determined according to income and not according to disease. Having witnessed first-hand the injustice caused by incomplete drug coverage under the Circular, hospital pharmacists rejected this scenario on the grounds that it would not solve the problem of inequity. In general, seniors' groups and the Quebec Hospital Association supported this option, as did the insurance companies, as it allowed them to retain clients for non-catastrophic benefits.

The fourth scenario consisted of a universal, mixed (public/private) regime. This regime would allow private insurers to coexist with the Quebec Health Insurance Board, the RAMQ. Employment status (employed, socially assisted, retired, or dependent) would be the basis on which individuals were assigned membership in either the public or a private plan. This scenario was supported by the private insurers because it allowed them to keep their market share without having to take on new clients who would be "bad risks." The pharmaceutical industry was also in favour of the most universal system possible: that is, the system that would cover the greatest number of people. The government was on board for two reasons. First, the user-fee income generated by such a program would help absorb the debt incurred by the previous program and allow the administration to more rapidly reach its zero-deficit goal (savings in the first year of the proposed regime were estimated to reach $240 million). In this way, the fourth scenario corresponded to the Treasury Board's primary criterion when examining any of the scenarios: namely, to keep public expenditures as low as possible. Second, a non-catastrophic program that ensured drug coverage for the entire provincial population would be a first in Canada and would fulfill the Parti Québécois's mandate of proving itself able to implement progressive social change with a genuine "Made in Quebec" program. The Parti Québécois had to move quickly, though, for at the federal level, the National Forum on Health was preparing to submit recommendations in favour of a new, Canada-wide prescription drug insurance program that would add drug coverage to the basket of Canada's publicly funded medical services (National Forum on Health 1997a).

In sum, forces external to the health-care system played a pivotal role in opening the window of opportunity for a major reform. Most important in this regard was the Parti Québécois's decision to insert into its 1994 election platform a commitment to reform. While that decision was a response to the fundamentally unfair regime then in existence, it was subsequently boosted by the Parti Québécois's wish to pre-empt the federal government from occupying that space. The presence of Jean Rochon as a political champion with commitment and clout helped to ensure that once the window opened, his party's commitment was not forgotten.

The result was that interest-related, institutional, ideational, and external (mainly financial) factors combined to give Quebecers a comprehensive reform—a reform that ensured that a wide range of prescription drugs would be available to all residents of the province as part of that province's public health-care system. At the time it was implemented, Quebec's plan was the only prescription drug insurance program in Canada to cover an entire provincial population. The federal government never did add drug coverage to its basket of universal, publicly funded health-care services. Although some other provinces subsequently broadened their coverage, Quebec's plan remains unique both in its public-private partnership formula and scope of coverage.

For-Profit Delivery: The Unthinkable Solution (1998–2000)

Our second case consists of for-profit delivery. In 1998, the Parti Québécois administration responded to a dramatic decrease in health-care resources and growing problems of accessibility by commissioning the Groupe de travail sur la complémentarité du secteur privé dans la poursuite des objectifs fondamentaux du système public de santé au Québec. Presided over by Roland Arpin, its aim was to explore how the private for-profit sector could help. Once having received Arpin's report (Groupe de travail 1999), however, the government shelved it. In this section, we examine the reasons for this non-decision, the only case of the six that did not give rise to a new policy.

As discussed earlier, in the mid-1990s, Quebec began to reduce health-care costs and effect a shift to outpatient care with the goal of attaining a zero deficit. This rationalization caused problems of access and wait times, and wait lists began to swell. Media reports on the inadequacies of Quebec's system and the merits of opening the door to the private sector were increasingly frequent. With the American system often cited as a model of accessibility, polls showed that public opinion was not hostile to introducing the private sector into health care (J.-F. Bégin 1998). More specifically, in 1998, 55 percent of Quebecers declared themselves willing to pay to obtain an earlier medical appointment and 74 percent believed that public-private partnerships would benefit the users of the health-care system (J.-F. Bégin 1998). Surveys in following years confirmed this trend: in 1999, 52 percent of Quebecers versus 41percent of Canadians were in favour of the idea of buying private services (Gagné 1999), and in 2000, 60 percent of Quebecers agreed that certain services should be delivered more rapidly to those who wished to pay for them (Sirois 2000). This proportion rose to 66 percent in 2002, when two of three Quebecers considered that those who could afford it should have the right to pay for a private health-care system (Moisan 2002). In short, institutional, ideational, and interest-related factors—not least increasing public pressure—were combining to give privatization, especially for-profit delivery but also for-profit insurance, more visibility on the governmental agenda.

At the political level, however, ideational factors caused for-profit delivery to meet with considerable ambiguity. Within the Parti Québécois cabinet was a faction that looked to the private for-profit sector to offset the failings of the public system and to thus make it easier for the government to pursue its goal of a balanced budget. Other cabinet members, however, including health and social services minister Jean Rochon, were fundamentally opposed to private for-profit insurance and the supposedly inevitable two-tier system that would result.

In response to pressures from the public and within the party, Rochon created a commission to examine the issue. In October 1998, in the middle of a provincial election campaign, Rochon charged Roland Arpin, a high-ranking career public servant, with evaluating the extent to which the private sector complemented the public sector in achieving the fundamental goals of Quebec's health-care system. More specifically, Rochon instructed Arpin to evaluate the nature and evolution of health-care spending in the private sector and to determine the role that the private sector should play in helping Quebec's public system meet its fundamental goals.

Rochon's strategy was singularly effective at determining the decision-making agenda. Wanting to put off privatization as long as he could, Rochon gave Arpin a mandate limited to the study of bridge-building between the public and private spheres rather than the redistribution of services per se. Arpin was not asked to make specific proposals, to evaluate the cost or the feasibility of any recommendations, or to suggest ways to promote privatization. Arpin's very appointment was strategic: while Arpin had great credibility in governmental circles on cultural and education policy, he was unknown to the medical world. By appointing him, Rochon bought time and demonstrated goodwill to cabinet members and to all those who were pushing for greater privatization—while reducing the import of the very commission he had created.

Following the re-election of the Parti Québécois in November 1998, Pauline Marois replaced Jean Rochon as minister of health and social services and confirmed the mandate of Arpin's group. The Arpin report submitted to Marois in July 1999 stated that even though the supply of private-practice medical services had grown slightly in Quebec, such services remained a very marginal part of the system overall (Groupe de travail 1999). The report opined that the private sector must be allowed a greater role if problems of access were to be solved, and made recommendations for planning the role of the private sector in health care. But in accordance with its mandate, the recommendations consisted of general principles rather than specific actions.

As health and social services minister, Pauline Marois was responsible for ensuring the legacy of her predecessor: it was difficult for her to brush the report aside. But in truth, the issue of privatization was a priority for neither the government nor Marois. Because the proposals of the report would have required significant actions to be implemented, it was relatively easy for the minister to avoid making a policy decision, especially since the issue was so controversial. One senior public servant referred to it as a Pandora's box: "This is a field where nobody wants the government to do anything that can't be undone. Because in health care, in Quebec, the moment you bring up the word *private*, you've committed high treason."

At the governmental level, therefore, ideational and institutional factors downgraded the import of Arpin's report. But ideational factors were important for the public as well. Several of our respondents pointed to the absence of public consensus around privatization as one of the reasons for the unpopularity of the concept. Health-care workers and the public at large often confused private financing and the private delivery of services, and the concept of public-private partnerships was similarly nebulous. Indeed, part of Rochon's reason for appointing the Arpin Commission was to educate citizens on the concepts and issues associated with privatization, to help them realize the extent to which the private sector was already present in health care, and to bring them to reflect on what services should be covered by the public versus the private system. But Quebec's powerful health-care unions proved to be staunch opponents to any discussion on the matter. Even the vague proposals of the Arpin report were poorly received by unions and social groups, which found them to be overly favourable to the private sector.

Following in the footsteps of her predecessor, health and social services minister Marois responded to a delicate situation by forming a commission of her own. In June 2000, Marois instructed the Clair Commission to produce an overview of the health system as a whole and to explore means to improve service organization and financing going forward. In this way, even though the actors did not agree to implement a new policy (the decision-making agenda), the issue stayed on the governmental agenda.

Waiting Lists: Spokes in the Wheels (2000)

Our third case consists of Quebec's policy response to growing waiting lists, a problem that confronted all Canadian provinces at roughly the same time. In the mid-1990s, a conjunction of factors lengthened waiting lists in Quebec's health-care system, especially for general and cardiac surgery. The issue was exacerbated by hospital closures, bed reductions, a massive early retirement program for health professionals, and the government's failure to invest monies realized from the closing of community hospitals into front-line care as originally planned. The resulting waiting-list crisis provoked concern and outrage, and both patient advocates and medical professionals complained vociferously: some 35,000 Quebecers, it was claimed, were awaiting surgery of some kind (Lessard 1995; Presse canadienne 1995). The media took up the cause, at one point producing daily profiles of wait-listed people at risk of death as a result of a delay in their treatment. Without reliable data on the state of wait times in the province, the government was defenseless against the mounting pressure. On several occasions, it responded by unexpectedly injecting funds into the system, not strategically but to buy short-term respite (Dufour 2000; Lessard and Bégin 2000). The problem was clearly present on the governmental agenda, but it would take several years for it to reach the decision-making phase.

Government awareness of the waiting-list problem can be traced to 1993, when the administration created two working groups to examine the issue (Comité de gestion des listes d'attente en cardiologie tertiaire and Groupe de travail sur la chirurgie générale et orthopédique au Québec).

The groups' findings were discouraging. It was not infrequent for local-level health-care institutions to use handwritten waiting lists that made it impossible to compare data between institutions, let alone glean the magnitude of the lists around the province. The allocation of operating room facilities often took place on the basis of physicians' personal influence rather than relative need, and the very definition of waiting lists differed from one institution to the next. These and other findings made it clear that Quebec lacked the tools to evaluate the magnitude of its wait lists, let alone produce a quick solution. Rather, it would be necessary to study the treatment trajectory of illnesses in their entirety to determine where the roadblocks were located.

In 1995, health and social services minister Jean Rochon moved the issue forward by creating the Action Plan for Access to Surgical Care and the Support Group for Access to Surgical Care (Ministère de la Santé et des Services sociaux 1995b). Under this program, health-care administrators began to gather waiting-list information on an irregular basis three to four times per year, but most data still failed to make their way to the ministry. At this point, the leading hypothesis was that ongoing reforms such as the decentralization of services and the shift toward ambulatory care would change the structure of the health-care system and fix problems of access. But by 1998 it was evident that the reforms were actually aggravating the problem, especially since the funds earmarked for front-line care had failed to materialize. At the same time, limits to the quality and reliability of the data compiled since 1995 were becoming apparent. By August 1998, the Support Group for Access to Specialized Surgical and Medical Care had clarified the issue: rather than compile for the sake of compiling, it would be necessary to develop systems and tools to assist administrators to manage and prioritize cases in real time.

Meanwhile, Montreal's regional board for health and social services had, on its own initiative, begun to work on waiting lists for heart surgery, orthopedics (hip and knee), and cataract surgery using the United Kingdom's National Health Service (NHS) model. In the spring of 1998, the regional board added the management of waiting lists to its strategic plan. The idea made its way onto the electoral platforms of Quebec's two main political parties before the fall elections, and by 1999, the reduction of wait times was a priority of the newly re-elected PQ government.

In the background, however, lurked important interest-related factors: reticence on the part of the medical profession and the health-care institutions to participate in wait-list management strategies. Many surgeons were convinced that the problem of waiting lists was principally caused by a lack of resources and that only the allocation of additional resources would solve the problem. According to them, waiting lists were nothing more than a short-term, labour-intensive means of managing a system that the government was choosing to deprive of necessary funds. Other surgeons worried that a wait-list management system would undermine their authority by taking the decision of when and on whom to operate out of their hands. Still others saw long waiting lists as a measure of their professional success. Institutions were also unenthusiastic about assigning staff to track the lists: with budgets already strained by cutbacks, the project seemed an additional burden that did little to resolve the real problem.

After some procrastination, Pauline Marois, who succeeded Jean Rochon as health and social services minister in 1998, decided that the only effective means of addressing the opposition to wait-list management was with transparency. But monopolized by the problem of emergency room care, the ministry continued to view the dossier as a technical rather than a political matter, and the actual choice of a policy was, for the time, left to ministry employees. Staff accordingly began to design the Service Access Management System (SGAS), a wait-list management system that aimed to generate reliable data, rank patients fairly, and determine acceptable wait times. Administrators studied the Saskatchewan Surgical Care Network and the Western Canada Waiting List Project and visited the Cardiac Care Network of Ontario. Their ambition was to develop a centralized system that would rank the importance and urgency of all surgeries in the province based on criteria elaborated by an expert panel.

Two interest-related factors, however, short-circuited this ambition. The first concerned the political urgency of the project: with all eyes on emergency room crowding, mundane data collection took a back seat and the wait-list project was not given the funding necessary to establish ranking criteria for all surgeries or to implement the system beyond the institutional level. The other was the resistance of the medical community. Physicians in Quebec tend to identify strongly with their specialization, and uniting all specializations with a view to developing a common prioritization matrix quickly led to gridlock. Getting doctors to agree on codes of best practice that determined who to operate on, when, and in what order proved to be similarly impossible.

Faced with these difficulties, Health Minister Marois decided in March 2000 that the system should prioritize tertiary cardiology (cardiac surgery, angioplasty, and diagnostic catheterization). Marois's decision had two immediate advantages. The first was institutional in nature: the strategy would allow the SGAS project to be implemented and evaluated in one medical specialization before additional funds and time were invested in others. The project could thus move forward, albeit in one specialization only, rather than be aborted due to the difficulties of establishing a cross-disciplinary consensus on the prioritization of care. The second advantage was interest related. By prioritizing one specialization, the government could succeed in reducing wait times for one of the groups most dramatically affected: patients awaiting heart surgery.

It is for these reasons that in 2003–2004, Quebec's SGAS system evolved to take clinical data into account when weighing cases and risk factors for tertiary cardiology. On the basis of the weight and urgency of each case, experts developed a ranking system that prioritized patients on lists for each participating institution. But whereas the system was originally meant to be implemented for all surgeries, it was extended only to radio-oncology at that time. Even for these two types of surgery, the system ranked cases only by institution and not across the province as was originally intended.

Philippe Couillard's appointment as minister of health and social services under the Quebec Liberals in 2003 briefly promised to resuscitate one of the original goals of the SGAS project: the publication of waiting-list data. When he first took office, Couillard proposed to make the lists available on the Internet so that Quebecers could shop for care. But while institutional waiting lists for certain surgeries are now posted on the Internet (Ministère de la Santé et des Services sociaux 2008), the information available for each region is not updated frequently enough to allow patients to use it to make an informed decision about where to obtain treatment.

In summary, the instauration of SGAS was a relatively weak and limited reform. Although a wait-list monitoring system was indeed introduced, establishments participated on a voluntary basis and the system applied only to a small number of procedures. To this day, wait-list management remains at the organizational level.

Alternative Payment Plans: Inching Toward Change (2000–2002)

Our fourth case consists of Quebec's venture into alternative payment plans with the establishment of family medicine groups (FMGs). Introduced in 2001, FMGs were first and foremost intended to revolutionize the paradigm and the philosophy of how primary care services were organized. This they proposed to do by changing case management practices and by introducing a multidisciplinary approach to front-line care. While reforming payment schemes was not a primary objective, FMGs were also intended to introduce new terms of physician remuneration, such as capitation. In practice, however, FMGs resulted in only moderate changes to Quebec's fee-for-service model, and while the new FMG structure is believed to benefit rural populations, the model is less popular in urban regions, especially Montreal.

The roots of alternative payment plans are over 30 years old. In the 1970s, primary care under Quebec's medicare system was mainly provided through local community service centres (CLSCs), most of whose doctors were salaried, and private practices, where physicians operated on a fee-for-service basis. In the 1980s, however, Quebec's Ministry of Health and Social Services slowed investments in the CLSC model. It had become clear that physicians were reluctant to join CLSCs: some 75 percent of the doctors paid by the public system operated in private practices where they earned more money and enjoyed greater autonomy. In an environment where treatment was growing increasingly complex, however, the multiplicity of independent providers was affecting the continuity of care. During the mid-1990s, cutbacks to the health sector laid the groundwork for emergency room overcrowding that was worsened by an aging population. By the end of the decade, overcrowding had reached crisis proportions. The Ministry of Health and Social Services held provincewide forums on the problem, and a hypothesis began to emerge: if services were better integrated upstream, that is to say, in primary care, patients would have an attractive—and less costly—alternative to crowded emergency rooms (Ministère de la Santé et des Services sociaux 1999).

The Ministry of Health and Social Services was not alone in believing in the merits of more integrated services. In 2000, the College of Family Physicians of Canada filed a report that proposed a model for primary care services based on family practice networks made up of interdisciplinary teams (Collège des médecins de famille du Canada 2000). The same year, the Quebec Federation of General Practitioners recommended reorganizing medicine into private practices operating within integrated networks (SECOR 2000). A consensus began to emerge: better continuity of care, greater coordination, and more primary physicians would improve health-care delivery and maximize available funds. By 2000, then, ideational and external financial factors had placed the reorganization of primary care firmly on the governmental agenda. Rather than take immediate action, however, the government was obliged to delay, as ongoing budget cuts precluded an injection of funds.

As an alternative, then, and in order to better define the choice of a policy, health and social services minister Pauline Marois appointed Michel Clair, a lawyer and former politician who had been the minister of revenue, the minister of transportation, and the president of the Treasury Board under the Parti Québécois, to head the Commission for the Study of Health and Social Services. Among other duties, the Clair Commission was charged with proposing solutions for reorganizing primary health-care services. The findings of the Clair group would come to define the decision-making agenda.

One of the measures that the commission took to fulfill its mandate was to visit establishments in Canada and abroad that had reorganized primary care services. Two cases in particular captured the attention of the commission members: General Practitioner Fundholders in Britain, and Health Maintenance Organizations in the United States, especially Kaiser Permanente. These two models had certain elements in common: first, a solid organization based on the sharing of material and human resources; and second, a sound understanding of the clientele and of service integration. The commission also studied whether creating partnerships between Quebec's CLSCs and local doctors' offices could help integrate a population-based approach without requiring patients to register with a specific doctor or CLSC. Lastly, the commission consulted the Quebec Federation of General Practitioners (FMOQ), looking for ways to integrate its recommendations. Using the information thus gathered, it elaborated a test model and met with the public to solicit feedback and build support.

In its final report submitted in December 2000, the Clair Commission recommended a system that would retain physicians in both CLSCs and private practices but would reorganize doctors into family medicine groups (FMGs)—voluntarily constituted teams of professionals responsible for providing services to a given population (Commission d'étude sur les services de santé et les services sociaux 2000). Participating physicians would share resources and support staff, and patients registered with the group would have access to any of its doctors, not just their own primary care physician. Remuneration would consist of three elements: capitation according to the number of patients registered, a base amount, and fee-for-service payment. Most importantly for the politics, FMGs would be responsible for providing patients with around-the-clock access to primary health care.

Once the Clair report was filed, the choice of a policy took place in record time. In February 2001, less than two months after the release of the report, health and social services minister Marois announced the government's intention to move forward with FMGs. The rapidity of Marois's response can be understood in light of the availability of new federal funds: the Primary Health Care Transition Fund, a federal sum earmarked for financing initiatives designed to improve primary care (Santé Canada 2007). Marois's successor, Rémy Trudel, entrusted the execution of the FMG model to ministry staff members who set up implementation and advisory committees and enlisted the participation of medical professionals, union representatives, and hospital managers. Members of the implementation committee studied Ontario's primary health groups, sketched out a model for groups of a given size, and designed mechanisms for accessibility, registration, continuity, case management, and interprofessional collaboration. But intent on the political advantages of rapid implementation, the ministry pursued implementation without first negotiating salary and operating conditions with the FMOQ. This approach was in stark contrast to Clair's recommendation to consult stakeholders closely in order to develop a flexible model. Indeed, the physicians complained that the ministry was developing the most detailed, centralized model possible without adequate discussion with them even though they would be the most affected by the reform (Dutil 2002).

Part of the reason for this purportedly unilateral approach on the part of the ministry was interest related and consisted of political pressures. The idea of around-the-clock access to primary care physicians had struck a chord with the public, and the ministry rushed to announce the implementation of FMGs during the 2001–2002 pre-election period. Politicians campaigning on the issue were intent on getting as many

FMGs as possible up and running: they pressured the ministry to push the project through even before negotiations were complete. Feeling coerced and pushed aside, however, the FMOQ insisted that it would not accept FMGs without first negotiating operating conditions and the terms of doctors' remuneration (Paré 2001; Sirois 2001).

One of the most contentious issues was around-the-clock access. While 24-hour access was for political reasons of prime importance to the ministry, physicians resisted, particularly as the registration aspect of FMGs required them to sign a contract with their patients: the contract introduced an unaccustomed level of accountability to a profession whose members often saw themselves as independent entrepreneurs. Furthermore, even though the FMOQ was in favour of the FMG concept, it also protested against what it termed the government's complex and bureaucratic means of implementing the new groups, namely, the requirement for each FMG to execute three kinds of formal association agreements.

The government's rush to claim victory, before negotiations had even begun, ultimately affected the reform itself. The legal complexity of the proposed new structures and the pressure to push through negotiations with the FMOQ meant that the policy originally chosen—the FMG model as proposed by the Clair Commission—was not, in the end, the policy that emerged. By the time that the FMOQ and the Ministry of Health and Social Services came to an agreement in 2002, registered patients' around-the-clock access to a primary physician was watered down to around-the-clock access for frail patients only.

Changes to the remuneration system that had been considered the cornerstone of the reform also failed to occur. Most of the remuneration paid to FMG physicians remained fee-for-service. FMG physicians also received $7 per patient registered, an additional amount to cover administration and communication costs, and a three-hour session fee for interdisciplinary tasks and non-clinical activities. When taken one by one, these sums do not appear excessive, but when totalled, they represented a 15 percent increase over the remuneration of a primary care physician who chose not to practice in an FMG. The ministry also paid the salary of two nurses and two administrative assistants per FMG and gave computer equipment to each group. An additional sum of $7 per visit was paid to physicians who cared for vulnerable patients. But because salary negotiations in Quebec were (and remain) centralized, any sum paid by the government to a general practitioner working in an FMG also had to be paid to other general practitioners in the province. This extension of benefits to all physicians, not just those working in an FMG, substantially weakened the structure of financial incentives designed to attract physicians to FMGs in the first place. The result has been that means of remunerating doctors—one of the goals of the reform—have not changed much since FMGs were created, but physicians' pay has gone up.

FMGs came up against another problem in Montreal, Quebec's largest population centre. In 2001, a stand-off between the president of the FMOQ and the minister of health and social services, Rémy Trudel, took place. Trudel insisted that there would be no exceptions to the standard FMG model, not even in Montreal. The FMOQ, in contrast, wanted to work out an alternative model adapted for Montreal, where solo practices, little or no case management, walk-in clinics, and a multiethnic clientele posed particular challenges (Fédération des médecins omnipraticiens du Québec 2001). While an agreement was eventually reached, the number of FMGs in the Montreal area never grew as anticipated.

In summary, FMGs were a reform with great promise that floundered in the implementation phase after the succession of four health and so-cial services ministers. The government was quick to follow up on the recommendations of the Clair Commission because there seemed to be consensus on the general values and central principles of Clair's model. Stakeholders saw FMGs as a solution to problems of accessibility and agreed on the need for more equity, improved continuity of care, better disease prevention, more health promotion, improved case management, and more interprofessional collaboration. But when it came to translating principles into action, interest-related, ideational, institutional, and finan-cial factors led decision makers to de-emphasize the element that was to have been a key characteristic of the model: changes to the remuneration system of Quebec's physicians. This reticence can be partly explained by the fact that the reform was more oriented toward the reinvigoration of primary care than toward the implementation of alternative remuneration models. Without a clear commitment on the part of the administration to move away from fee-for-service payments, the reform remained marginal.

Regionalization: The Wedding-Cake Model of Governance (2003)

The first step toward the regionalization of health services in Quebec took place in 1971, when the Ministry of Health and Social Services gave the province its first regional-level structure in the form of 12 regional health and social services councils. In 1991, Marc-Yvan Côté followed the recom-mendations of the Rochon Commission and replaced the councils with 18 regional health and social services boards whose territorial boundaries followed the same lines as Quebec's administrative regions. The regional boards had full power to plan and organize services and allocate resources (Québec 1991). The idea was to create regional entities whose boundaries made intelligent use of local sociopolitical characteristics, thus facilitat-ing the efficient organization of services and care. The next major step toward regionalization took place in 2003 when, just a few months after the provincial election, the new Liberal administration adopted Bill 25 (Québec 2003). This bill significantly altered the responsibilities of the regional level by transferring the management and the organization of health and social services to the new local-level health and social services centres created by the same law (see Table 6.1). In contrast to the 1991 reform, the priority of Bill 25 was to decentralize, not to regionalize per se.

With this brief history, we see that regionalization has been a low-key but integral part of Quebec's health and social services system for the past 35 years. As far back as the Castonguay-Nepveu Commission of 1966, government-commissioned reports have influenced how the concept of regionalization has evolved. Indeed, the drive to decentralize services has helped to determine the very shape of Quebec's health-care system. But because regionalization has been part of the government agenda for such a long time, it is difficult to determine the precise precursors of the reforms of 2003. Instead, it is more realistic to conceive of regionalization as an ongoing matter that has changed as regional structures have evolved. What is certain is that a climax took place in the 1990s, when growing costs culminated in the large-scale restructuring of the health-care network. It was at this time that the regional boards undertook the first mergers of local establishments by merging certain CLSCs and CHSLDs (residential and long-term care centres).

After the events of the 1990s, the next significant step toward regionalization was the 2000 appointment of the Clair Commission. The Clair Commission was responsible for holding public debates on the challenges

TABLE 6.1
Changes in Responsibilities of Three Levels of Government before and after 2004

	Before 2004	*After 2004*
Provincial level	Ministry of Health and Social Services	Ministry of Health and Social Services
Regional level	16 regional health and social services boards (regional boards) and 2 regional councils	15 health and social services agencies, 1 regional board, 1 regional health and social services centre, and 1 Cree council
Local level	• 328 public institutions, each with its own governing board (as of May 2004)	• 95 health and social services centres (HSSCs) • 96 public institutions not merged with HSSCs (mainly teaching hospitals, rehabilitation centres, and youth centres with regional or supra-regional missions as of September 2009; Ministère de la Santé et des Services sociaux, 2009)

facing Quebec's health and social services system and for suggesting ways to better organize the system. In the first debates, speakers accused the regional boards of meddling in the management of local institutions and called for the boards to be abolished. Later, stakeholders and experts counter-argued that the regional boards played an important role in the management of the health-care system and should be preserved. By the end of the public hearings, the Clair Commission had come to recognize interest-related and institutional factors and recommended against changing the number or territorial boundaries of the boards on the grounds that "the regional boards and the regions that they serve are the result of delicate political negotiations" (Commission d'étude sur les services de santé et les services sociaux 2000, 211). In this way, the commission respected the boundaries of Quebec's administrative regions, which also govern the organization of the province's education and environmental programs. The commission did, however, advocate implementing decentralized, integrated primary care services based on a population approach.

At the urging of health minister François Legault, the Parti Québécois government responded to the Clair report in 2001 by adopting Bill 28 (Québec 2001). Bill 28 did not revamp Quebec's governance structures per se but nonetheless made significant changes to management methods, accountability measures between various levels of the system, and the composition of boards of directors.

It was not until 2002 that regionalization reached the decision-making agenda on a larger scale. Health care was a central issue in the 2003 election campaign, and all three of Quebec's principal political parties promoted their own vision of how the governance of the health-care system could best be regionalized. The most radical of these visions came from the Quebec Liberal Party, which called into question the representative nature and accountability of the regional boards. It criticized them as intermediary structures that offered no services and that lacked regulatory and taxation powers (Parti libéral du Québec 2002). The Liberals promised, if elected, to abolish the boards and entrust the coordination of services to local institutions.

The Quebec Liberals beat the incumbent Parti Québécois at the polls in April 2003 and promptly appointed Dr. Philippe Couillard, a neurosurgeon, as minister of health and social services. Eager to fulfill his party's electoral promises, Couillard decided that decentralizing services to the local level would be one of his first priorities. Framed around the desire to improve accessibility, integration, and the continuity of care, the reform's less explicit goals included greater accountability, greater effectiveness, and lower costs as per the principles of New Public Management philosophy.

Summer 2003 thus became a period for reflection on the organizational model that would best articulate the goals of the reform. Researchers studied Canadian and foreign experiences with decentralization and found their greatest inspiration in Alberta's model. This model was organized on two levels, a provincial level and a regional level, and had greatly integrated the province's health-care services. But the team objected to the scale of Alberta's mergers, which it felt would be excessive in Quebec.

The local service network model that eventually emerged from this research process was the fruit of the participation of a range of stakeholders. The model was designed to integrate institutions on a local and territorial basis as originally recommended in the Clair report. It was soon crafted into legal form as Bill 25, which the Liberal party submitted to Quebec's National Assembly in November 2003. Bill 25 was organized around two principal measures. First, it converted 15 regional boards into health and social services agencies.[4] The territorial boundaries remained unchanged. Second, Bill 25 merged Quebec's local health and social services establishments into 95 health and social services centres (HSSCs) responsible for offering, managing, and organizing a full range of services to the population on their territory. To fulfill this responsibility, HSSCs were instructed to develop local service networks by negotiating agreements with the various establishments and providers in their territory, including pharmacies, medical clinics, family medicine groups, and community organizations. Each local service network would be ultimately responsible for the health of the population to which it provided services and was accountable to the agencies for its performance (Ministère de la Santé et des Services sociaux 2004).

In early December 2003, a parliamentary commission on the bill took place. Much of the criticism centred on the merger of institutions whose missions, visions, and operating philosophies differed substantially. The original bill required that all hospital centres without exception be merged into HSSCs, and members of CLSCs were fearful that a hospital-type mentality would come to dominate traditional primary care activities. The government agreed to allow some exceptions to the mergers, for example if the population served by the institutions in question presented sociocultural, ethnic, or linguistic singularities. In that way, the project resolved institutional issues and integrated ideational factors to garner stakeholder support.

Implementation of the reform began in early January 2004. The newly created agencies were instructed to "draw up and propose an organization model based on one or more local services networks covering all or part of the agency's area of jurisdiction" (Québec 2003, 2). Agencies were given just three months to propose their organization models, a process that required intense negotiations and political compromise in several regions (Contandriopoulos et al. 2007). The regional proposals were submitted in April 2004. In June 2004, health minister Couillard announced the creation of 95 HSSCs, some of which were more reflective of opportunism than of a genuine commitment to take local social and economic realities into account.

In hindsight, there is no doubt that this reform altered the powers of the regional level of Quebec's health-care system. The management and organization of health and social services were transferred from the regions to the HSSCs and, in return, the agencies' responsibilities for accountability, financial coordination, human resources planning, and accreditation were strengthened. These changes were later confirmed by Bill 83 (Québec 2005), which further adjusted the responsibilities of each level of governance.

One of the most interesting characteristics of the reform was its rapidity. This rapidity can be largely attributed to politics and political change: the reform was a priority of the newly elected Liberal government. Pressures by interest groups forced the government to abandon its project to abolish the regional boards, but by rechristening them regional agencies, the administration kept face and respected its electoral promise. The result is that unlike several other provinces, Quebec still operates a three-tier service organization model that has retained regional-level institutions and guarantees the autonomy of the boards of directors of local-level health and social services institutions.

Insofar as devolution is concerned, however, the 2003 reform is clearly a step back. It is not accidental that the regional agencies lost their management, coordination, and service integration duties to the local level in exchange for continued planning responsibilities and the new prerogative to supervise management and accountability agreements. This redistribution of responsibilities suggests that hidden behind its move to decentralize, the government actually intended to bring greater centralization to the health-care system and thus break with Rochon's 1980s model for political and democratic regionalization (Martin, Pomey, and Forest 2010). In the end, the provincial government's decision to invest the agencies with strong managerial responsibilities positioned the provincial level with greater control over Quebec's health-care system.

Needs-Based Funding: When Morality Meets Politics (2004)

Our final case consists of the evolution of budget allocation methods for regional-level health-care structures funded by the Ministry of Health and Social Services and for local health-care establishments funded by regional structures. In 2004, years of policy debate came to fruition when, in the spirit of New Public Management philosophy, new budget allocation methods were adopted to promote equity across regions and to facilitate the transition of the system from disease-centred to prevention-centred medicine that respected the principles of population health. Even though the reform took place after our predefined period of study, its amplitude and importance after so long a gestation period persuaded us to extend the period of study for this one case. As a result, this section analyzes why the policy failed to move forward for a number of years and then finally proceeded, albeit in a limited manner, in 2004.

Prior to the decision of 2004, health-care institutions in Quebec were mainly funded on the basis of past budgets. It is true that the *Act Respecting Health Services and Social Services* specified that the Ministry of Health and Social Services would fund regional boards on the basis of the number of residents in the region and that the regional boards would then distribute those funds among health-care institutions in their territory. But in practice, population-based funding took place only marginally. Year after year, the ministry renewed the budgets of the regional boards according to what the boards had spent the year before. This did nothing to encourage efficiency or to ensure equity between regions: some areas lost population while others gained, and the fact that budgets were not adjusted accordingly resulted in growing discrepancies in the services rendered in different parts of the province. The situation only worsened as the health-care system evolved toward a more community-based approach to the delivery of care.

The first signs of a needs-based budget allocation system reaching the governmental agenda lie as far back as December 1987. At that time, the Rochon report advocated allocating resources on a regional basis. This suggestion was tied to the Rochon Commission's proposal to create regional health and social services boards. A former proponent of program-based funding, Liberal minister of health and social services Thérèse Lavoie-Roux backed the proposal and brought greater clarity to the concept of client-focused programs. It was not until 1991, however, that regional boards replaced regional health and social services councils. Meanwhile, budgets continued to be allocated on a historical basis: they were merely recalculated to conform to the territorial boundaries of the newly created boards.

In 1993, the Ministry of Health and Social Services created the Working Group for the Allocation of Financial Resources, charged with creating a frame of reference for allocating the budgets of Quebec's health-care system. The working group's mandate was to address policies, orientations, service organization, resource allocation, and accounting. But the group's recommendations centred on changing the information systems of hospital centres so as to better track costs and activities (Groupe de travail sur l'allocation des ressources financières 1993). It was difficult to change budgeting methods, the group argued, as long as data on expenditures continued to be fragmentary and inconsistent from one institution to the next. For institutional reasons, therefore, budgeting for establishments continued to occur mainly on a historical basis. The ministry did, however, begin to use population-based data to distribute development funds and assign budget cuts.

There was another reason for the delay in moving needs-based funding to the decision-making agenda: an interest-related one. The explanation lies in the nature of Quebec's electoral system (Select Committee on the Election Act 2005):

> Under the current system, regions that have sustained a loss of population continue, because of certain concessions, to elect the same number of members as before, which ensures that their representation in the National Assembly remains constant. Members from urban constituencies therefore tend to represent proportionately more people than do Members from rural constituencies.

This quirk in Quebec's electoral system meant that an impartial, population-based funding system risked cutting health-care dollars in regions that were losing population. In other words, needs-based funding promised to be politically unpopular in the very regions where votes were most valuable. As will be seen in chapter 7, a similar situation in Newfoundland and Labrador influenced decisions in that province as well.

In the event, political reticence would somewhat give way to financial factors. The budget cuts of the 1990s and the government's failure to invest the savings thus realized into front-line care, as originally intended, reduced hospitals' spending power. While some institutions found creative ways to respect their new budgets, others ran up large deficits. So when hospital spending began to grow again in the late 1990s, most of the money went to filling the deficits of those hospitals that had in a manner of speaking been the least financially successful. Of course, the disadvantage of this strategy was that it penalized hospitals that were more adept at managing their funds. In order to avoid this situation happening again, the Parti Québécois government and health and social services minister Pauline Marois introduced new legislation on balanced budgets in 2000. The *Act to Provide for Balanced Budgets in the Public Health and Social Services Network* (Québec 2000), submitted in March and adopted in June, prohibited health-care establishments from running budget deficits. Notwithstanding the new legislation, some health-care establishments continued to accumulate significant deficits and indeed felt justified in doing so.

This situation finally compelled the ministry to truly turn to a budget allocation method that used efficiency measures and/or a population-based approach. At the urging of the deputy minister of health and social services, Pierre Gabrièle, a committee was created to re-evaluate budgeting methods for hospital centres. A second committee was created to re-evaluate budgeting methods for CLSCs (local community services centres) and CHSLDs (residential and long-term care centres). Denis Bédard, former secretary of the Treasury Board and professor at Quebec's School of Public Administration in Montreal (École nationale d'administration publique), was appointed president of both committees. Chosen for his prominence in the field and his expertise in finance, Bédard's appointment testified to the government's intention to find a real solution.

Bédard's committees faced important challenges. As difficult as the calculations were sure to be, the hospital budgeting committee hoped to estimate future performance by comparing the costs of treatment of a given pathology between two institutions and adjusting budgets for increased efficiency. But the CLSC and CHSLD environments were characterized by a dearth of standardized data, forcing the committee to base its calculations on a number of unknown variables. How many seniors needed shelter? How many young people needed housing? What costs were reasonable to treat cases that varied in severity and number? And perhaps the most difficult question: how to predict service use over time.

Bédard's report on hospital centres was submitted in December 2001, and the report on CLSCs and CHSLDs followed six months later (Comité sur la réévaluation du mode de budgétisation des centres hospitaliers de soins généraux et spécialisés 2002; Comité sur la réévaluation du mode de budgétisation des CLSC et des CHSLD 2002). Both reports recommended that budgets be allocated on a program-by-program basis for all three levels of operation: ministry funding of regions, regional funding of health-care institutions, and health-care institutions' funding of services. For hospitals, commissioners wrote, the ministry should fund regions according to the population's needs and the average consumption of services, adjusted for costs engendered by the exchange of services between regions (Comité sur la réévaluation du mode de budgétisation des centres hospitaliers de soins généraux et spécialisés 2002).[5] Regions should allocate hospital resources on a program-by-program basis adjusted for factors like teaching activities, research activities, and the remoteness of the location. Finally, hospital institutions should allocate their resources by program using a normative approach that considered the services provided (volume and complexity) and standardized costs.

As for CLSCs and CHSLDs, the volume of consumption of services should first be estimated at the ministerial level for each program, provincewide, and then multiplied by average standardized costs. The budget for each program should then be distributed among regions using a population-based approach that standardized consumption levels after adjusting them for regional factors. Regional budget allowances should be adjusted to compensate for the net effect of service exchanges between regions. The regional boards were to use the same normative approach to distribute resources among health-care establishments, based on the volume of comparable services and standardized costs adjusted for factors that affected a given establishment.

Bédard's committees used a threefold argument to promote their recommendations. First, budgeting under the proposed system would be based on an objective understanding of changes in beneficiary profiles, services, and costs, making it easier to more accurately predict the health-care system's financial needs. Second, the population-based approach would ensure an equitable distribution of resources. Third, the use of standardized costs would stimulate efficiency and improve performance.

But political reluctance to upset influential non-urban voters continued to delay the implementation of the reform, and in the end, needs-based funding only moved from the governmental agenda, where it had been for 15 years, to the decision-making agenda with the 2003 election victory of the Quebec Liberal Party. Armed with a majority of seats, the Liberals lost no time in fulfilling their election promise to regionalize care. In December, with a majority in the National Assembly, the Liberals passed Bill 25 replacing the regional boards with regional agencies in charge of creating local health and social services networks. The new structure provided an excellent cover to move forward on needs-based funding. The new health and social services minister, Philippe Couillard, appointed associate deputy minister of health and social services Pierre Malouin to head the new Permanent Consultation and Coordination Committee for Resource Allocation, charged with creating a needs-based budget alloca-tion formula. Malouin had developed a similar formula for the Ministry of Education, which turned out to be too simple to apply to the more complex field of health care. But by dividing the work among subcommittees, the permanent committee eventually developed a formula that found favour with the Quebec Hospital Association and the associations of CLSCs and CHSLDs. This agreement freed the ministry to choose a policy.

By this time, it had become evident that the new budgeting system could not be applied overnight. According to the formula, some regions had large surpluses that could not be redistributed all at once without throwing the system into panic. This was the case of Montreal, where the annual surplus was in the order of $200 to $225 million. For institutional reasons, therefore, the administration gave itself five to seven years to bring budgets in line with needs-based calculations by shaving money off development funds every year and leaving operating funds intact. Minimum levels of services and minimal teams were also developed for remote regions where readjustments would have otherwise been too dra-matic—and the political fallout too severe. The Liberal strategy also had the advantage of securing the support of interest groups who suspected that their regions would lose out in the long run but who were placated by the promise that funding would be cut only gradually. Opposition was also muted by the technical nature of the funding calculations, which at the development stage made it impossible to know the exact extent of the adjustments to come.

Perhaps more than anything else, however, the lack of opposition to the Liberal reform can be attributed to an ideational factor: its portrayal as a question of inter-regional equity. This overtone of "moral reform," as one informant described it, made the changes difficult to oppose. And yet one of our respondents suggested that rhetoric aside, needs-based funding was little more than a modern disguise for per capita budgeting. After the reform, only a few agencies actually began to use needs-based calculations to allocate resources to the establishments in their territory.

So despite the reform's ambitions, its application was limited in scope. Notably, the new resource allocation formula based on key indicators did not apply to physical health, which is of course a major item in health-care budgets. Monies for physical health programs continued to be allocated on a historical basis. Because of this particularity, only a small proportion of the budget was actually allocated according to population indicators. Nonetheless, the reform may have laid the groundwork for more population-based funding in future years. In the interim, the politics of protecting the status quo—influenced largely by Quebec's electoral boundaries—at the detriment of equity demonstrates that "when morality meets politics," it is not easy to make a decision.

ANALYSIS OF THE DECISION-MAKING PROCESS: IS THERE A PATTERN?

A feature we notice about policy-making in Quebec is the large role played by experts through the vehicle of reports and commissions of inquiry on subjects that informed the policy-making process. The reports were so influential that we can consider their authors as policy entrepreneurs and the reports themselves as powerful policy tools. Indeed, we would hardly exaggerate were we to coin the phrase, "No report, no reform." In every case studied here, the policy decision or non-decision (a decision in itself) was preceded by the publication of one or more reports, a notable characteristic of which was the careful political calculation the government gave to choice of commission or committee head who was principal report author. Analysis of all six cases shows that the import of each report and the eventual choice of a policy, however limited, was to a large extent associated with the political authority of the individual chosen to head the commission and write the report. Interestingly, most of these reports involved individuals who either had been, were, or were to become insiders to the health decision-making process.

For example, the report for the prescription drug insurance program—the most substantial reform among the 30 cases studied for this book—was authored by Claude Castonguay, a former minister of health and social services, a past commissioner, and an ex-insurance executive with a wide sphere of influence (Comité d'experts sur l'assurance médicaments 1996). Similarly, in the case of waiting lists, the successive committees on general surgery, orthopedics, and cardiology were headed by individuals well known in Quebec's medical community. Their reports facilitated the choice of a wait-list management system, even though financial constraints and a lack of leadership later caused decision makers to abandon the plan to centralize the lists. As for regionalization, the origins of the government's change in mentality with respect to how regional-level services should be organized lay in the Rochon report, with the Clair report's reflections on governance, accountability, and the organization of primary care services serving to crystallize the ministry's 2003 decision. Both Rochon and Clair commanded tremendous authority in medical and governmental circles. The Clair report was also seminal in the creation of family medicine groups and the concomitant introduction of alternative payment plans, a program that quickly claimed the support of minister of health and social services Pauline Marois because of its political popularity. Regarding needs-based funding, the Bédard reports of 2002, while unremarked by the public, once again guided the decision-making process at the government level: by 2004, discussions on their findings had cajoled resistant stakeholders into supporting new, albeit less innovative than originally intended, budget allocation methods. Finally, like the appointment of Bédard, the choice of Roland Arpin to head the commission on privatization was deliberate, but in a negative sense: Arpin was unknown in the world of health and social services and held little credibility in the field. His legitimacy in administrative circles was impressive, and his administrative expertise assured the community that his work would be thorough and reliable, but his lack of influence and the imprecise nature of the directives to his working group (both of which were deliberate on the part of health minister Rochon) meant that Arpin's final recommendations remained too general to permit implementation.

It is on the role of interests that we suggest, tentatively, that there may be significant differences between Quebec and other jurisdictions. On the one hand, the array of interests with noticeable influence may have been wider in Quebec than other provinces. The interaction of regional interests and researchers knowledgeable about regionalization influenced the 1991 reform "positively" and limited the "damage" of the 2003 reforms. The unions played a role in blocking the forces of privatization (for-profit delivery) even though polling data showed Quebecers were relatively open to such possibilities. Such influences were not at the expense of traditional provider interests, however. Physician groups formally exercised much influence on the issues that most affected them, or had the potential to do so. This was observed in the alternative payment plan case and in the wider FMG reform where FMOQ was able to veto changes. It was not observed but effective in removing any thought of regionalizing medical budgets. Physician influence was seen as well in the ability of the medical federations to limit the speed with which progress was made on wait times. Although part of the provincial state, hospital interests also resisted reform on wait times with real effect. In the case of prescription drugs the range of interests included insurance, pharmacist, and pharmaceutical interests as well as the voices of unions and leftist groups. The legitimization of all these interests arguably had two effects: it made it hard to achieve substantial reform given the array of different interests, and yet made large reform possible where there was some harmony of interests.

Although not a prominent feature in the adoption of reforms in Quebec, knowledge was part of the context against which more colourful elements wrestled to influence change. The exception was the case of needs-based funding, where a legacy of poor data collection made it impossible for the reform to fulfill its potential. In three of the reforms studied here—the cases of waiting lists, regionalization, and alternative payment plans—high-ranking bureaucrats and policy-makers indicated that they were inspired by the experiences of other provinces. In the other three cases, Quebec seems to have preferred "home-grown" solutions that actually distanced it from the other provinces. Furthermore, our interviewees made no reference to the role of federal-level structures in the policy-making process except in the case of prescription drug insurance; the rumour that the federal government was preparing a national prescription drug program (Natural Forum on Health 1997a) largely accounts for the rapidity of Quebec's decision (though not the content), as the Parti Québécois wanted to adopt its program first. Even in the case of alternative payment plans, when federal Health Transition Funds were used to shape the family medicine group model, Ottawa appears to have had very little influence.

Our analysis of the six issues showcases a last important feature of policy-making in Quebec: the preponderant role of the minister of health and social services, particularly when the minister in question was also a physician. At the risk of overgeneralizing, we can perhaps coin a second phrase: "No doctor, no reform." Five of the six most important reforms proposed in Quebec over the period of study were suggested by physicians: first Dr. Rochon (prescription drug insurance, waiting lists, for-profit delivery), then Dr. Couillard (regionalization, needs-based funding). The credibility of these physicians and their capacity to win over the public had an incontrovertible impact on their ability to pursue their ideological and ethical convictions. Of course, there were countervailing forces: as we have seen, other factors served to downscale or shelve all reforms except the prescription drug insurance program. Nonetheless, only one reform of six—FMGs and alternative payment plans—was proposed by someone other than a minister who was not also a physician. It is important to note, though, that new legislation was not required to create FMGs and that the new model, while certainly unique, was hardly revolutionary: it fell in line with experiments that had already taken place on Quebec territory. Furthermore, insofar as the public was concerned, a reform that promised Quebecers around-the-clock access to their family doctor did not require the same degree of political credibility as did other changes.

This conclusion as to the importance of doctors to Quebec's reforms is not intended to disparage the qualifications of health minister Pauline Marois. But the track record of Marois's successor, Rémy Trudel, nonetheless demonstrates that the appointment of a minister unknown to the world of health and social services constitutes a major handicap for the execution of reform (David 2001; Lessard 2001).

CONCLUSION

Over the last two decades, Quebec's health-care system has been profoundly marked by the work of two ministers of health and social services: Drs. Jean Rochon and Philippe Couillard. Jean Rochon came first and acted early: even before Rochon's appointment as minister, the Rochon report had sketched out a vision of public health care that would channel not only his reforms, but those of his contemporaries and their successors as well. Originally based on progressive ideals of equity, social justice, and public participation, that vision has been diluted as a changing political and financial landscape led to the debate on for-profit delivery of (and payment for) health-care services—a debate that still shakes the province today. This change in direction can be traced to the emergence in the late 1990s of problems of access to care, problems that were broadcast by the media and were instrumental in convincing Quebecers that private funding and the private provision of care could alleviate long waiting times (see the opinion polls in J.-F. Bégin 1998; Léger Marketing/Journal de Québec 2007). The election results of 2003 and 2007 were proof positive of Quebecers' change of position: in both years, the Liberals were elected on platforms that did nothing to reject privatization (Parti libéral du Québec 2003, 2007) and, in 2007, the much newer and more conservative Action démocratique du Québec captured the official opposition on the strength of a campaign that advocated increased personal responsibility and greater privatization of health care (Action démocratique du Québec 2007).

Former health and social services minister Couillard also had great influence over the evolution of Quebec's health-care system, which since Couillard's spearheading of Bill 33 has been moving determinedly away from its anti-private underpinnings.[6] A recent sign in this direction lay in the 2007 appointment of Claude Castonguay, himself a former Liberal minister of health and social services, to pen recommendations on the state's role in providing access to care and financing and providing services. This appointment promised to bring the history of Quebec's health-care reforms back full circle, for Castonguay. In this instance Castonguay was appointed not by the minister of health and social services but by close friend and minister of finance Monique Jérôme-Forget (Québec 2007). He is the same figure who promoted the universal prescription drug plan that first united private and public insurers 10 years before. Fulfilling expectations, Castonguay's report, released in February 2008, recommended that the *Canada Health Act* be modified and that the private sector be allowed an expanded role in the delivery of care (Groupe de travail sur le financement du système de santé 2008). Following the December 2008 provincial elections, however, again won by the Liberals with the Parti Québécois in the role of the official opposition, the new minister of health and social services Dr. Yves Bolduc seems to be far from officially supporting the greater privatization of services. Meanwhile, Couillard left politics and joined a group of private investors working to develop private health-care services. By all indications, this debate is far from being over.

NOTES

1. The commission cost $6 million and lasted two years (Duplantie 2001).
2. Things finally came to a head when the *Chaoulli* case (Supreme Court of Canada 2005) crystallized the consequences of the lack of access to services at the legal level. In a spectacular decision that made headlines across the country, the Supreme Court of Canada responded to the *Chaoulli* case in 2005 by striking down Quebec provincial legislation that had banned the sale of private insurance policies for medical procedures covered by public medicare (Madore and Tiedemann 2005; Supreme Court of Canada 2005). In response, the Government of Quebec passed Bill 33 authorizing the sale of private insurance for selected medical procedures to be provided in private clinics. Extensive media coverage of the case allowed privatization proponents to make headway as a population discouraged with the status quo started to show itself ready to embrace for-profit delivery as a solution (Léger Marketing/Journal de Québec 2007; Lessard 2005).
3. The six diseases covered under the Outpatient Circular were cystic fibrosis, cancer, severe psychiatric disorders, insipid diabetes, tuberculosis, and hyperlipoproteinemia.
4. Since the inception of regional boards in 1991, Quebec has been organized into 18 health and social services regions. Three of those regions (Nunavik, Baie-James, and Nord-du-Québec) assume responsibility for aboriginal populations and were exempt from the modifications legislated by Bill 25. A total of 15 regional boards were therefore transformed into agencies. The Centre régional de santé et de services sociaux de la Baie-James, the Régie régionale de la santé et des services sociaux du Nunavik, and the Conseil Cri de la santé et des services sociaux de la Baie-James retained their original status.
5. The commissioners also recommended that provincewide, ultra-specialized services be charged to the regional boards of the patients' place of residence, and that the exchange of local and regional services be compensated globally within each region.
6. Adopted in November 2006, Bill 33 modified the *Health Insurance Act* to allow an individual to enter into an insurance contract to cover the costs of insured services required for certain surgeries designated by law. The bill also created a legal framework for the exercise of certain medical activities

in specialized medical centres (activities also designated by law). In addition, the bill specified the conditions under which a hospital could associate with a medical clinic to provide specialized medical care to hospital patients (Québec 2006).

Chapter 7

Between a Rock and a Hard Place: The Difficulty of Reforming Health Care in Newfoundland and Labrador

Stephen G. Tomblin and Jeff Braun-Jackson

Introduction

One theme of this volume is that larger efficiency-related health-care reforms were significantly correlated with hard times and fiscal stress. The argument is not that fiscal crisis necessarily led to such reforms but that, without crisis-induced pressures, efficiency reforms of any substantial magnitude were relatively rare.

Economic hardship was a constant in Newfoundland and Labrador from 1990 to 2003, the years we cover in this study, although less so in the first few years of the millennium. Like other provinces, Newfoundland and Labrador was affected by the severe downturn in the business cycle of the early 1990s and its fiscal consequences. In Newfoundland and Labrador this situation was compounded by the disappearance of the northern cod fishery beginning in the mid-1980s and the subsequent federal moratorium on the fishery in 1992. The cod fishery had been the economic backbone of many outports for over a century. For the great majority of these often remote fishing villages, there was little or no prospect of attracting new industries to replace what was lost. Many of the affected people, especially older workers who had spent all their labour force years in the fishery, had little prospect of finding a job in St. John's or elsewhere in the province.

In these circumstances the overriding priority of the Government of Newfoundland and Labrador was to deal with the adjustment pressures. An estimated 35,000–40,000 people were directly affected in a province with a total population of less than 535,000.[1] As the magnitude of the challenge was beyond the wherewithal of the provincial treasury, the federal government became involved. For a decade, federal, federal-provincial, and provincial adjustment programs were the priority, ranging from income support for education and skills upgrading, to buying back fishing licenses and providing financial support for relocation.

Even with massive federal financial support, the fiscal position of the province was precarious during much of the 1990s. Thus, other things being equal, it was logical that any health-care reform that would add to budgetary expenditures would be an uphill battle, whereas reforms that offered the possibility of efficiencies and savings for the provincial treasury would be welcomed. As all six case studies examined in this volume contained some element of potential efficiency, this chapter on Newfoundland and Labrador might have been a story of efficiency-driven reform. This is a tale of little reform, however. The reason is that the fisheries crisis and the dismal provincial fiscal situation, as large as they loomed, were not the only factors shaping outcomes. Much more was at play.

The political rules of the game, in particular, influenced what transpired and what did not. On a representation-by-population basis, the areas most affected by the crisis in the fishery were also heavily overrepresented in the provincial legislature. In such a context, any government wishing to remain in power would naturally have felt an obligation to focus on the "old regime" and adjustment processes available for the fishery (i.e., for rural communities). Change or lack of change was to be determined by the power and autonomy of the ideas, interests, and institutions connected with the old regime and its capacity to survive and make sense of changing realities. In Canadian political science there has been much debate about state autonomy and the extent to which modernization should produce "inevitable" policy changes. In state-centred theory, however, it has been argued that the institutions and the political games constructed or inherited by premiers should not be underestimated (Cairns 1988). Prescriptive calls for modernization reforms and new forms of integration by modernization thinkers have proven in practice to be neither automatic nor inevitable (Tomblin 1995).

The political game has reinforced an approach to province-building weighted toward natural resources. The service sector—including health—in Newfoundland and Labrador has clear urban biases and interest group challenges; it is fragmented, scattered, and competitive. In provinces with strong rural traditions, the service sector has always been a harder sell. Only recently has there been more priority placed on lowering tuition, increasing immigration, and recruiting professions essential for health and other types of technical-industrial transformation—and these discussions tend to appear at the margins of political discourse. The political incentive to push health-care reform onto the radar screen was lacking as was the logic in building the kind of bureaucratic structures, knowledge networks, and partnerships essential for defining and promoting health restructuring. Context mattered.

The embedded institutional traditions influenced the behaviour of key stakeholders, especially physicians. The recruitment and maintenance of rural versus urban doctors were part of an inherited system that created competing ideas, processes, and assumptions. Rural physicians tended to be "international" and paid a salary, while "domestic" urban doctors were more likely to be nationally trained and paid on a fee-for-service basis. In the area of primary health-care reform, rural doctors and communities championed policy changes, whereas urban centres faced more policy constraints. These cultural, geographical, and political economy divisions contributed to a lack of consensus among physicians on health-care reform.

The people of the province, as important stakeholders, were by and large willing to accept the status quo. The introduction of medicare in 1969 had given those in remote and rural areas access to physicians for the first time in their lives. People in urban centres had enjoyed theoretical access to physicians, but on an out-of-pocket fee-for-service basis that had in practice limited their access. Medicare removed these cost barriers. While access to physicians improved in all provinces, the degree of improvement was probably greatest in Newfoundland and Labrador.[2] Fast-forwarding to the 1990s, the people of the province were in some sense more conscious of the benefits of medicare than concerned about what might be lacking.

The Newfoundland and Labrador Medical Association was also a key stakeholder. Its members, too, were satisfied with the status quo so long as they could frame the debate with respect to physician remuneration and scopes of practice.

Geography and climate also mattered. Whether they live on the island of Newfoundland or the Labrador Peninsula, the people of the province experience brutal weather. Their homes are many miles from Canada's political and economic heartland. These factors have helped create in Newfoundlanders and Labradorians a unique culture with a distinctive way of seeing things. This perception has been reinforced by a sense that mainlanders had "taken them for a ride" on major economic development projects such as Churchill Falls. Reform ideas that originated on the mainland were often therefore treated with suspicion (Elkins and Simeon 1980). The fact many regions of the province lacked good Internet service compounded the problem of isolation.

In a nutshell, the crisis in the fishery was the dominant issue that shaped the environment within which health-care issues were considered. But the interaction of politics, history, geography, and culture also help explain the limited reform that occurred. These embedded traditions shaped the historical pace and direction of health policy ideas and processes in the province. Coping effectively with a crisis requires the renewal of governance and encouragement of new forms of political-policy connections that reflect changing circumstances and new interdependencies. It also requires investing resources and building local knowledge and capacity based on "best practices." In Newfoundland and Labrador, the service economy is not recognized in the same way the fishery is, which has created problems for those trying to mobilize new health ideas, interests, and institutions. Within such a context, it has been difficult to shift power or contest the status quo.

Our purpose here is to document the nature and extent of reform in Newfoundland and Labrador from 1990 to 2003 and to analyze why reforms did or did not occur. Six province-specific research questions will guide the case-by-case analysis:

Why did the Government of Newfoundland and Labrador

1. establish regional health authorities (RHAs) to assume responsibility for the management and delivery of a significant range of health services?
2. not establish a needs-based funding formula for regional health authorities?
3. pilot a number of alternative payment plans for primary care physicians, typically based on salary, but not expand them?
4. not establish either a wait list management system or a wait list tracking system?
5. not create a policy framework that made possible or made difficult the development of private for-profit delivery of medically necessary services that had historically been delivered in private not-for-profit hospitals?
6. not establish either a universal or targeted prescription drug plan?

This chapter is divided into three sections: The first focuses on the political and policy-making contexts that underscored the policy landscape. The second section provides an analysis of the reform decisions and nondecisions. The final section concludes with an evaluation and explanation of why health policy reform was either very limited or entirely absent in Newfoundland and Labrador.

THE POLICY-MAKING CONTEXT IN NEWFOUNDLAND AND LABRADOR: HISTORICAL OVERVIEW

Managing debt has shaped policy-making in Newfoundland for decades. Two years after the 1931 Statute of Westminster granted Newfoundland legal freedom, the Dominion of Newfoundland was unable to fulfill its debt obligations. This led to an arrangement under which its constitution was temporarily suspended and the government placed under a British-appointed Commission. Three options were put to the people in a 1948 referendum: return to responsible government, continuation of the Commission, and confederation with Canada. The referendum did not produce a majority for any of the options. The Commission option had the least support and was accordingly dropped. In a second referendum Newfoundlanders chose Canada, albeit with a small majority (Hillier and Neary 1980).

Joey Smallwood had been the leader of the pro-confederation forces during the referendum period, and his Liberal party won the general election in 1949 to form the first provincial government. Smallwood was popular and his Liberals won the next five provincial elections, generally with little effective opposition.

Having been the leader of the forces that fought for the Canada option, Smallwood claimed the political credit for the infusion of federal cash transfers that went with Confederation, both the grants to individuals (old age pensions, baby bonuses, and unemployment insurance) and to governments (such as specific-purpose matching grants and unconditional Equalization grants). This infusion of new money raised standards of living but was not a formula for home-grown prosperity and jobs. Smallwood personally attempted to "modernize" the economy by encouraging development projects. Some failed (such as a refinery at Come-By-Chance and a linerboard mill in Stephenville) at considerable cost to the province. A deal struck with the Government of Quebec relating to Churchill Falls proved an even larger blunder.

Raymond Blake argues that economic development was not really the objective behind Newfoundland and Labrador's entry into the Canadian federation in 1949. It was the time of the Second National Policy, and the real goal was social benefits. According to Blake (1994, 6),

> The Maritimes had opted for union in large part because it was promised great economic opportunity.... Newfoundland never demanded economic development, its people were never promised it, and Newfoundland never received it. Instead, it was promised greater social benefits and it is in the area of social welfare policy that Newfoundland gained, in the short term.

Union with Canada was seen as a rather pragmatic response and not the product of policy debate and analysis.

Smallwood was a populist. He dominated his cabinets, leaving little effective authority with his ministers. There was little emphasis placed on policy or social networking, knowledge construction or exchange across state-society boundaries. He did not encourage the development of functional knowledge centres and policy networks outside of government that are normally associated with social and policy learning, nor did he go out of his way to develop the bureaucracy (Bradford 1999; Howlett, Ramesh, and Perl 2009). He related to the people directly, not through intermediate bodies like churches, businesses, unions, or social organizations. This centralized "strong leader" government is a legacy that remains at the time of writing. While premiers Clyde Wells and Brian Tobin experimented with economic planning, community accounts, different forms of regionalization, social strategic planning, and so on, Newfoundland and Labrador is not known for its public policy experimentation and new forms of civic engagement.

Smallwood eventually lost support, and in 1972 his government was defeated. For the next 17 years the Progressive Conservatives ruled, first under Frank Moores and then Brian Peckford. The Progressive Conservatives inherited a province that was still the poorest in Canada. The unemployment rate in Newfoundland and Labrador during their era was consistently 15 to 20 percent, generally double or close to double the national average.

The years of Progressive Conservative government were marked by disagreements with Ottawa about constitutional issues including ownership of offshore resources. Peckford, in particular, was a strident provincial nationalist who promised prosperity based on provincial control and management of Newfoundland's natural resources. In 1984, the Supreme Court of Canada ruled that the federal government owned the offshore resources in question. This might have put the kibosh on Peckford's strategy, but he found an ally in Brian Mulroney, the new federal Progressive Conservative prime minister. In 1985, the two leaders signed the Atlantic Accord, which provided for joint management and revenue sharing of the offshore.

Peckford was an old-style province builder; his brand of politics was about gaining control of the development of essential natural resources. Comparable to Peter Lougheed, or W. A. C. Bennett, he sought to increase the power and autonomy of the provincial state over the resource economy. Peckford expanded public bureaucracies and reinforced new ideas, institutions, and interests connected with his provincial vision, but this vision was not service centred. The policy agenda focused almost solely on natural resource development.

The people of Newfoundland and Labrador may have been attracted to Peckford's sizzle. But with unemployment still very high, they tired of waiting for the steak and returned the Liberals to government in 1989. The Liberal party remained in office until late 2003, which coincides with the period of analysis here. Premier Wells was the first of four Liberals to hold the premiership. Wells favoured a strong federal government that could continue to redistribute in favour of the less wealthy provinces. Wells is well known for his role in blocking the Mulroney government's Meech Lake constitutional reforms. But what is most relevant here is his government's response to the recession of the early 1990s and the closing of the fishery. As was the case in other provinces, the Wells government asked the people to swallow some unpleasant fiscal medicine. In the health sector this led to a rate of increase in per capita spending that was close to zero in constant dollars over five years. Not surprisingly, this period was marked as well by significant out-migration.

On the other hand, Premier Wells was a policy reformer. Compared with his Progressive Conservative predecessors, Wells was more of a centralist and policy wonk who was clearly committed to health transformation and policy innovation. He helped push the knowledge and service-based economy onto the public agenda. The premier constantly expressed the view that the status quo was not an option, and that there was a need for fundamental policy change. The regionalization of health care, discussed in the next section, appealed to Wells not just as a means of reducing costs. Wells was a tireless advocate of centralizing health care, and other policy fields as well, based on a regional vision. Regionalization in sectors such as education, municipal governance, health, and economic development became the dominant political mantra. It is also important to point out that Premier Wells was an advocate of regional integration across provinces, and he became a new partner in the Atlantic Premiers Council.

The re-election of the federal Liberals in 1993 improved the federal-provincial relations atmosphere for Wells in that the new prime minister, Jean Chrétien, had also been a strong opponent of the Meech Lake Accord. But Ottawa's priority at that time was fixing the treasury. Whatever additional short-run pain the Canada Health and Social Tranfer (CHST)–related cuts in federal transfer payments to provinces may have caused, by the end of the decade Newfoundland and Labrador's fiscal position had improved. By 2000, the flamboyant Brian Tobin, who had replaced Wells as premier in 1996, had departed and after an interlude Roger Grimes, was elected party leader and hence became premier. Grimes appointed a Royal Commission focusing on Newfoundland and Labrador's place in the Canadian federation (Government of Newfoundland and Labrador 2003). The table of contents of the commission's report covers three pages but mentions the word "health" only once in passing. This near silence is a metaphor for our analysis here: health care never acquired the priority in Newfoundland and Labrador that it did in other provinces.

Case Studies

For each case study, data were obtained from face-to-face and telephone interviews conducted between September 2004 and March 2005. A total of 30 individuals were interviewed for times varying from 40 to 110 minutes. They included politicians, union leaders, public servants, health professionals (physicians and nurses), members of regional health authorities, and members of interest groups who participated in the health policy community during the period 1990 to 2004/05. Data were also gathered from legislative debates from the Newfoundland and Labrador House of Assembly, government websites, government royal commissions and reports, and media databases such as the *Globe and Mail*.

Regionalization

The only area where formal, integrated reform was achieved in Newfoundland was regionalization. In the early 1990s the Government of Newfoundland and Labrador, like many other provinces, identified the possibility of regionalized health districts as a mechanism to manage increasing health-care expenditures and escalating fiscal challenges.

The concept of regionalized health care can be traced to Smallwood's government in 1965. At that time a Royal Commission on Health was established to report on the state of the health-care system in the province and make recommendations for improvement (Government of Newfoundland and Labrador 1966). At the time, Canada-wide hospital insurance was not even a decade old, and publicly funded medical care had not yet been created. Among the report's findings, the commission recommended that the provincial Department of Health become the overarching planning authority, and that the province be divided into regions with services within each region provided by a regional health board responsible to the minister of health. The report also recommended the establishment of a provincial health council to provide a consultative forum to assist with health planning (Government of Newfoundland and Labrador 1966).

During the 1970s, the province continued to feel pressures resulting from the combination of rising expenditures for social programs including health care, and the goal of improving access to care and the overall health of Newfoundland and Labrador residents. Two significant reports were issued, the first being *A Concept of Regionalization of Health Care Services in the Province of Newfoundland* (Newfoundland and Labrador Health Board Council 1972). The report examined different models and methods for adoption of a regionalized health-care structure. It ultimately recommended that four or five regions be established to oversee research and planning, organization, administration, and evaluation of health services. The Council's report stressed that boards must have financial responsibility and autonomy to successfully implement the proposed models. Following the Health Council's report, a Health Study Group was created to provide an overview of health-care delivery in Newfoundland and Labrador (Government of Newfoundland and Labrador Health Study Group 1973). The findings of the report supported the Health Council's recommendation that regional boards have some degree of financial responsibility. The report further recommended that a pilot project be implemented to evaluate regionalization. The pilot project, however, was never initiated, perhaps because the province was not yet dealing with a full-blown fiscal crisis. Regionalization lost momentum and fell off the government's agenda.

Beginning in the 1990s, the national economic downturn resulted in increased fiscal challenges. For Newfoundland and Labrador, these challenges were exacerbated in 1992 as the collapse of the northern cod fishery decimated employment and handicapped the province's ability to pay for basic services. Also in 1992, the provincial budget announced a freeze on health-care spending resulting in, among other things, the elimination of 450 acute care beds and 850 jobs (Botting 2000). During a Health Ministers' conference, the concept of regionalization was put forward as a viable option to deal with escalating health-care costs, which renewed interest in comprehensive health system restructuring in Newfoundland and Labrador.

The combination of economic pressures facing health care—rising costs, a national fiscal crisis, anticipated reductions in federal transfers to the provinces, and the provincial freeze on health-care spending—forced the Newfoundland and Labrador government to explore alternative service-delivery configurations, pushing regionalization onto the government agenda. The Wells government appointed Lucy Dobbin, a former CEO of St. Clair's Hospital in St. John's, to chair a commission to review how hospital boards could be collapsed. The commission's report, released in March 1993, considered the effect of regionalization on the quality of health services, the coordination of acute and long-term care services, and the ability to take advantage of economies of scale (Dobbin 1993). Hubert Kitchen, the minister of health, noted that "the new board structure will provide the opportunity to enhance patient care services and will allow us [the government] to improve efficiencies in resource utilization. In general, this approach will provide a climate for more innovation and cost effective delivery of quality health care services" (Botting 2000, 21).

In 1994 the government established institutional health boards across the province to provide hospital and other institutional services to patients. Board members were responsible for hiring staff and coordinating services. They were accountable to the Department of Health. In 1998, the government further announced the creation of a second type of health board known as community health boards. These boards were charged with providing a broad spectrum of community health services including health promotion, health protection, and single access points of entry for home care, home support services, nursing homes, drug rehabilitation services, and mental health services (Botting 2000).

A total of four community health boards were established. Two additional health boards were designated as integrated boards. These boards, located on the Northern Peninsula and Labrador, combined the services of both the institutional and community health boards. The establishment

of community health boards by government reflected the shift in thinking from acute care to wellness and prevention. In other words, instead
of the health-care system simply treating illnesses, medical professionals
began to lobby for wellness and promotion campaigns to get people to
change their behaviours as a means of reducing the incidence of particular diseases. The boards' overall objective was to promote "individual
responsibility for one's own health" (Botting 2000, 17).

Despite the wellness rhetoric, the need to address the fiscal crisis and
achieve cost savings remained the issue at the heart of the decision-making
agenda. The health boards were creatures of government with respect
to their structure, size, and function. Board members were appointed ;
the government feared that elected boards would be enslaved to local
interests.

The policy choice stage was limited to a select group of participants, namely, bureaucrats, politicians, and health-care professionals.
Regionalization was generally viewed as a political decision. Citizens,
labour groups, and community interest groups were excluded from the
discussion. Nonetheless, the contributions of key individuals from government, hospitals, and health institutions endowed the initiative with
a "made in Newfoundland and Labrador" feel.

While the government maintained tight control of the debate, it made
efforts to respect the privileged position of physicians. The decision to
regionalize was made without alienating physician groups, by specifically
excluding issues related to physician compensation from the development
of regional service delivery systems. Regionalization was embraced by the
provincial government because it did not affect the hegemonic position of
physicians in the health system, it did not cost more than the old health
system, and it could be marketed to citizens as a method of achieving
efficiencies and improving patient care.

Needs-Based Funding

Formal health-care funding models were initiated in Newfoundland
just prior to its entry into Canada in 1949. At the time, hospitals could be
found only in the province's few larger urban centres. This combined with
scarce physicians' resources and epidemics of various diseases prompted
the government to examine new ways to allocate health-care funding to
increase access for patients. From this crisis emerged the Cottage Hospital
system, in which physicians and nurses became government employees, and medical facilities were established in outports and other rural
communities. For a nominal annual fee (originally $10 for a family and
$5 for an individual), the rural population had access to these facilities
without charge.

The expansion of Newfoundland and Labrador's health-care system continued with the introduction of universal hospital insurance in 1957 and medical insurance in 1969. By the end of the 1960s, Newfoundland and Labrador residents had access to universal health care that was similar to that enjoyed by all Canadians. In this regard, it is worth noting that the focus of health care remained the biomedical model, rather than a public health model of health promotion and disease prevention. Facilities during this period were funded based on line-by-line budgets, which were approved by the Department of Health for each individual hospital or health-care facility.

At the beginning of the 1970s, a fundamental shift occurred as health-care practitioners began to lobby for broad health-care reform that would focus on community health and disease prevention programs. The health practitioner lobby included a proposal to change the funding systems to provide for more local control of service delivery. This proposal was partly successful in that a global funding model was adopted for each institution. This enabled management within each institution to allocate funds rather than having line-by-line decisions made in St. John's. The qualification was that the new model still granted discretion to the Minister to override local decisions. Since the beginning of the 1990s, discussions and debates have focused on the adoption of a population-based funding model to replace the current system, which allows ministerial discretion.

The Newfoundland and Labrador Health Boards Association (NLHBA) was a prominent driver in bringing the issue of needs-based funding models to the institutional and interest agendas. Beginning in 2001, the NLHBA actively lobbied the provincial government to adopt a set of needs-based funding principles to guide budgeting for integrated health boards. The NLHBA recommended that the previous annual budget be used as a baseline, with the expectation that budgets would be adjusted over a period of three to five years according to a set of funding principles agreed to by government. During that time, an equitable funding model would be created. This concept was based in part on the needs-based funding model developed in Alberta where budget stability had been achieved by using a minimum guarantee over the previous year's budget (Newfoundland and Labrador Health Boards Association 2001).

The NLHBA's key recommendation was that the total basket of health money for one year should be allocated on the basis of population-based funding and delivered by the integrated health boards. The boards would also deliver fiscal allocations for assured access and provincial service funding—allocations that were not population based. Assured access would provide special funding for sparsely populated RHAs to compensate them for higher service delivery costs. Provincial services funding would include the basket of tertiary medical services provided by the Health Care Corporation of St. John's.

The NLHBA recommended that the amount of money for population-based funding be divided into pools representing the various services funded in proportion to the most recent calculations of spending. The following programs and services would be included in population-based funding pools: acute inpatient; ambulatory care including both salaried and fee-for-service physicians operating clinics; long-term care; protection, prevention, and promotion; the Cancer Control Program; community living and various support services; children, youth, and family services; and mental health and addictions (Newfoundland and Labrador Health Boards Association 2001).

The NLHBA successfully brought the issue of needs-based funding models to the government agenda. However, the issue never moved beyond this stage and was ultimately resisted by government for a variety of reasons.

First, a population-based funding model would disconnect political control from the distribution of health resources. In the context of the "top-down" legacy of Joey Smallwood's government, elected officials, even decades later, wanted to maintain a degree of political control over how health resources were distributed. From this perspective, it is not surprising that a government would be disinclined to cede power and authority over the distribution of resources through the introduction of needs-based funding models.

Second, in a province that has traditionally relied on a powerful executive to make decisions, with little input from outsider groups and the public, lack of capacity and policy networks posed a serious impediment to the introduction of complex funding formulas. The Government of Newfoundland and Labrador had not made it a priority to develop the capacity for accurate databases to supply the information that was required to sustain a viable population-based funding model for health care.

Finally, government shied away from population-based funding methods because the adoption of such a model threatened to exacerbate tensions between urban and rural communities. There was concern that in a population-based funding model, a large majority of funding would be invested in St. John's, given that it was the only large urban centre, leaving rural communities significantly underfunded. Additionally, needs-based models implied hospital closures and job losses for rural outports. Government apprehension stemmed from a recognition that hospitals are significant economic drivers in small rural communities. There was a great deal of confusion over the assumptions that informed needs-based approaches, and what the impact would be on competing community interests. For all of these reasons, there was little political interest in embracing needs-based funding reforms on a provincial basis (Newfoundland and Labrador Health Boards Association 2001).

In summary, despite lobbying efforts from the NLHBA, political considerations and a lack of policy capacity led to the decision not to implement needs-based funding models for regional health authorities. The Department of Health and Community Services (renamed in 1997) continued to submit all budget requests to the Treasury Board and the Department of Finance, and to allocate funds to the health boards. Political executives were motivated, for the most part, by the mobilization of public opinion rather than objective indicators of health. The province's small population and rural geography made a population-based funding model a difficult sell for the politicians in the province. The boards themselves, however, adopted their own needs-based funding models within their respective jurisdictions (McKillop, Pink, and Johnson 2001).

Alternative Payment Plans

Given that Newfoundland and Labrador is a relatively poor province with a mainly rural, sparsely distributed population, the province has long faced challenges with the recruitment and retention of physicians. These problems had intensified by the 1990s due to increased urbanization and new technical procedures available in larger centres. As a result, Newfoundland and Labrador has been open to experimenting with various models of remuneration and alternatives to traditional fee-for-service. In general, the Newfoundland and Labrador Medical Association supported alternative payment plans, and from 1990 to 2003 a number of alternative payment arrangements were piloted in the province. However, none of those programs were sustained or expanded beyond the pilot period.

Prior to 1990, a Royal Commission noted that fee-for-service payment models were not flexible and did not adequately address patient needs (Government of Newfoundland and Labrador 1984). The commission recommended that new payment models be developed to influence the supply and practice locations of physicians to address persistent challenges with recruitment and retention. Renewed interest in primary care reform surfaced in the early 1990s as fiscal conditions became more troublesome, and governments and health-care associations alike began to look for innovative ways to deliver health services at a reduced cost. However, in the beginning stages of this renewed interest in broad primary care reform, issues related to physician compensation were not addressed.

In 1993, the Newfoundland and Labrador Hospital and Nursing Home Association published *Guidelines for Hospital Boards to Improve Recruitment and Retention of Physicians in Rural Newfoundland and Labrador*. The report pointed out that there were some instances where salaried and fee-for-service physicians working in the same hospital or community had considerable differences in income for the same amount of work.

For the most part, in the early 1990s the provincial government and the Newfoundland and Labrador Medical Association (NLMA) worked collaboratively. The NLMA was included in the membership when a co-ordinating committee for physician recruitment was established by the minister of health and community services. The province also successfully negotiated a four-year agreement with the NLMA in 1998, which included wage increases for both salaried and fee-for-service physicians. But there was no evidence of renewing governance based on a more collaborative interprofessional framework or generating new forums for professional-civic engagement and knowledge exchange.

The relationship between the NLMA and the provincial government was amicable until the late 1990s, when the two parties began to part ways as a result of several disputes. In 1997, the province imposed a cap on the number of new doctors who could set up their practice in St. John's, as part of a strategy aimed at getting more physicians to practice in rural and remote communities. Physicians who chose to work in the capital region were penalized for working in overserviced areas, and were paid 50 cents on the dollar for their services. The NLMA fought vigorously against this practice. Despite the growing animosity, it continued to support alternative payment arrangements and attempted to work with government on primary care initiatives.

In 1998, Newfoundland and Labrador physicians spearheaded a pro-ject known as the Clarenville experiment, which focused on improving quality of life and scope of services for physicians practicing in the rural Clarenville and Bonavista areas. The physicians proposed that fee-for-service be replaced by a salary paid on an hourly basis by the regional health authority. Medical care would be managed by the regional health board, and physicians would establish a new not-for-profit organiza-tion to oversee the project's development (Rich 1999). The organization would contract with providers in communities to provide services under a block funding payment arrangement. Doctors participating in the project would be responsible for providing primary care to hospitals and clinics, with the assistance of nurse practitioners and other health professionals who would also be paid by the RHA. Given the likely start-up costs and benefits associated with health-care transformation, the NLMA pressured the government for additional resources to cover office expenses, recruit-ment of team members, and research and evaluation of outcomes. The government insisted that the project be cost neutral.

An agreement for the Clarenville experiment was close to fruition in the summer of 1999, when talks stalled. The entire project was physician-driven and featured a behind-the-scenes approach to negotiation that was, for the most part, adversarial, pitting the government against one of the most powerful interest groups in the province. But since the project did not receive much public attention, or federal financial support, the government did not feel compelled to move forward.

In the spring of 2001, the two parties made one final attempt to reach an agreement. The physicians made some concessions, even agreeing to a tax ruling to maintain their self-employed status, but government continued to put new parameters on the project to exercise more control. There were also some conflicts between the young physicians' plan in rural Clarenville and the larger medical association, and this made it difficult to get very far toward a resolution. It was a showdown over the amount of control the government wanted to maintain and the inability of physicians to mobilize a broad public-professional network or coalition. Negotiations fell apart as the relationship between the two groups deteriorated. In the end, the NLMA backed away ("Newfoundland Rural PCR Talks Stalled" 2001). By July 2001, the project was moribund.

The following years were marked by a strained relationship between the government and the NLMA. The province continued to allocate funding to recruit salaried physicians and to explore more effective ways to compensate physicians. In 2001, the NLMA requested that the government provide an additional $15 million to address gaps in funding related to family physicians and on-call issues. The government rejected the request, noting that it could not afford that amount. The minister of health and community services added fuel to the fire, stating that even if an extra $15 million were available, the government would not allocate it to primary care physicians as there were more critical issues to address such as cardiac care, home support, and drug therapies. In response, the NLMA initiated a job action, withdrawing all physicians from government committees, and began to pressure government to renegotiate the memorandum of understanding to raise fees for family physicians and to broaden compensation for on-call coverage.

In 2002, all physicians, including surgeons, were set to negotiate a new contract with the province. However, negotiations broke down quickly as physicians pressured government for pay increases, having accepted a two-year wage freeze in their previous contract. The physicians went on strike for more than two weeks. In the end, both the NLMA and the government agreed to binding arbitration to strike a new collective agreement. The agreement included a parity award of $23.9 million with respect to fee-for-service compensation to bring Newfoundland and Labrador physicians up to 95 percent of the pay levels of Maritime physicians, and an 18 percent increase for salaried physicians over three years.

Although the issue of alternative payment plans was on the government agenda, the Clarenville experiment brought into sharp focus the obstacles to decision-making. Physicians were reluctant to accept changes to their scope of practice and alternative payment plans that would be administered and controlled by the provincial government. The government, for the most part, did not want to challenge the hegemonic position of the NLMA. Given the continued issue of recruiting and retaining physicians, and the challenging fiscal conditions, the provincial government preferred to maintain the status quo. Projects related to alternative compensation for physicians never achieved the sustained attention that is required to implement permanent reform.

For-Profit Delivery

In Newfoundland and Labrador, the provincial government made public commitments to upholding the medicare model. However, while there was overt support for a publicly funded service delivery model, Newfoundland and Labrador did not create any policy frameworks to deter the development of private, for-profit health service delivery systems along the lines, for example, of what was done in Saskatchewan in 1995. From 1990 to 2003, the possibility of an enhanced private sector role in the delivery of health services did indeed exist legally in Newfoundland and Labrador. In fact, provincial laws in Newfoundland and Labrador were more open to foreign investment than in most other Canadian provinces. The loose regulatory parameters generally favoured a potential role for private investment. Yet in that part of the health-care system covered by the *Canada Health Act*, the prospects for private investment existed more in theory than in reality.

Between 1990 and 2003, the issue of introducing for-profit medical services in Newfoundland and Labrador only dimly pierced the policy radar. The government did not introduce any legislation, nor did it hold any public hearings or commission any research to formally investigate options to address the issue. It neither encouraged nor discouraged private investment. In short, little attention was paid to the idea of privatization. It was not a high priority on the government's health-care agenda.

Reinforcing the notion that privatization was an insignificant item on the health agenda was the government's decision in 1997 to offload transportation costs to private businesses or directly to individuals. Since all tertiary health procedures were carried out in St. John's, patients living outside the capital had to travel for major surgeries, radiation treatment, and more complex diagnostic procedures. This made it difficult for patients to access certain medically necessary procedures, and local newspapers were filled with horror stories about people who had suffered because of the centralized system for tertiary care.

This lack of attention to privatization at the government agenda stage can be attributed to a variety of factors, but most simply it came down to economics. The fiscal conditions in Newfoundland and Labrador and widespread poverty did not create a climate that would lend itself to the introduction of market-based solutions for health service delivery. Economic conditions aside, there were other factors that contributed to Newfoundland and Labrador's decision not to change legislation to prevent the possibility of privatized health services. There was no one inside government who chose to champion this cause. There was little pressure from entrepreneurs wishing to invest, and other interest groups largely ignored the issue. There were some discussions about introducing the private ownership of MRIs and other diagnostic services. It was decided, however, that permitting for-profit delivery for these services would make it more difficult for the government to control costs. It is worth noting that the government did make some small decisions during the late 1990s. The most significant of these was the government's initiation of several public-private partnerships for the construction and administration of long-term-care facilities in Corner Brook, Burgeo, and St. John's. The provincial government provided some funding, and the management and construction of the facilities was executed by the private sector with support from private investments. The decision to undertake private-public partnerships allowed the Liberal government to construct long-term-care facilities more quickly to accommodate need, rather than waiting until the province had the fiscal capacity to borrow money to do the projects publicly.

In the period studied, the government did little to either promote or prevent an enhanced role for the for-profit sector in the delivery of medically necessary health services. With the exception of some small public-private arrangements introduced in long-term care, the issue of privatization simply failed to gain any significant traction at the government decision-making stage. No formal legislative or institutional decisions were made about the for-profit delivery of medically necessary services. The fiscal climate and widespread poverty in the province, combined with a lack of leadership, meant that privatization was a non-issue.

Wait Lists

Beginning in the mid-1990s there was a growing sense of crisis across Canada regarding wait times and pressure for governments to focus attention on the problem, to define it accurately, and to implement evidence-based solutions to curb the crisis of wait-time queues. In Newfoundland and Labrador, while a series of problems propelled the issue onto the government agenda, provincial officials opted not to create a wait-list management or tracking system as part of their strategic health plan.

A range of factors help explain Newfoundland and Labrador's inaction on wait-list reform during these years. First, the overarching sense of nationalism that had emerged under the provincial Progressive Conservative governments of Frank Moores and Brian Peckford continued to influence policy decisions, and encouraged suspicion about embracing outside policy initiatives that did not account adequately for local circumstances. Second, the top-down leader-centred approach to provincial governance made it difficult for the province to develop the policy networks that were necessary to support external calls for reform, or to contest from within the power of status quo expectations, regimes, and policies. Skilled leadership and money were requisites for developing a system to manage wait times, and both were in short supply. Finally, while there were challenges in providing timely access to services, there was no state of crisis, as there may have been in other provinces, and little political incentive to create a new service delivery model to accommodate wait-time expectations.

In the early to mid-1990s, wait-time reform ranked low on the priority list for government. The closure of the northern cod fishery in 1992, the national recession, and the reduced federal grants associated with introduction of the Canada Health and Social Transfer in 1995 compelled the Wells government to enact a policy of economic austerity. The government reduced the provincial civil service, froze wages for public sector workers, and capped expenses for hospitals. In this context, even maintaining current service levels presented insurmountable challenges for decision makers.

These measures, however, intensified the problem of wait times and pushed the issue onto the decision-making agenda. Public frustration with lengthening wait times, and media coverage of long wait times for surgical and diagnostic procedures such as MRIs, drew the attention of politicians and decision makers to the need for a management system to ensure timely access to care. In particular, two highly publicized cases about small children who were not able to access MRIs in a timely manner caught the attention of provincial health officials (Priest 2005a, 2005b, 2005c).

In 2002, the Department of Health and Community Services published the paper *Health Scope: Reporting to Newfoundlanders and Labradorians on Comparable Health and Health System Indicators* (Government of Newfoundland and Labrador 2002a). The document examined wait times for cardiac surgery, radiation therapy for breast cancer and prostate cancer, and specialist physician visits. The intent of the report was to raise questions not only about current circumstances, but what might need to be done to change the status quo. The findings supported the need to regulate and integrate wait lists from different health-care silos across the province.

The evidence brought forward in the report also supported political requests for increased federal funding. While there may not have been a "wait-times crisis" in Newfoundland and Labrador, the province continued to experience fiscal pressures in part due to federal transfer cutbacks. To this end, growing queues provided evidence of budgetary challenges and reinforced the need for more funding from Ottawa.

Although no formal reforms were adopted to manage wait lists, some informal, reactive measures were implemented by government and health-care practitioners. Given that Newfoundland and Labrador is a small province, many physician, specialist, and tertiary care services are confined to the St. John's region, making it easier and more natural for those physicians to organize themselves informally. Wait-list reform was essentially an urban problem, attracting the attention of certain branches or silos of medicine (e.g., cardiac care, knee replacement). For cardiac care, in particular, surgeons in St. John's pooled their resources to develop an informal system for provincial wait lists. To relieve the pressure, in 1997 the government provided funding to send patients outside the province to receive cardiac care. Additionally, in 2001 funding was allocated to reduce wait times for cardiac surgery and cardiac catheterizations.

Yet these powerful interests had little reason to push for more fundamental change. While in interviews some cardiac surgeons expressed a sincere desire to publish wait times for procedures, the fiscal reality of the province served as a powerful deterrent. With its poor fiscal capacity, small population, limited number of physicians, and specialists and tertiary medical care confined to the capital region, the province struggled just to maintain current health service levels. Embedded governance practices and traditions worked against any calls for a more formal, province-centred model of waiting-list reform.

Prescription Drug Reform

Newfoundland and Labrador did not have a universal drug program. Policy debates on public prescription drug coverage focused on maintaining the capacity to fund the existing, targeted programs, rather than on expanding programs to cover more drugs for more people. Only the province's most vulnerable groups were eligible for prescription drug coverage. While the government intended to implement a broader needs-based approach to drug coverage, "needs" have been historically framed by political competition and debate rather than by systematic data collection.

The Newfoundland and Labrador Prescription Drug Program provided catastrophic coverage for specific, vulnerable population groups through three separate programs: the Income Support Program, the Senior Citizens Drug Subsidy Program and Ostomy Subsidy Program, and the Special Needs Program. This combination of programs subsidized drug costs and dispensing fees for residents receiving social assistance, seniors who received Guaranteed Income Supplements from the federal government, patients with cystic fibrosis, and Food Bank clients.

Barriers to reform at the provincial level included a lack of consensus about what constitutes catastrophic care, and issues of equity in the delivery of catastrophic care. At the federal level, the historical exclusion of pharmaceuticals from the medicare bargain (hence no integrated governance or institutional system to promote a common approach to problem definition) and the reluctance of the federal government to assist the provinces in providing broader drug coverage to more people imposed significant barriers for drug reform. Being a small province with a small population, Newfoundland and Labrador did not have the opportunity to buy drugs in bulk, and therefore the lack of federal facilitation presented challenges.

In 1997, Newfoundland and Labrador agreed to participate in the Atlantic Drug Formulary, but this interjurisdictional cooperation did not extend to the bulk buying of drugs. The intention of the formulary was to encourage cooperation among the four Atlantic provinces. Among other things, this entailed sharing resources to review new drug therapies coming onto the market, but it did not mandate that each province adopt a common set of drug benefits. Decisions to implement the recommendations made by the Expert Advisory Committee of the formulary were dependent on the different fiscal circumstances of each of the four provinces. Generally, the creation of the formulary did not result in substantive changes for any of the Atlantic provinces.

The issue of prescription drug coverage appeared periodically on the Newfoundland and Labrador government agenda. The trigger in some cases was a report from federally appointed bodies such as the National Forum on Health, the Romanow Commission, and the Kirby Committee. Each in its own way encouraged the idea of Canada-wide coverage, whether for all prescription drugs or catastrophic costs only. In other cases, interest groups engaged the media to highlight inequities and inconsistencies in the current coverage programs (Sullivan 2005).

However, during the 1990–2003 period Ottawa did not act on any of these reports to the extent of proposing an extension of Canada-wide insurance to include drugs. Nor did Newfoundland and Labrador (or any other province for that matter) think that the existing federal financial contribution for medicare was sufficient to cover the costs of extending prescription drug coverage to all individuals in the province.

Fiscal challenges prevented the Newfoundland and Labrador government from making any headway on drug coverage issues, as the province struggled just to maintain the status quo for catastrophic coverage. The population was too small for the government to buy prescription drugs in bulk, collaboration through the Atlantic Drug Formulary produced no results, and assistance was not forthcoming from the federal level. While some groups were critical of current coverage programs, their efforts to reform drug coverage were unorganized and added little steam in the quest for reform.

ANALYSIS

Regionalization was the only one of the six policy cases in which the Government of Newfoundland and Labrador undertook reform. Plainly, the economic crisis and related severe fiscal difficulties were pivotal to putting this item on the government agenda since regionalizing held the possibility of efficiencies. Indeed, the advantages of such an initiative were being discussed at the time at meetings of provincial health ministers. The idea was by no means new to the province; in fact, the decision process was the culmination of many years of debate within Newfoundland and Labrador. The model created in the early 1990s was top-down with board members appointed by and accountable to the government. The decision to establish separate institutional and community boards was evidence that the final decisions were unique to the provincial circumstance. The decision to exclude physicians from the authority of the boards reflected the government's recognition that physicians would not readily accept this kind of oversight.

Several interacting factors propelled regionalization. Economic challenges were the primary driver of reform, but other factors also influenced the decision to proceed with regionalization beyond the pre-emptive desire to achieve cost savings. On the non-economic side of the regionalization coin, there were few reasons to oppose this proposal and little resistance from outside groups, physicians in particular. The concept of regionalization had garnered the support of the Newfoundland and Labrador Medical Association because it did not directly affect the status of physicians or their billing practices. Moreover, there was historical familiarity with the concept. The provincial government was able to tailor regionalization to suit the unique needs of the province and sell it to the public as a "home grown" solution.

As for the other five cases, no single factor can be isolated to explain why Newfoundland and Labrador was not able to achieve any reform. It could be argued that each of these cases, like regionalization, held the promise of economic efficiencies. However, in the case of alternative payment plans and for-profit delivery, the promise of such gains required short-term increases in spending. On the wait-times file, too, it would have been difficult to contemplate adding bureaucratic expenses to advance this issue when hospital budgets were being cut and staff laid off. As for the needs-based funding case, we noted that such a reform would disadvantage rural areas. The government may have concluded that the only political way of acting on this would have been to safeguard the potential "losers" and this, too, would have meant more spending. In sum, in a time of fiscal crisis it would have been difficult for the government to find additional money to fund reforms, whatever the fiscal dividends might be in the long term. Moreover, it is not hard to imagine Finance and Treasury Board ministers and officials expressing doubt that these dividends would ever appear.

In many cases, the top-down tradition of decision-making and resource allocation was another obstacle to reform. Needs-based funding would have meant allocating large sums of money annually by formula rather than political decision. Reform proposals for wait times and for compensating primary care physicians similarly held out the prospect of replacing political control of expenditures with more formulistic approaches. Implementing the proposed reforms would involve complex analysis (especially needs-based funding and wait times but also alternative payment plans), and the province had limited capacity to engage on these issues.

A recurring theme in each of the case studies is the relationship between economic challenges, geography, and history. With respect to geography, the sparsely distributed population and the divide between the "outports" and the "townies" created political and physical obstacles to reform. The balance between urban and rural Newfoundland was of particular concern in the needs-based funding case but arose as well in wait times. In both situations the losers would have included the parts of the province most devastated by the fisheries crisis.

Evidently, the political priorities of the province did not include health-care reform, at least not to the extent in other provinces. The Liberals formed a majority government in 1989 with a slightly smaller share of the popular vote than the Progressive Conservatives. They were re-elected with more of the popular vote and more seats in 1993, 1996, and 1999 than they had secured in 1989, suggesting that they were not out of touch with the people and priorities of the province. Indeed, in the Progressive Conservative party platform for the 2003 general election, which saw the Conservatives defeat the Liberals, there was scarcely a word about the issues discussed in this chapter. In a nutshell, it was not only the Liberal party that saw the political priorities of the province the way it did.

CONCLUSION

A theme of this volume is that crisis is often associated with reform. But whether health transformation occurs after a crisis depends on the nature of the discourse and the rise of new powerful ideas, interests, and institutions capable of challenging and defeating the status quo and putting a new action plan in place. Newfoundland and Labrador lacked the political resources, service-based economic/policy traditions, university-centred knowledge networks, and traditions of democracy to move forward on health-care reform. Technical-political decision-making was fragmented, insular, and competitive. All of this made it difficult to respond to any crisis.

The reform that did occur was not health-care focused. It is true that Newfoundland and Labrador had similar shortcomings in its health-care system as the rest of Canada. But these shortcomings were not perceived as big issues relative to the collapse of the fishery and the challenges of adjustment. The end of the fishery not only affected communities and individuals. It also threatened the broad balance in the province between some of the more remote communities and St. John's in particular. Like other smaller jurisdictions, the province lacked the range of talents to cope with complex changes in health care. Politics aligned with economics, as the most skilled individuals gravitated to the issue of highest priority.

Of the six case studies examined in this volume, the government undertook reform on only one issue: regionalization. Regionalization was the exception to the rule in part because it held out the promise of savings. The fiscal challenges imposed by the collapse of the fishery made cost savings imperative. The devolution of power to the regional areas allowed the government to legitimize the reconfiguration of services while achieving the much-needed cost savings. The province had decided to regionalize many of its non-health activities, and health care was caught up by this momentum.

In summary, Newfoundland and Labrador was an outlier. For a variety of reasons, the province was unable to achieve even the small degrees of reform that occurred in the other provinces. Certainly fiscal and economic challenges played a significant role in either limiting or facilitating (in the case of regionalization) reform. However, a fiscal crisis plays a different role in a province that is constantly struggling to keep its head above water. Instead of prompting further reform, the economic hardships in Newfoundland and Labrador effectively made health care a lower priority than it was in other provinces.

NOTES

1. For current population figures, see www.stats.gov.nl.ca/.
2. The matching grant formulas for both hospital insurance and medical care had included some degree of implicit equalization. That is, they covered a higher share of eligible expenses in relatively low-income provinces like Newfoundland and Labrador than in high-income provinces. When Established Programs Financing in 1977 and then the Canada Health and Social Transfer in 1995 replaced hospital and medical insurance, this advantage for the lower-income provinces was preserved.

CHAPTER 8

CANADIAN HEALTH-CARE REFORM: WHAT KIND? HOW MUCH? WHY?

HARVEY LAZAR, PIERRE-GERLIER FOREST, JOHN N. LAVIS, AND JOHN CHURCH

Each of the five provincial chapters tells a story about reform and is thus an end product in itself. But because these five provinces are broadly representative, accounting for three-quarters of Canada's population, the 30 case studies also provide the basis for a narrative about the whole of Canada. In this chapter we draw on the experiences from all five provinces to answer three questions. What kind of health-care reform occurred in respect of six health-care policy issues in the five provinces during the 1990–2003 period? How much reform occurred? What factors accounted for the answers to the first two questions?

The six policy issues were purposively selected as representative of the broader health policy reform challenges that Canadians faced during the 1990–2003 period. By selecting at least one issue from the governance, financial, delivery, and program content domains, we included the different aspects of decision-making faced within the health sector. The sample purposively included at least one issue from each of the three largest publicly funded expenditure categories: the hospital, physician, and pharmaceutical sectors. The selection also ranged from the overarching national macro-policy framework level (prescription drug coverage as a possible extension of the framework and whether for-profit delivery was compatible with the framework) to meso-policy issues that combined efficient delivery with equity of access. Moreover, although all of the cases were large and important issues in their own right, some were also linked to even broader reform challenges. For example, the case study on alternative payment plans was also a window into the broader issue of primary care reform. Thus, in analyzing the nature and extent of reform for these broadly representative six issues, we shed light on the nature and extent of health-care policy reform more generally.

That said, the focus here is on *policy* reform in the health-care sector. Reform also occurs through the creative efforts of health-care profession- als and health-systems managers largely, if not entirely, independently of government. That kind of reform is not the focus of this book. The second point is that reform is not necessarily a good thing. Where a health system is satisfying well its intended purposes, the absence of reform may be viewed as much welcome "stability." Where a health system is not meet- ing its intended purposes, however, the same lack of reform may be seen as "rigidity." The desirability of more or less reform is thus dependent on the context in which it is being considered.

What Kind and How Much Reform Occurred?

In order to determine what kind and how much policy reform occurred, we needed a frame of reference. To answer these first two questions, we looked for an appropriate standard against which we could test the kind of reform that had been experienced and measure its magnitude. It was understood that there was no standard that everyone would consider appropriate. But there was one that the research team thought that many readers would consider fair and transparent. We also believed that readers who had reservations about the choice would be able to "translate" our empirical results into whatever alternative standard they thought more reasonable. The standard selected was the consensus of the reforms pro- posed in the reports of the various commissions, task forces, and advisory bodies appointed by provincial and federal governments from the late 1980s until 2003 (sometimes referred to as "grey literature"). This meant we would compare the reforms that took place with the policy reform ideas that had been set out in well-researched, major reports of that era.

Annex 1 provides an analysis of the reports based on studies under- taken by Kevin O'Fee (2002a, 2002b). The annex spells out how the grey literature consensus was determined for each of the six issues. O'Fee concentrated on systemwide reports. The provincial reports came in two waves. The first emerged in the late 1980s and early 1990s amid economic recession and fiscal restraint. These reports emphasized the transfer of decision-making and service delivery to the regional level. The overriding theme was that such devolution was the key to improving health service delivery and reducing unit costs (O'Fee 2002a, 3).This led to proposals for "regionalization, deinstitutionalization, and hospital restructuring" (ibid.). Objectives like comprehensiveness, accountability, responsive- ness, improved quality, and system integration were viewed as long term and as being more attainable in the aftermath and as a consequence of regionalization and rationalization.

The second wave was published in the late 1990s and early 2000s, by which time fiscal pressures had eased somewhat. Second-wave reports had similarities in their emphasis on revisions to governance structures, financial arrangements, a variety of delivery-related issues (such as advancing primary health-care reform, wait-list management, and the role of the private for-profit sector), health management information systems (which had implications for both governance and delivery), and coverage (both expanding and restricting). The reports stressed common themes: long-term sustainability, accountability and transparency, access and quality. With relative consistency, primary care reform was seen as the fundamental building block for reforming the entire health-care system. This was closely followed by an expressed desire to clarify lines of responsibility within the governance of the health system and to make relationships among providers, health authorities, and governments more precise and, in many cases, more contractual in nature (O'Fee 2002a).

With regard to the kinds of reform, we make two distinctions. One is between reforms that were directionally consistent with the grey literature consensus and those that went in a markedly different direction. The former are referred to as *consensus reforms* (or just plain "reforms") and the latter as *counter-consensus reforms*.

The consensus reforms generally (not always) supported strengthening the macro-policy framework associated with the principles of the *Canada Health Act* and related provincial health insurance statutes. To the extent that the grey literature expressed itself on publicly administered insurance, it was to favour its expansion. With respect to delivery, the consensus favoured strengthening existing delivery agents (such as the system of primary care) rather than replacing them. Thus, the consensus position did not involve a greater role for markets either through private for-profit insurers competing with publicly administered insurance or through private for-profit providers competing with private not-for-profit providers. Counter-consensus reforms generally aimed at increasing the role of private insurance and private for-profit delivery.

As our work proceeded, a second way of distinguishing among kinds of reform emerged, as will be described in chapter 9. This distinction is on the proximity of the public to a reform. In general, the public interacts with the health-care system in two ways: people pay for services, and they receive services. As receivers of services, members of the public experience reforms directly. As payers of taxes, insurance premiums, and out-of-pocket fees, citizens also engage directly with the health system. In the main, these direct interactions correspond with the "delivery arrangements" and "program content" domains.

There are also many aspects of the health-care system that do not touch the public directly but that have implications for services received and costs. These aspects of health care involve the "governance" and "financial" domains. Note that the financial domain here refers to the financial arrangements of the system like how revenue is raised to pay for programs and services, how hospitals are funded, and how health providers are remunerated.[1] Under these distinctions, regionalization is part of the governance (or governance arrangements) domain, needs-based funding and alternative payment plans for primary care physicians are part of the financial (or financial arrangements) domain, wait times and for-profit delivery are considered as part of the delivery (or delivery arrangements) domain, and drug reform is treated as part of the program content domain. The significance of these distinctions will become clear in the discussion that follows.

As for how the amount of reform is "measured," if all of the elements in the grey literature were met for a particular issue, this is referred to as "comprehensive" reform. Other degrees of reform are described as "significant," "moderate," "limited," or "none" depending on how many and which of the elements in the grey literature benchmark were translated into policy by a province. Each of these degrees of reform is defined in annex 1 for each of the six issues. These same terms are also defined and applied for counter-consensus reform issues.

This method of assessing the extent of reform is sensitive to the comprehensive standard, not the starting point. Thus, hypothetically, a province that began the 1990s performing at close to the comprehensive definition for a particular policy issue and then moved to that standard during the 1990–2003 period would be assessed as having achieved comprehensive reform even though the amount of incremental reform was not large. A second province that began well below the comprehensive definition in 1990 and moved very substantially over the decade but not all the way to the benchmark would be assessed as having achieved less than comprehensive reform despite having made a larger policy change.

It should also be noted that this methodology does not entail taking a snapshot of the policy stance of the five provincial governments for the six policy issues in 2003. It is therefore logically possible for additional reform to have occurred or for the amount of reform to have been reduced between the time a policy reform decision was assessed and 2003. In fact, in a couple of cases there was more than one reform in an issue between 1990 and 2003. Adjusting the methodology to take these changes into account would have added to the complexity of our approach without likely altering the broad findings.

With regard to the benchmarks, the only issue that called for a publicly visible "big bang" was the idea of extending prescription drug coverage to all Canadians (which, framed in this more expansive way, can also be considered a change to existing financial arrangements, not just a change in which drugs are covered). For all other issues, the benchmark was aimed at modifying the internal workings of provincial health systems (e.g., altering incentives for physicians, changing how regions and hospitals were funded, or creating a more systematic approach to dealing with long wait times). Some of these issues did not engage the general public but were of vital interest to those working inside the system. If carried out to the comprehensive level, these reforms would certainly have been seen as massive by the insiders affected.

Overall, provincial governments focused on trying to construct more effective and efficient health systems within the prevailing health-care model, rather than moving their systems toward a new model. But this broad stance was not adopted by all. There were also advocates of more for-profit delivery with a mixture of motives. Some advocates doubt-less wanted to transform the current system into one in which for-profit delivery would play a major role. Others believed that some private for-profit delivery would enhance competition and in so doing improve the efficiency of what would remain a mainly not-for-profit system. There were still others who thought that a more accommodating regulatory en-vironment would provide the delivery system with access to new financial resources and thereby relieve some of the fiscal pressure on government. In any case, the consensus of the grey literature was not supportive of more for-profit delivery, which is why policy innovations in this direction are described here as counter-consensus reforms (annex 1).

Table 8.1 summarizes our findings on the nature and degree of reform. It shows that provincial reforms in 18 of the 30 cases were directionally similar to the grey literature consensus. Only four involved counter-consensus reforms. In the other eight cases, there was no reform. If Newfoundland and Labrador is excluded since there was no reform in five of the cases in that province, 17 of the remaining 24 cases involved reforms that were directionally similar to the grey literature proposals, four were counter-consensus, and three involved no reform.

Several broad observations can be made about the table. First, over the period studied, in relation to the comprehensive reforms proposed in the commission and task force reports, relatively little reform occurred in the five provinces taken as a whole. Sixteen of the 30 cases were assessed as "limited," "none," or "counter-consensus limited." Only one case was as-sessed as comprehensive, and one at the border between comprehensive and significant. *Meagre* is the adjective used here to describe this finding.

The similarities and differences among provinces are considered in chapter 9. Here a few province-specific points stand out. There was more reform in Saskatchewan than in other provinces, with Alberta not far be-hind. In contrast, Newfoundland and Labrador was an outlier. Not only was there less reform in that province but also less interest in reforming health care owing to higher political and policy priorities. Quebec com-missioned many reports on reform issues, but the actual amount of policy action was assessed as "limited" or less in five of the six cases. But Quebec prescription drug reform was the largest reform among the 30 cases.[2] Ontario followed a step-by-step incremental approach with the word "moderate" perhaps best describing the results in that province.

TABLE 8.1
Nature and Extent of Provincial Policy Reform Decisions Relative to Grey Literature Standards, 1990–2003

Province	Issue					
	Regionalization	Needs-Based Funding	Alternative Payment Plans	For-Profit Delivery	Wait-List Management	Prescription Drug Coverage
Alberta	Significant	Significant	Moderate	Counter-consensus moderate	Limited	Limited
Saskatchewan	Significant	Significant	Limited	Significant	Significant/ comprehensive	Counter-consensus limited
Ontario	None	None	Moderate	Counter-consensus moderate	Moderate	Moderate
Quebec	Counter-consensus limited*	Limited	Limited	None	Limited	Comprehensive
Newfoundland and Labrador	Moderate	None	None	None	None	None

Note: *Quebec had a substantially regionalized system at the beginning of our assessment period. The regional power grew during the 1990s as authority was shifted from both the ministry and local institutions to the regions. By the early 2000s, much of the power that had been devolved from Quebec City to the regions had been reclaimed by the centre and thus the position of the regional level relative to the centre was in decline.

EXPLAINING THE OUTCOMES: WHAT ACCOUNTS FOR MEAGRE REFORM?

Recapitulating Theoretical Considerations

What accounts for the conclusion above that the reform performance was meagre? There is no single theory in the health policy, public administration, or political science literature that captures the complexity of governmental decision-making. Malcolm Taylor, for example, in his classic analysis of the seven decisions that created Canada's health-care system, discusses eight different theories and the extent and limits of their explanatory power (2009, 492-98). As noted in chapter 2, we anchored a significant part of our approach in the agenda-setting model developed by John Kingdon (2003) and made heavy use as well of an approach that distinguishes among ideas, interests, and institutions and factors exogenous to the health system.

The Kingdon model is non-linear, meaning that it does not contemplate the idea that decisions move logically forward from one stage to another in a straight-line progression to a final decision. Kingdon finds the process "messy." Fundamental to his approach is that "problems," "policy," and "politics" are separate streams of activity populated by different people or organizations. Most of the time, they flow in parallel. But periodically an event occurs that causes either the problem stream or the politics stream, or both, to merge with the policy stream. These events create what Kingdon calls a "policy window" in which there is an opportunity to couple a problem and/or politics with a policy solution. These windows do not stay open for long, but they are the moments to make reform happen.

The study team began, for the interview part of the research, with separate sets of questions for the governmental agenda phase (how and why an issue began to attract the attention of government), the decision agenda phase (why a government decided it had to make a decision, including a decision not to do anything), and policy choice.

Much of our focus was on the policy choice phase of the decision process. Our methodology was built on the work of many political scientists. As noted in chapter 2, we use the terms *independent variable*, *variable* (unless explicitly modified by the word "dependent"), *factor*, and *influence* interchangeably. The independent variables are generally linked to one of four categories of variables: institutions (such as the government structures or "rules of the game" within which decisions were taken, policy legacies, and policy networks); interests (winners and losers); ideas (such as values and knowledge); and factors external to the health sector. This model is often referred to as the 3I model for ideas, interests, and institutions, or 3I plus E (for exogenous factors) model.

There was no presupposition, however, that all of the important explanations for what governments decided would necessarily be encompassed by these four categories of variables. Nor was it assumed that all of the variables would play similar roles in shaping outcomes. In short, these very broad clusters of variables were a starting point but not intended to prejudge actual observation.

Indeed, as the research team compiled and then analyzed and assessed the findings in relation to our research questions (particularly the question "What factors accounted for reform?"), we made important adjustments. Based on this learning, some of the four categories were decomposed into eight categories: insider interests, values, knowledge, institutions, fiscal crisis or near fiscal crisis (hereafter fiscal crisis), public opinion / civil society, media, and technological change.

We initially coded the influence of governments as "elected government officials," a subcategory of insider interests. But there were certain conditions under which we thought such coding would be misleading. Specifically, newly formed first-time governments under certain circumstances did not behave as insiders. When these conditions occurred, they were coded to a ninth category, "change in government/leader" (explained more fully below).

Eight of the nine categories were in turn divided on the basis of whether they included factors that were endogenous or exogenous to the decision process. Technological change turned out to be a small influence in relation to our 30 cases and is not considered further in this chapter. Its role is reflected in chapter 9 where the analysis is more disaggregated than it is here.

Distinguishing between Endogenous and Exogenous Factors

In a well-functioning democracy, authoritative decision-makers are those with the legal power to decide issues that are constitutionally within the realm of their authority. The decision-makers can be cabinet members, ministers, or public servants delegated to decide by a minister or by statute. In rare cases the decision-maker may be the legislature. It is not only their legal authority but the act of deciding that makes these persons or bodies authoritative. It is normal to think of those vested with such authority as insiders—endogenous to the decision process. Their advisors, whether from the public service or otherwise, and those with relatively easy access to deciders or advisors, are treated as endogenous as well.

Yet we concluded that for purposes of understanding health reform, such an approach concealed more than it conveyed. As we examined the results of our research, we were struck by the fact that most large reforms (those assessed as comprehensive or significant) were undertaken by newly formed, first-time governments that had committed to reform prior to taking to taking office. The commitments were made either during an election campaign or during a leadership contest within the governing party. In either case, the broad reform commitments were taken prior to forming the government and acted on swiftly—in the first half of that first mandate—upon taking office. In a sense these new governments were the new brooms to "sweep out the old ways" and bring in a different course of action. Accordingly, we chose to distinguish between governments that met these criteria and all other governments. The former category was defined as "change in government, or leader of a governing party, that committed to reform during the election campaign or leadership contest that first brought the newly formed government to power, and that acted expeditiously on its commitments after assuming office." We use the shorthand "change in government/leader" below. It is an exogenous factor.

Only one of the nine categories was exclusively endogenous: insider interests. Four were wholly exogenous: change in government/leader, fiscal crisis, public opinion/civil society, and media. The four remaining categories—values, knowledge, technological change, and institutions—included factors that were both endogenous and exogenous. While in some cases the distinction between endogenous and exogenous variables was self-evident, in others it was less so. We have already explained the reason for distinguishing newly formed governments that met certain criteria from other governments. The reasoning that led to the distinctions in three other less-evident situations is set out below.

First, the Canadian people were viewed as outsiders to the decision process. It is true they are insiders to the health system as patients (especially) and also as payers (through taxes, premiums, and out-of-pocket expenses). But paying for or receiving health services does not give the public insider access to the policy-making process. As will be seen below, the Canadian public has had a considerable influence on reform but as an outsider to the decision process, an exogenous factor.

Second, groups representing health-care providers were viewed as endogenous. Some of these provider groups, particularly medical associations, had considerable influence on policy outcomes. Other insiders, such as nurses and other unionized health workers, had little direct influence on policy despite their access to decision makers or advisors. These relatively weak provider groups often joined with outsider groups like anti-poverty organizations and bodies representing seniors to create "health coalitions." Despite having insiders in their ranks, these coalitions were treated as exogenous.

Finally, backbenchers on the governing side of the legislature were treated as endogenous because they had access to decision makers via the party caucus. Opposition members of the legislature were treated as exogenous.

Weighting of Factors and Four Ways in which Factors Influenced Reform

The factors that influenced reform differed in the magnitude of their impact. It was simply not practicable to assign a precise weight to each factor. It would have been misleading, however, to give all the same weight. What we settled on was a simple division between "major" factors and all others.

All factors, major and otherwise, were also coded on the basis of the role they played relative to the grey literature benchmark consensus: factors that facilitated consensus reform (pro-reform), hindered consensus reform (anti-reform), mediated between pro- and anti-reform variables (referred to as "middle territory" below for the sake of simplicity), or facilitated counter-consensus reform.[3] As mentioned in chapter 2, anti-reform influences and those that favoured counter-consensus reform both indicate opposition to reforms proposed in the grey literature. However, anti-reform suggests attachment to the status quo whereas counter-consensus reform indicates opposition to the status quo and movement in a different direction than that proposed in the grey literature consensus.

RESEARCH RESULTS

Annex 2 shows, on a province-by-province and case-by-case basis, the number of times different independent variables were identified as having had explanatory power in relation to the outcomes in the 30 case studies. In total, 313 influences were observed, of which 105 were analyzed as "major" influences. Table 8.2 shows the number of times each of the categories was found to be a major factor in the 30 cases. It is the first of several tables that, when considered together, begin to answer the question about what accounted for reform.

The reliability of the data in the tables that follow is based on two factors: the common approach to data collection and analysis used in the 30 case studies, and the consistent approach to weighting independent variables across the 30 studies. To help ensure this consistency, this chapter's authors reviewed the 30 cases and discussed the findings of each with the individual case study authors in an iterative process. We assigned roughly similar weights to influences of roughly similar magnitude across the 30 studies and also accounted for differences in magnitude of influence.

Notwithstanding all of the above, we recognize that accounting for government decision-making is as much art as it is science. The numbers in all the tables should therefore be viewed as conveying relative influence in a qualitative sense, not in a quantitatively precise sense.

With all of this methodological explanation, we proceed to a discussion of each of the categories and the role they played in determining outcomes.

TABLE 8.2
Number of Times Categories of Independent Variables Were Major Influences on Reform Decisions in 30 Cases

Independent Variable Category	Number of Major Influences
Exogenous	
Change in government/ leader	13
Fiscal crisis	13
Public opinion and civil society	9
Media	4
Exogenous and endogenous	
Values	16
Knowledge	12
Institutions	11
Endogenous	
Insider interests	27
Total	105

Analysis of the Nine Categories

1. Change in Government/Leader

The reasoning underlying the influence of the "change in government/ leader" category is straightforward. Substantial policy reforms invariably create losers as well as winners. Losers may have longer memories than winners, especially if the winners consider the reform their just desserts whereas the losers feel the outcome is fundamentally unfair. Undertaking substantial policy reforms thus potentially involves political risks. Governments are most likely to undertake such reforms when risks can be best "managed." An example of managed risk may be found in the following scenario: an opposition party commits to certain reforms during an election campaign and is elected to office with a majority; the premier appoints a policy champion and presses forward swiftly while the electoral mandate is still fresh. If the government is able to take action—introduce legislation, promulgate regulations, take administrative action, or make a policy statement that is generally considered binding (depending on the nature of the commitment)—in the first half of its mandate, this may leave time for the wounds of the losers to heal. A similar example may arise after a struggle for power within a governing party, as the newly elected leader seeks to put his or her stamp on the government by doing something substantially different.

When a new government assumes power, it inherits the laws, policies, and administrative practices that previous governments have helped to create. The new government has the opportunity to change things. If it does not act swiftly, it becomes a part of the existing status quo. But there is sometimes a window after it has first been elected in which it may behave as an outsider trying to fix the problems its predecessors have left behind.

The "change in government/leader" category was made up of two variables. One was the public commitment to reform that was made prior to or during the election or leadership contest. The commitment must be in the platform of the party or leadership contestant. The second variable was evidence that the election/leadership commitment retained priority with the newly formed government post-election. The most concrete evidence of this commitment was a sense of urgency leading to rapid policy action once the government gained office. The test for urgency was that the government must take action within the first half of the new mandate. An opposition political party or contestant for party leadership that committed to a big reform and, once in office, attempted reform swiftly but only on a small fraction of what had been promised was not the new sweeping out the old. We found that the appointment of a policy champion both created and reflected a sense of urgency. In that case, the prospects of substantial reform were enhanced. The policy champion could be the health minister or a non-elected person working out of the office of the premier or health minister. The premier could effectively appoint himself (e.g., Premier Klein on the issue of for-profit delivery). However done, the policy champion's job was to navigate the decision process quickly and sure-footedly. Not all newly formed first-time governments that followed this path achieved as much reform as they had planned, but in the 30 cases we studied it was part of the "formula" that produced the most reform.

Table 8.3 shows both the phase and the direction of reform for the 13 major variables attributed to this category. Eleven of these variables were directionally supportive of reform and two of counter-consensus reform. All 13 had their impact at the governmental agenda/decision phases, not on policy choice. The 11 pro-reform factors included four related to regionalization and four to needs-based funding—all eight in the early 1990s in Saskatchewan and Alberta (Romanow and Klein governments). The APP case in Saskatchewan also involved a major pro-reform commitment. The other two pro-reform factors related to the Parti Québécois's comprehensive prescription drug reform in the mid-1990s. The counter-consensus reform factors related to regionalization in Quebec in 2003 (Charest government). Note that despite major commitments, and quick action to meet reform commitments, three of the 13 major variables did not produce large reforms or produced counter-consensus reforms (APP in Saskatchewan and regionalization in Quebec).

TABLE 8.3
Distribution of Major "Change in Government/Leader" Independent Variables on Reform Decisions in 30 Cases

Phase	Direction				
	Pro-Reform	Middle Territory	Anti-Reform	Counter-Consensus Reform	Total
Governmental/ decision agenda	11	0	0	2	13
Policy choice	0	0	0	0	0

Six points of interest arose from our analysis of the data. First, the effect of these political commitments was reflected at the agenda-setting phase of the decision process. These commitments were broad enough to leave considerable scope for alternative policy designs.

Second, five of the seven large (i.e., comprehensive or significant) reform decisions were acted on in the first half of the first term of a newly formed government that had committed to such reforms in the election or leadership contest that brought it to power. The reforms involved three governments: the NDP government led by Romanow, first elected to power in Saskatchewan in 1991; the Klein Progressive Conservatives in Alberta, which won their own mandate in 1993; and the Parti Québécois (PQ) government elected in 1994 under Jacques Parizeau but with Lucien Bouchard at the helm when the reform was introduced. The Romanow and Klein governments both made significant reforms on regionalization and needs-based funding within the first half of their first term, and the PQ's comprehensive reform of prescription drugs was also achieved within the same time frame. The three political parties in question had made broad commitments for such reforms in the elections that brought them to power. The association between this variable and large reform is strong.

Next, these three governments accomplished much more reform in the first half of their first term than in the rest of their remaining years in office. And they were not one-term governments. The Romanow-led NDP won two more elections (1995 and 1999), and the NDP won a fourth term in 2003 under a new leader after Romanow retired. The Klein-led Progressive Conservatives won four general elections in succession. The PQ, first elected under Jacques Parizeau in 1994, was re-elected four years later under the leadership of Lucien Bouchard.

Fourth is that most newly formed, first-time governments did not make health-care reform commitments on a scale that would qualify as comprehensive or significant. At the provincial level, there were six changes of governing party between 1989 and the end of the third quarter of 2003. In addition, excluding interim caretaker premiers, seven changes of leadership occurred within governing parties.[4] Only four of these 13 newly formed governments committed to large reforms. They were the three governments noted above (Romanow 1991, Klein 1992–1993, and Parizeau-Bouchard 1994) and the Quebec Liberal government led by Jean Charest that took office in 2003.

Fifth, not all large commitments were met. For example, the Romanow government did not succeed in reforming remuneration for primary care physicians to the extent that it had planned. The combination of resistance from the Saskatchewan Medical Association and the loss of reform momentum proved hard to overcome. The loss of momentum was in itself linked to the amount of reform that had occurred early in Romanow's first mandate. Each reform—the reduction in drug benefits, regionalization, hospital closures and conversions, and changes to hospital funding—had a rationale that fitted with the NDP's "wellness" objective or its fiscal imperative. Taken together, however, these measures were apparently as much change as the public could handle at one time, including NDP members and supporters. As for the Klein government, its reform objectives were slowed after its initial burst of policy innovation. This resistance ranged from the Alberta Medical Association's objections to the large cuts in physician pay to the broader public resistance to for-profit delivery of publicly funded services. The improvement in fiscal conditions (discussed below) also took some of the energy out of reform. A third example is the Quebec Liberal Party's undertaking to eliminate regional boards during the 2003 general election campaign. Premier Charest appointed Dr. Philippe Couillard as minister of health and social services and allowed him much latitude both as minister and policy champion. Couillard was committed to doing away with regional boards. Although the government moved swiftly, it also encountered many layers of opposition, including from insider experts and regional voices. When the political process had run its course, the regional level retained a role, albeit with a different name, "regional agencies," and a reduced mandate.

Finally, it is also noteworthy that newly formed governments that did not make strong election commitments did not achieve large reforms. This applied to the Rae and Harris governments in Ontario and the several Liberal governments in Newfoundland and Labrador.

The category of change in government/leader helped open windows of reform. But it was rarely alone. More often than not it did do so when accompanied by a second exogenous factor.

2. Fiscal Crisis

A second major influence was fiscal crisis (more fully crisis or near-crisis fiscal conditions), which was present for close to half of the period under study.

During the 1970s and 1980s, provincial spending on health services grew rapidly. The 1980s were also marked by deteriorating provincial government finances with health-care costs contributing generously to that deterioration. When recession set in again at the beginning of the 1990s, the result was to load an additional fiscal burden onto a starting base that was already shaky. High unemployment was the first concern of the general public in the early 1990s, and the federal Liberals made jobs a centrepiece of their 1993 election platform. But among elites there was a broad consensus that the fiscal situation was the greater priority (Ekos Research Associates 1994, exhibit 3.1). Government budgets had to be balanced and government debt reduced to take the pressure off of monetary policy. If government tightened fiscal policy through spending cuts, the Bank of Canada would be able to relax monetary policy. Such a change in the macroeconomic policy mix was hypothesized as the surest approach to rekindling growth, eventually leading to jobs and a virtuous cycle (Economic Council of Canada 1988, 22-25).

At the federal level, this in fact turned out to be how events played out. The restrictive 1995 federal budget—including its very large reduction in cash transfers to the provinces, much of which was notionally intended for provincial health systems—was a turning point for Ottawa. Within a few years, federal finances improved greatly.

The fiscal challenge was severe for most provinces. In 1991, the newly elected Romanow government in Saskatchewan was warned by its financial advisors that unless it moved swiftly to improve provincial government finances, it would have trouble selling new Saskatchewan debt instruments as old ones matured. Among other things, this led the government to reduce health spending. Part of the tightening was accomplished through hospital closures and reductions in drug benefits. Since hospital closures generated understandable criticism, including from the government's own supporters and militants, needs-based funding was one way of deflecting criticism. In a period of tough fiscal times, it made explicit that resources would be directed to where they were most needed. Without crisis, the Saskatchewan government probably would have created regional health authorities, but at a slower pace than it did.

In Alberta, a large drop in oil and gas prices in the late 1980s and early 1990s resulted in a downward spiral into a governmental fiscal deficit. The deficit and related accumulation of debt was unacceptable to the government with its conservative approach to public finances. The government incentive to act swiftly and reverse the trend was reinforced by a warning from the right-of-centre populist Reform Party. The Reform Party had successfully elected Alberta MPs at the federal level and threatened to run provincially if the Progressive Conservative government did not tackle the deficit as a first priority.

In Newfoundland and Labrador in 1989, Clyde Wells inherited a fiscal situation that was as precarious as Saskatchewan's. The decline in the cod fishery followed by its closure added a major third dimension to the already chronically high provincial unemployment rate and the cyclical unemployment associated with the Canada-wide recession. Striking hospital support workers and striking nurses were legislated back to work in 1990 and 1999, respectively. Public sector wages were frozen for several years. There was no room for health-care initiatives except those that were thought likely to save money.

Harsh fiscal conditions resulted in reductions in provincial wage and salary budgets in Ontario during the period of NDP government (1990–1995). So-called Rae days (forced additional days of unpaid leave for public servants) is a reminder of the mood of the time and the government's clash with public sector unions. Quebec's fiscal situation was no better than Ontario's. Physicians' incomes were tightly controlled. When the PQ was elected in 1994, it put the government on a deficit elimination track. The decision to opt for a mixed public/private financing solution to the prescription drug case was a result of the deficit targets.

By the beginning of the 1990s, provincial governments had come to accept that it was not realistic to expect a reduction in demand for publicly insured provincial health services. The only way, therefore, to slow significantly the rate of increase in health spending was to cut back on the supply side, which was seen by some to have grown excessively in the 1970s and 1980s (Taylor 2009, 474-78). In provincial politics, this was reflected in the decision of almost all provincial governments to more or less freeze per capita health-care spending in constant dollars from 1992 to 1996 (described by CIHI as a period of "retrenchment and disinvestment" [2012, 1]). Alberta was the outlier as it went much further than other provinces in cutting back (CIHI 2012, Table A.3.2.2).

Although the details of the response differed from one province to another, a common reaction was the closing of some hospitals, the merging of others, and the imposition of expenditure caps on physician compensation (Barer, Lomas, and Sanmartin 1996, 219-24). Intake into medical schools was reduced. Some nurses were laid off, and others had their status converted from permanent (i.e., with fixed employment terms) to casual (i.e., without fixed employment terms). Supply was thus reduced even though there was no reduction in demand. Indeed, by the time Ottawa announced its austerity budget in 1995 and cut back sharply on its cash transfers to the provinces beginning in fiscal year 1996/97, the provincial governments were already four to five years into their freeze. Provincial governments had by then intervened so aggressively on the supply side of health services that they had to absorb the impact of the federal reductions outside the health expenditure "envelope." The federal cuts precipitated a prolonged period of tense and dysfunctional federal-provincial relations, much of it acted out in public.

By the late 1990s, the public finances of federal and provincial governments had improved significantly. But the stress on intergovernmental relations did not disappear as quickly. These tensions cast a shadow over Canadian politics until the 2004 First Ministers' Health Accord, which served effectively as the "peace treaty" that brought that episode to a close (First Ministers' Meeting 2004).

From the viewpoint of health system reform, the fiscal crisis had two quite different kinds of effects in relation to the six issues we studied. On the one hand, it served as a counterweight to expanding the range of publicly insured services. In Newfoundland and Labrador, fiscal crisis made the expansion of prescription drug coverage a non-starter. The cuts to prescription drug benefits in Saskatchewan were motivated entirely by fiscal crises. These two cases are reflected in the governmental/decision agenda row in the upper half of Table 8.4 in the "anti-reform" and "counter-consensus reform" columns, respectively.

Fiscal crisis did not prevent Quebec and Ontario from expanding their drug coverage, but it did shape the specific policy choices made by the governments of these provinces. The large role retained for private insurers in Quebec's prescription drug reform was driven heavily by the government's commitment to a balanced budget. Ontario's Trillium Drug Program was targeted at persons in households with high prescription drug costs relative to net household income through an income-related sliding-scale deductible. These two cases are shown in the policy choice row in the upper half of Table 8.4. They are in the "middle territory" column to reflect the fact that the provinces were balancing pro-reform and anti-reform factors.

TABLE 8.4
Distribution of Fiscal Crisis Independent Variables on Reform Decisions in 30 Cases

Nature	Phase	Direction				
		Pro-Reform	Middle Territory	Anti-Reform	Counter-Consensus Reform	Total
Counterweight to program expansion	Governmental/decision agenda	0	0	1	1	2
	Policy choice	0	2	0	0	2
	Both	0	2	1	1	4
Efficiency-enhancing	Governmental/decision agenda	7	0	0	2	9
	Policy choice	0	0	0	0	0
	Both	7	0	0	2	9

The bottom half of Table 8.4 involves nine cases. Seven are pro-reform and relate to regionalization, needs-based funding, and alternative payment plans that were experienced to varying degrees in Alberta, Saskatchewan, and Newfoundland and Labrador. The other two cases relate to for-profit delivery. They are coded as counter-consensus because they pointed toward a more market-oriented strategy for achieving efficiencies.

3. Public Opinion and Civil Society

Public opinion was determined through research studies (Maxwell et al. 2002; Mendelsohn 2002; Soroka 2007) and the myriad of public opinion polls available for the study period. The influence of civil society groups was determined by analyzing news coverage and information on websites. It should be noted that this category also includes policy entrepreneurs advising government on a single issue whether at the request of government or self-motivated.[5] (It does not include individuals who were appointees of provider groups; for example, a physician advising government on behalf of a medical association is viewed as representing physician interests.)

During the study period, a majority of Canadians strongly favoured maintaining medicare and fixing it where necessary (Mendelsohn 2002, 1-3). The views held by civil society groups generally coincided with the majority of Canadians as reflected in the public opinion data. At the broadest level, key civil society groups served as a voice for preserving medicare and expanding its scope. In fact, civil society groups aimed to protect and reinforce the dominant values of the period—the values associated with medicare.

Civil society groups can be divided into those with a wide lens (e.g., Council of Canadians), those with a health lens (e.g., Canadian Health Coalition), and groups that advocated for people with specific diseases. The latter were players in the Quebec and Ontario prescription drug cases.

The Council of Canadians has a wide mandate that reflects the views of the political left. Its website summarizes highlights from earlier years and reflects its interests. In 1995, for example, the council gave Prime Minister Chrétien a failing grade on social policy "for the Canada Health and Social Transfer cuts of $7 billion that put medicare, post-secondary education and vital social services at risk" (Council of Canadians 2011). In 2002, the website highlighted the council's message to the Romanow Commission "that health care must be properly funded, that it should be expanded to include pharmacare and homecare, and that it must be protected from international trade agreements" (ibid). That year the council held public events in 15 cities across Canada either before or at the same time as the commission's hearings. It also held events outside the annual meetings of the Canadian Medical Association when the CMA appeared to be endorsing more for-profit delivery in electing presidents who were strongly identified with that position.

The Canadian Health Coalition is "a public advocacy organization dedicated to the preservation and improvement of Medicare" (Canadian Health Coalition 2012a). Its membership comprises "national organizations representing nurses, health care workers, seniors, churches, anti-poverty groups, women, students and trade unions, as well as affiliated coalitions in nine provinces and one territory" (ibid.). It views health care from the perspective of the political left and centre-left. The coalition is interested in a broad range of health issues. Its website in 2012 highlighted nine issues, including the First Ministers' 2004 Health Accord, pharmacare, enforcement of the *Canada Health Act*, health-care financing, wait times, and continuing care. Given the substantial role of health unions in its makeup, it not surprisingly took a stand against a larger role for private for-profit delivery arguing that privatization of health services was a "guarantee" that Canadians would "pay more get less" (Canadian Health Coalition 2012b). During our assessment period, the coalition maintained ties with academic researchers whose views often overlapped its views. These connections helped the coalition to generate lucid criticisms of policy changes or proposed changes that did not align with its positions (Canadian Health Coalition 2012c).[6]

While the national efforts of both the Council of Canadians and the Canadian Health Coalition were impressive, it is doubtful that their efforts had a substantial impact on the federal government regarding such issues as pharmacare or home care. The federal Liberals came to power in 1993 with a commitment to enforce the *Canada Health Act*, which they and other critics claimed the Progressive Conservative government had not done. Whatever influence civil society groups may have had on the more forceful stance of the Liberals was probably marginal and short-lived. During the Chrétien years, they would have been seen as political opponents, groups that chose to "stay out of the tent and criticize rather than enter and compromise."[7]

The story is more complex when we hone in on the impact of this category of variables on the cases. On the one hand, we found little linkage between public opinion and three reform issues—regionalization, needs-based funding, and alternative payment plans.[8] This is because much of the decision-making on those issues was carried out without public knowledge or was not particularly visible to the public. Chapter 9 elaborates on this lack of transparency.

In contrast, in the 15 case studies that involved issues of delivery and program content, there was more transparency, and public opinion and civil society groups were more involved. Specifically, six of the seven pro-reform observations in the upper half of Table 8.5 were associated with the delivery domain. Public opinion played a major role in putting wait times on the governmental agenda in Saskatchewan and Alberta. The Friends of Medicare in Alberta and the Ontario Health Coalition could not prevent the Klein and Harris governments from placing for-profit delivery on the agendas of their respective governments. But they slowed the decision process. It took the Klein government seven years to implement reform. He was forced to water down his initial position significantly as a result of the local pressures brought to bear by the Alberta Friends of Medicare. In Ontario, it took eight years for the Progressive Conservative Party to achieve reform, by which time Ernie Eves had replaced Harris as party leader and premier. AIDS Action Now, an advocacy group in Ontario, was instrumental in putting drug reform on the governmental agenda and in persuading Premier Rae that his government had to make a decision. Policy entrepreneurs (included within the public opinion/civil society category) were important in the policy choice in two cases: the Ontario Cardiac Care Network and the Saskatchewan Surgical Care Network.

Seven of the nine major independent variables under the public opinion and civil society category supported reform (see Table 8.5). This was not a surprise. Rather it was a reflection of our selection of issues and method of analysis. Five of the six reform issues were associated with ways of improving or expanding the existing model for hospital and medical services, or improving the context in which the model operated. The sixth issue was for-profit delivery. Since the grey literature was against for-profit delivery, opposition to it is interpreted as pro-reform. There was no reason for public opinion or civil society groups to oppose reforms intended to improve a model that they knew well and supported.

TABLE 8.5
Distribution of Major Public Opinion/Civil Society and Media Independent Variables on Reform Decisions in 30 Cases

Independent Variable Category	Phase	Direction				
		Pro-Reform	Middle Territory	Anti-Reform	Counter-Consensus Reform	Total
Public opinion/ civil society	Governmental/ decision agenda	5	1	0	1	7
	Policy choice	2	0	0	0	2
	Both	7	1	0	1	9
Media	Governmental/ decision agenda	3	0	0	0	3
	Policy choice	0	0	0	1	1
	Both	3	0	0	1	4

4. Media

The media were not a major influence or indeed a factor of much import in any of the provincial case studies on regionalization, needs-based funding, or alternative payment plans. This result is consistent with our earlier observation that these issues were decided without any noticeable influence from public opinion and civil society groups.

The issues where the media were most influential were wait times and, secondarily, prescription drug reform. All five case studies of wait times noted some media influence on reform; in Alberta, Saskatchewan, and Ontario, the media were a major influence. The media were also a major factor in the prescription drug reform in Ontario. The impact of the media in these cases helped to put the issues on the governmental agenda and to advance them to the decision agenda. The media, however, had no observable influence on the specific policy choices that were made.

As for the issue of for-profit delivery, the media played a role but a lesser one. The resistance of the Friends of Medicare in Alberta enjoyed media coverage as did the federal government's opposition to Premier Klein's initiative. Klein himself was a sufficiently outgoing proponent of privatization that he, too, made for good copy.

5. Values

Values, knowledge, and institutions are the next three categories discussed. It will be recalled that we decided to divide "ideas" into two separate categories—values and knowledge—so that the role of evidence could be distinguished from values. Table 8.6 enables us to compare how each of these categories affected policy reform. As institutions include policy legacies, and the line between legacies and values can be blurred, we have also incorporated institutions into Table 8.6.

The egalitarian values that played a large role in the development of Canada-wide medicare continued to exert influence during the period studied. Given the meagre amount of reform that was undertaken, it will come as no surprise that these values played a bigger role in protecting medicare than in changing its fundamentals. Indeed, the fact that values were employed to protect medicare suggested that there were competing values. While private for-profit delivery was not, and is not, precluded under the *Canada Health Act*, it was seen by some as an assault on medicare, especially by the civil society groups mentioned above. The next chapter will discuss the role of values in different provinces and on different issues. Our focus here is on the Canada-wide setting and the fact that values played a much larger role in the governmental agenda and decision agenda phases of decision-making than at the policy choice stage.[9]

Matthew Mendelsohn's work for the Commission on the Future of Health Care in Canada speaks to the role of values. Mendelsohn examined all available public opinion polls on health care between 1985 and 2000 and reached the following conclusions (2002, 1-2):

> Despite this perceived decline over the past decade and dissatisfaction with a number of key aspects of the system, this report shows that Canadians continue to prefer the Canadian model. They have reached a mature, settled public judgment, based on decades of experience, that the Canadian health care model is a good one. Some public opinion polls elicit off-the-cuff, transitory responses to recent events, while others represent informed and relatively stable preferences that reflect people's deeply held views. The latter can be thought of as "public judgment" rather than just "public opinion,"[10] and although Canadians are still grappling with what to do in the future, they have reached a public judgment about the past: they like Medicare and think it should be preserved.[11]

Mendelsohn's conclusion was reinforced in a series of dialogues organized in 12 different cities across the country on behalf of the commission. These sessions showed that "Canadians are passionate about health care and very concerned about its future. They want to keep the core principles of the Medicare model that accord with their strongly held values of universality, equal access, solidarity, and fairness" (Maxwell et al. 2002, vi).

The medicare model had much support. Not only was it important to Canadians individually and collectively, but it was also reflected in "institutions" such as the *Canada Health Act* and related provincial public health insurance legislation. The federal Liberal Party, and the NDP at both the federal and provincial levels, claimed parental rights and rarely missed an opportunity to stress how important medicare was to Canadians. Unionized health-care workers, the Canadian Health Coalition, the Council of Canadians and their numerous affiliates were politically active in support of these values as were large swaths of the research community. In some sense, the combination of values upheld by the public, the legislation in which the values were embedded, the interest groups and politicians who promoted and defended medicare, the public servants who were attached to it for reasons both self-interested and altruistic, and their numerous supporters from the research community, was akin to a vertically integrated industry. It could be called Medicare Inc. The one sure issue on which all the political actors involved in Medicare Inc. could agree was the need to protect what was most precious to them: public funding for hospital and medical services that were accessible to all with priority given to those whose medical needs were most urgent. Enlarging the reach of medicare was a goal for many, but not all. Otherwise, the program was untouchable. Those who questioned any aspect could count on rapid retribution.

During the Chrétien and Martin years (1993–2006), the governing Liberal Party of Canada made no firm commitments to the provinces and territories to expand the boundaries of medicare, focusing instead on enforcement of the legislation. Shortly after winning office in 1993, the Chrétien government warned provinces about breaches of the *Canada Health Act* and subsequently imposed penalties on five provinces (Madore 2005, section F). For its remaining years in office (until 2006), the Liberal government "went to ground" on enforcement (i.e., worked on enforcement through private consultation with provincial governments) except for its dispute with Premier Klein about some of his privatization ideas.

In his 1995 budget, Finance Minister Paul Martin announced a planned cut of $7 billion annually from Ottawa's transfer payments to the provinces, much of it notionally intended for health care. This decision alienated provinces. It also reduced the prospects of expanding the scope of the health services to which the *Canada Health Act* might apply since its scope depended on provincial cooperation. It might be thought therefore that the legitimacy of the Liberals as the party of Canada-wide medicare would have been in shambles. But the Liberal government held cards in both hands. In its right hand were the high-value cards worth many billions of dollars as a result of its cuts in transfer payments to the provinces and territories. In the late 1990s and the very beginning of the 2000s, it was parsimonious about returning these funds to the provinces. But from its left hand the Liberal government was dealing out cards with lower face values, tens of millions of dollars, large enough to keep the dream of expanding medicare alive. By funding pilot projects, commissioning reports, and holding major conferences, and by its ongoing rhetoric, the federal Liberals encouraged Canadians to hold to the idea that medicare was a fair and just way of financing and delivering services and a concrete expression of Canadian values. The "sharing values" were not just abstractions but had political, institutional, interest group, and civil society connections; these values were therefore very important factors in health-care politics. Indeed, for some Canadians the legacy had status as a national symbol of Canadian distinctiveness (Mendelsohn 2002, 2; Soroka 2007, 23-24).

The values of medicare—the risk-sharing embedded within it—also had an offensive posture. This posture applied to the idea of enlarging the Canada-wide publicly financed health insurance system to include uncovered needs such as prescription drugs and home care. It applied as well to reforms that were expected to improve the delivery system such as regionalization, needs-based funding, and alternative payment plans for primary care physicians. But the evidence shows that the expansion or improvement of medicare did not resonate with the wider public to nearly the same degree as did protecting the existing system (Abelson et al. 2004, 190). In this sense, the main goal and role of the values category during the 1990–2003 period remained one of protecting and improving the status quo.

6. Knowledge

The knowledge category includes information and analysis found in major reports, interjurisdictional learning, and the knowledge arising from activities of the research community. Given this breadth, "knowledge" played a role in almost all reform cases, and in some cases there was more than one knowledge-related observation. It played a major role in 12 cases, 10 of which supported reform (Table 8.6).

There is much overlap among variables in the knowledge category. For example, new findings of an individual researcher or research team may be published in a journal. The principal author may provide the same results, packaged differently, to a provincial task force or legislative committee that in turn may integrate them into its report. The researcher may be contacted by public servants from other jurisdictions to brief them. His or her work may also identify data gaps that get taken up by provincial authorities and the Canadian Institute for Health Information (CIHI). This category also overlaps with the insider interests and institutions categories in that these actors often undertake or fund research which they then use to advocate or resist policy reform. Our analysis was not sufficiently fine-grained to allocate a part of the impact to the interest group or institution and a part to research.

Bearing in mind these qualifications, the knowledge variable that was cited most frequently in the 30 cases was "major report," usually from commissions or task forces commissioned by governments (annex 2, Table A2.1). Governments normally provided some kind of public reaction to the report recommendations since they had commissioned the work. Reports often packaged existing information and knowledge in a way that attracted media attention. In most cases this coverage helped generate public discussion of both the report and government feedback. But once the reports were released, the authors had limited time and resources to sustain their message. Moreover, as should be clear by now, their recommendations almost invariably proposed much more reform than governments were willing to embrace at the time.

The limited short-run impact of major reports is not surprising since such reports may be commissioned for more than one reason. A report may be commissioned as a stepping stone to building public support for large changes in health policy. It may be used to give profile to a set of issues during a period when policy action is judged to be impractical but a government wishes to keep the reform flame alive. It may be aimed at a specific task, such as the report that framed the policy choices that resulted in comprehensive reform of prescription drug policy in Quebec. From a different perspective, it may also be employed to sideline an issue, as the Arpin report was seemingly designed to do with respect to for-profit delivery in Quebec. After major reports, "research/information" and "interjurisdictional learning" were the other two knowledge variables most cited in the case studies.

Two points related to the role of knowledge are noteworthy here. First, knowledge played a larger role in policy choice than it did during the governmental agenda or decision agenda phases of the reform process—the opposite of what we found on values. In general, knowledge was not an opener of policy windows.

Second, the finding that knowledge was mainly influential after a reform window had opened speaks to the challenges of using knowledge to advance reform. Many reform ideas that accumulated over the years did not lead to reform. There is a range of possible reasons: the policy research community may not have connected well with the "problems" and "politics" streams; it may have connected at the wrong times or failed to sustain its connections; or it may have done all the right things but lost out in the rough and tumble of political decision-making. In some cases there may have been limited receptor capability in government due to limited resources or as a matter of choice. Nonetheless, governments made large investments in knowledge creation during our study period, and Canadians need to do better in incorporating it into the decision process.

TABLE 8.6
Distribution of Major Values, Knowledge, and Institutional Independent Variables on Reform Decisions in 30 Cases

Independent Variable Category	Phase	Direction				
		Pro-Reform	Middle Territory	Anti-Reform	Counter-Consensus Reform	Total
Values	Governmental/decision agenda	10	0	0	3	13
	Policy choice	1	0	0	2	3
	Both	11	0	0	5	16
Knowledge	Governmental/decision agenda	2	2	0	0	4
	Policy choice	8	0	0	0	8
	Both	10	2	0	0	12
Institutions	Governmental/decision agenda	3	0	1	0	4
	Policy choice	6	1	0	0	7
	Both	9	1	1	0	11

7. Institutions

Some institutions of interest are specific to the health sector and others are not. In the latter category are overarching institutions, including federalism and the Westminster system, which might have influenced our 30 case studies. On the Westminster system, Carolyn Tuohy (1999) has written that for major health reforms to occur, among other things, the "political system must provide a consolidated base of authority for policy action" (11). Given the relatively limited direct influence of the federal government and federal-provincial relations on our six reform issues, it is the consolidation at the provincial level that is relevant for our purposes. During the period studied, all provincial governments enjoyed majorities in their legislatures (including one case of a stable coalition), and the party system generally left little or no room for independent action on health by individual MLAs (except for a brief period in Alberta). Yet the fusion of executive and legislature was not a major theme in any of the five provincial chapters or in the 30 case studies that underpinned them. The fusion was taken for granted (as was the first-past-the-post electoral system that had helped to create majority governments).[12]

As for federalism, our cases showed little direct impact at the overarching level from 1990 to 2003, unlike earlier periods in the development of health services.[13] Concerning the six policy issues assessed in this book, federal law was permissive but not directive. The federal transfer legislation, initially Established Programs Financing and then the Canada Health and Social Transfer, in conjunction with the *Canada Health Act*, neither precluded nor required the reform directions in the grey literature consensus. It simply insisted that the existing Canadian model for hospital and medical services be preserved and where possible improved, but not replaced. In this sense, the impact of federalism was toward preserving the status quo. It should come as no surprise, therefore, that the federal government and federal-provincial relations were seen as a major influence on policy reform outcomes in only three of the 30 cases. And in two of these cases—the Alberta for-profit delivery and Quebec prescription drug reform—the federal role was not the decisive factor in the outcome. Where it was decisive was in the introduction of the limited 1998 Alberta Child Health Benefit Program, which was funded indirectly through the federal government's National Child Benefit. This was, however, a small reform. Put more positively, the *Canada Health Act* was not an impediment to the reforms that served as the basis for this book. Its flexibility permitted a wider range of reforms than was in fact undertaken.

This conclusion has to do with the direct effects of federalism only. There is a plausible argument that there were indirect but not inconsequential effects that our research methodology did not show. Two are noted here. One is derivative of the political strategy used by the federal Liberal government from the time it took office in 1993 until its defeat 2006. Its political priorities in respect of health care put it in conflict with a majority of provinces most of the time and with the federal opposition parties of the right. As noted above, during its first 18 months in office, the Chrétien Liberals enforced the penalty provisions of the *Canada Health Act*, resisted provincial demands for an equal role with the federal government in the interpretation of the *CHA*, and rejected the provincial request that the National Forum on Health be co-chaired by a premier. The 1995 budget was highly divisive as was the way in which it was communicated. The subsequent battle between the provinces and Ottawa about the level and adequacy of federal funding for health care was dysfunctional, which exacerbated tensions in the federation (Lazar et al. 2004a, 141-44; Marchildon 2004; Standing Senate Committee 2002b, section 1.2). While that battle was being waged, the federal government was communicating the view that medicare was a national icon and that opposition parties on the right had a "hidden agenda" that would undermine it. The federal Liberals also used their considerable communications resources to minimize the political damage from their cuts in transfers by turning attention to these other issues. This tactic may well have succeeded to the extent that civil society groups, public opinion, and the media generally focused on these federal-provincial-territorial issues and public sector/ private sector divides when the actual substance of reform was at the provincial level. Unintentionally, Ottawa may have lessened the time and attention that civil society groups, the public, and the media gave to the actual reform agenda.

Second, the decision of provincial premiers in the late 1990s to fight the reduction in federal transfers reduced the incentive for provincial governments to undertake certain kinds of reform. Specifically, any province that undertook a major expansion of insurance coverage without a large federal financial contribution would have undermined the provincial argument that their health systems were underfunded. One effect of this situation was to leave in limbo proposals for extending medicare to include prescription drugs and home care—issues that the federal Liberals chose to talk about but not act on.

With regard to the health-specific institutions, we note two types that were relevant to reform outcomes. First were ad hoc policy networks associated with the two most technical issues—needs-based funding and wait times. In the reform of needs-based funding, informal networks of experts with technical knowledge played a significant role in Alberta and Saskatchewan. On the wait-times issue, the creation of the Ontario Cardiac Care Network between 1988 and 1990 was heavily influenced by an effective policy network of a precursor organization, the Metropolitan Toronto Triage System. These two organizations were the pioneers of wait-list management in Canada. Almost a decade later, the Western Canada Waiting List Project—a collaborative undertaking by seven regional health authorities, four medical associations, four provincial ministries of health, and four health research centres—ran from 1999 to 2004. The Saskatchewan Surgical Care Network drew on the contacts associated with that enterprise and others. These policy networks account for five of the nine pro-reform policy choice influences in the institutions section of Table 8.6.

Second were the bilateral management committees made up of representatives of provincial medical associations and ministries of health. The management committees were in early stages of development during the study period and influenced only a few decisions (e.g., the decision agenda and policy choice in Alberta).[14]

Table 8.6 compares the ways in which values, knowledge, and institutions (excluding indirect effects of federalism, which is a principal theme of chapter 12) influenced reform outcomes in the 30 cases. In all three categories, the factors were mainly pro-reform. Values were most influential at the governmental agenda / decision agenda phases of the decision process, while knowledge and institutions played a relatively larger role at the policy choice phase. Together these two points suggest that the effects of knowledge and institutions were very similar. In fact, in several cases, policy networks (institutions) transmitted the knowledge that led to policy outcomes.

8. Insider Interests

This section focuses on organizations that decided on policy reform, that influenced it, or that attempted to do so by virtue of their access to the decision process. The analysis includes organizations representing physician interests, hospitals and other care institutions, nurses and other health professionals, as well as elected and appointed provincial officials who decided or advised on health policy. These organizations often combined advocacy and bargaining roles. The discussion below does not focus on single-issue interest groups. Their role is set out in the individual case studies and was discussed above under the "Public Opinion and Civil Society" heading.

Provincial Medical Associations. As the six policy reform issues dealt with in this book were within provincial legislative competence, not only constitutionally but also practically, the focus here is on provincial medical associations. The role of the Canadian Medical Association is discussed in chapter 11.

To understand the role of provincial medical associations during the years we studied, some historical perspective is useful. Although provincial medical associations (and their precursors) opposed the creation of publicly financed medical insurance during the 1950s and 1960s, once the federal *Medical Care Act, 1966* was enacted, a process of accommodation evolved between the associations (in the case of Quebec two "medical unions"[15]) and provincial governments (Tuohy 1999, 207-34). Initially, arrangements between medical associations and governments addressed mainly increases in the fee-for-service schedule for physicians. In the 1980s, the dispute about physicians' right to extra-bill soured the relationships. Once the *Canada Health Act* and related provincial legislation had been passed, however, the accommodation process between provincial medical associations and provincial governments began anew. The logic of focusing on fee schedules alone, however, did not work for government (Lomas, Charles, and Grew 1992). Government needed some way of controlling aggregate costs, which required keeping tabs not only on the fee schedule but also on the number of physicians authorized to bill the province and the intensity with which those physicians, on average, provided each service. As these needs were addressed, relations between medical associations and provincial health ministries became closer and more intertwined. It is this post-*CHA* renewal process and its outcome that were the backdrop to our case studies.

By the 1990s, "master agreements" set out the relationships between provincial medical associations and provincial governments (usually health ministries) in most provinces. Some read like international agreements in their formality. While the agreements functioned mainly as instruments for collective bargaining, secondarily they became vehicles through which provincial governments could systematically obtain physician input into planned policy and program changes affecting physicians. The medical associations therefore had insider access to proposed policy reforms affecting physician compensation and working conditions. By the early 2000s the medical association in each province had established itself as the sole legal representative of the medical profession. In Quebec, separate bodies represented primary care physicians and specialists. Although these unusual relationships between state and insider interests were not guaranteed to last in perpetuity, the relationships became wider and deeper. Some provinces created bipartite or tripartite committees in conjunction with their respective medical associations to oversee the relationships.

The 2000 Memorandum of Agreement between the Ontario Medical Association (OMA) and the Ministry of Health and Long-Term Care (MOHLTC) illustrates the scope of the understandings. It provided that a Physician Services Committee would oversee a process to monitor and evaluate the items laid out in the agreement. The committee was made up of representatives of the MOHLTC and the OMA, with a co-chair from each party and a facilitator chosen jointly. One provision of the committee's mandate shines light on the scope of the ministry-association partnership: to "develop recommendations, either on its own initiative or as a result of reports and recommendations received from committees reporting to it, to the MOHLTC and the OMA leading to the enhancement of the quality and effectiveness of medical care in Ontario."[16]

Among the other four provinces we studied, the arrangements varied. In Alberta, during the years when there were regional authorities, the master agreement was tripartite involving the provincial medical association, the government, and the representative of the regional health authorities. Like Ontario, the Alberta arrangements had a committee structure to "manage, oversee and provide general guidance to the relationship and the budget process" (Alberta 2003). The Saskatchewan master agreement relied on committees with specific-purpose mandates. It called on the board of the Saskatchewan Medical Association to establish committees, and to chair on such issues as "rural and regional programs and incentives." In Quebec, there were two principal agreements, one with the Fédération des médecins omnipraticiens du Québec and one with the Fédération des médecins spécialistes du Québec.[17] The government's role was somewhat broader in Quebec than in other provinces. The two federations had long accepted that physician remuneration should increase at the general rate of increase in the public sector. Much effort accordingly went into the fee schedule and issues around utilization (Lomas Charles, and Grew 1992, 81-103). In Newfoundland and Labrador, the government was represented by the treasury board minister, not the minister of health, signalling that the agreement more tightly focused on issues of financial remuneration.

It is within this framework of structured relationships between medical associations and provincial governments that we examine the influence of medical associations on three of the policy issues. The alternative payment plan (APP), regionalization, and wait-times cases each had the potential to alter sharply the public payment/private delivery bargain. APP threatened to narrow the entrepreneurial freedom of physicians. If fee-for-service was eliminated as a form of remuneration, it might be uneconomic for doctors to operate solo practices and small medical partnerships. In any case, it would detract from the self-image of the physician as a self-employed professional. Regionalization might have shifted medical budgets to the regional level with unknown impacts on physician compensation and professional autonomy. The wait-times case also had implications for the professional autonomy of individual physicians.

In the APP case, there were differences within the physician community. When the public payment/private delivery bargain was initially reached in the 1960s, it was recognized that "continuation of private, fee-for-service as the predominant mode (of payment) would be the result" (Tuohy 1999, 204). Although this remained the case during our period of study, with the great majority of physicians including almost all older primary care doctors preferring fee-for-service, some younger family physicians favoured alternative payment systems. A key role for associations representing doctors' interests therefore was to work out an internal consensus to bridge these differences. The consensus position that medical associations typically brought to the discussion with government officials was one that would allow physicians to choose between the traditional fee-for-service (FFS) method and one or more of the alternatives such as capitation or salary, including methods that blended FFS with one of the alternatives. This position fell well short of the grey literature proposals that favoured rapidly ending fee-for-service but was a step in that direction; the magnitude of the step varied among provinces but in no case amounted to a large reform between 1990 and 2003. Governments understood the range of views within the medical profession and did not push for comprehensive reforms. They made the political judgment that they had to work with the doctors rather than alienate them.

In Newfoundland and Labrador, there was good cooperation between the Newfoundland and Labrador Medical Association (NLMA) and the Ministry of Health in the 1990s. The NLMA tended to support alternative payment systems for family doctors, and a deal with the province that would have actively encouraged alternative payment schemes on a voluntary basis was close to fruition in 1999. In the end relations soured, mainly over money, and no reform was implemented.

The Quebec case was similar. The province and the Fédération des omnipracticiens du Québec (FMOQ), the federation representing family physicians, reached a tentative agreement that would have seen doctors reorganized into voluntarily constituted family medicine groups responsible for providing services to a given population. Compensation of participating physicians was to consist of three elements: capitation according to the number of registered patients, a base amount, and fee-for-service payment. This understanding collapsed when, in anticipation of the coming 2003 general election, the government attempted to rush the implementation of the arrangement before working through the details with the FMOQ.

In Ontario, the reform policy was also voluntary. Family Health Networks, established in 2001, provided a choice of blended payment (capitation based on age and sex profile of patients with some FFS and bonus elements) or reformed FFS.

The Saskatchewan Medical Association strongly resisted some of the ideas that the Romanow NDP government had been considering when it attempted to move forward its agenda for primary care reform. By that time the government was in the second half of its first mandate and attracting much criticism for the reforms it had implemented. The SMA had not shown a significant interest in the regionalization and needs-based funding cases and it was under pressure from its members to take a stand on protecting the inviolability of FFS. The fact that FFS was central to the Saskatoon accord that had signalled the end of the physician strike three decades earlier may also have been a factor. Whatever the explanation, the SMA blocked early progress of alternative payment plan reform, and Saskatchewan remained a laggard on this issue throughout the study period.

In contrast, it was the Alberta Medical Association that put APP on the governmental agenda in that province. In fact, the AMA had a major influence on all phases of the decision process. In other provinces, the medical associations were most heavily engaged at the policy choice phase and secondarily the decisions stage. Provincial medical associations urged that alternative payments be available as an option for doctors who were ready to sign on to newly forming group practices. But they also insisted that this option be voluntary. Government should not compel a shift away from fee-for-service.

Speaking for all physicians, the Canadian Medical Association declared that "individual medical practitioners have the liberty to choose among payment methods" (CMA 2002, 36). The four provinces in our five-province sample that acted on this issue accepted this limitation on the policy changes they implemented. On the APP issue, it is thus fair to say that the provincial associations representing physicians played a decisive role, probably *the* decisive role, in establishing the nature, extent, and pace of reform once the policy window opened. A paper that covers the later years of our study period reaches similar conclusions (Hutchison et al. 2011, 278):

> Several provincial governments are negotiating primary health care reform initiatives with the provincial medical association representing family physicians on the basis of voluntary participation and pluralism of organizational and remuneration models. This approach recognizes that for Canada, system-level innovation in primary health care is possible only with the support or, at a minimum, the acquiescence of organized medicine.

For the APP issue, most provincial medical associations were involved and influential in all phases of the decision process.

With respect to the idea of transferring medical budgets to regional health authorities, the influence of medical associations may not have been visible, but it was real. The first wave of grey literature consensus included the idea that physician budgets should be managed at the regional level. Had this occurred, there is no telling how it would have played out for physician remuneration and autonomy. At minimum, it would have made life more complicated for the provincial medical associations bargaining on behalf of physicians. Instead of dealing with one provincial body only (two in Quebec), the associations would have had to deal separately with each regional health authority, which would have been problematic considering that different regions often have different priorities. In any event, this idea turned out to be a non-starter politically. Governments knew that physician groups would object. The grey literature consensus on this point was "dead on arrival." For all practical purposes, it never reached the governmental agenda.

The issue of wait times also had the potential to affect the physicians' core bargain with government, specifically the private practice part that resisted incursions into their professional autonomy, by imposing externally determined rules or norms for deciding which patients should have priority in diagnosis and treatment. This idea did not progress far in most provinces during the study period for several reasons unrelated to group pressures, such as the lack of agreed measures for wait times and inadequate data. But insider interest groups were also influential. Some physician groups and hospital boards were skeptical of the idea of actively managing wait times, dragging their feet if not publicly opposing it. On the other hand, a small number of individual physicians in Ontario and Saskatchewan played the role of policy entrepreneurs championing the reform cause. Ultimately, working with others in the relevant provincial policy networks, these physicians helped achieve results that more doubting physicians would come to accept as professionally tolerable. In contrast, in provinces where there was no champion from the medical community to counter resistance from associations representing physicians and hospital boards/management, reform was more limited. Both in the provinces where substantial reform was achieved and those where it was not, the physician community, if not the medical associations, was instrumental in influencing the nature and extent of reform once the policy window had opened.

In sum, on issues that mattered most to physicians, provincial medical associations were able to protect physician interests. In some cases this was achieved by keeping the reform window shut. In others, they did so by persuading governments to advance their goals through incentives rather than through regulation. In still others, the medical associations recognized the need for action and attempted, with considerable success, to move to the front of the parade and lead a proposal toward an outcome that physicians supported.

Hospital Interests. To varying degrees, all six issues had the potential to affect hospital interests significantly. The focus here is on three issues in which hospitals stood to be most heavily affected. First, proposals to regionalize could change hospital governance and lead to closure of some hospitals. Needs-based funding could affect how, and how generously, hospitals were funded. Wait times had implications for hospital and physician autonomy in managing wait lists (and potentially hospital budgets if they were tied to performance in wait-list management).

Excluding the state-owned and operated rural cottage hospital system in Newfoundland and Labrador and hospitals operated by the federal government for war veterans and Aboriginal Canadians, almost all Canadian hospitals had been established mainly by religious orders, charities, or municipal governments as private not-for-profit entities. With the implementation of publicly funded hospital insurance, provincial governments became involved in the manner in which hospitals managed records and accounts. This was necessary to be sure that the provinces were claiming the appropriate amount from the federal authorities as shareable expenses under the *Hospital Insurance and Diagnostic Services Act*. Provinces also had accepted the federal government's right to audit hospital expenditures, which added to the provincial government's interest in making sure that hospitals maintained their financial books appropriately. When Parliament passed the *Established Programs Financing Act* in 1977, the link between provincial spending and federal contribution was severed. But by that time, provinces had become very concerned about the rate of growth in health spending as an issue on its own, and not just to satisfy cost-sharing relationships with Ottawa. While hospitals and their political allies had recourse to the political process to support their case for more funding (through their MLAs, political party connections, local office holders, and the press), provincial authorities had the final say in determining the annual operating budgets of hospitals.

At the beginning of our study period in the 1990s, there were differences between hospital governance in Quebec and in the other provinces. Three decades earlier, in 1960, Quebecers had elected the Quebec Liberal Party to office. Under the leadership of Jean Lesage, the National Assembly enacted hospital insurance (1961) and hospital (1962) legislation. In 1966, the government appointed a Commission on Health Care and Social Services. The Castonguay-Nepveu report recommended that health care be fully managed and funded by the provincial state and that all care and services should be universal and free of charge (Commission d'enquête sur la santé et le bien-être social 1967). The commission subsequently recommended that program administration should be carried out at the regional level. By the early 1970s, health and social services were delivered through a system of 12 regional administrative départements with common boundaries for all government ministries. Thus, at the beginning of our period of analysis, Quebec hospitals were, in at least two respects, in a different place than hospitals in most other provinces. First, they were state institutions. Second, they were part of a system of governance that was administered regionally.

All provinces were under fiscal stress in the early 1990s, and several provincial governments were in receipt of reports at that time recommending that health services be organized at a regional level. Quebec was again first off the mark. During the study period, two major reforms were undertaken that affected Quebec hospitals. First, in 1991 the Regional Councils for Health and Social Services that had been created in 1971, and that administered provincial health and social service programs, were replaced by boards that were vested with the authority not only to implement the policies established by the Minister but also to plan, organize, and evaluate programs and policies within the region. Having power concentrated at the regional level was useful during this period of hospital rationalization, but by the late 1990s it was seen by critics, including hospital and medical interests, as superfluous. During the 2003 Quebec general election, the opposition Quebec Liberal Party committed to eliminating the regional level entirely and replacing it with local health and social service networks. The commitment enjoyed substantial support but also attracted strong opposition. Once in office, the newly elected government of Jean Charest took quick action to implement its promise, ran into stiff opposition and subsequently decided on a compromise. Authority was shifted downward to new local networks, and the regional boards were eliminated. New regional agencies were, however, created. The initial mandate of the regional agencies was to help establish the local networks. The building blocks for the networks were local hospitals, community service centres, and residential and long-term care centres. The new regime allowed some hospitals that did not integrate readily with other local institutions to remain free-standing but part of the Quebec state.

The other four provinces also undertook some reforms that affected hospital interests profoundly from the perspective of governance and funding. On regionalization and needs-based funding, Saskatchewan moved first and Alberta soon thereafter. Both closed many hospitals in the process of establishing regional health authorities (in Saskatchewan "districts" initially) for the purposes of planning, coordinating and integrating services, and allocating resources, especially for hospitals and other care institutions. In Saskatchewan, leaders associated with small hospitals outside the main population centres tried to slow the reform train, but fiscal crisis meant they never had a chance. In Alberta, Premier Klein's government excluded known opponents of regionalization from his roundtable consultation process. In both cases, the regional health authorities became the new boards. Both provinces experimented with partially elected boards, but by 2003 boards were again fully appointed. Both provinces also replaced global budgeting with a formula-driven, needs-based approach to funding the regions. Regionalization and needs-based funding in these two provinces constituted four of the seven large reforms in our sample of 30 cases.

In Newfoundland and Labrador, the process of regionalizing hospitals and other institutions was announced in 1993 and implemented in 1996. Some hospital interests, especially in St. John's, resisted but the project nonetheless was advanced. Subsequently, the Newfoundland and Labrador Hospital and Nursing Homes Association proposed a needs-based funding model. In this case, it was the Government of

Newfoundland and Labrador that resisted, seemingly because it preferred to retain the flexibility and discretion to allocate among competing claims (Tomblin and Braun-Jackson 2005).

Ontario did not choose to regionalize during the 1990s or early 2000s but it too, through its Health Services Restructuring Commission, closed some hospitals and merged others. What it did not do was displace the hospital boards.

The details in annex 2 show that hospital interests were more often than not against reforms, especially on the regionalization and wait times issues. Focusing on the four major variables only, two involved hospital interests slowing wait-time reforms (Quebec, and Newfoundland and Labrador), one unsuccessful case of resistance to regionalization (Saskatchewan), and one unsuccessful pro-reform effort to encourage needs-based funding (Newfoundland and Labrador). One outcome of this period was that organizations that spoke for hospitals as distinct interests ceased to exist after the regional authorities were established in Saskatchewan, Alberta, and Newfoundland and Labrador. Hospitals were integrated into regional systems of governance.

In sum, the model of private not-for-profit hospitals began to change when publicly funded hospital insurance became available in the late 1950s. Public funding put hospitals on a more secure financial footing, but in the process hospitals lost some autonomy. The nature and extent of that loss differed among the provinces. For example, the exigencies associated with federal-provincial cost-sharing constrained hospitals from charging patients for standard beds.

Regionalization reforms during the 1990s and early 2000s further eroded the idea of hospitals as autonomous, independent entities. The details varied among provinces. But in becoming increasingly part of a system of regional services, hospitals in Saskatchewan, Alberta, and urban Newfoundland and Labrador also increasingly became part of the provincial state, as had Quebec hospitals much earlier. Ontario was the lone province among the five not to regionalize hospital services. This did not prevent the Ontario government from closing some hospitals and merging others. Those that remained, however, retained considerable autonomy. Ontario hospitals were in a grey zone, far from fully autonomous but by no means integrated into the provincial state.

Major Pharmaceutical Firms. From 1990 to 2003, prescription drugs were the third-largest use of funds for health care after the hospital sector and physicians. Spending on prescription drugs was also growing at a faster rate than for hospitals and physicians. Yet pharmaceutical firms have scarcely been mentioned to this point in the book except in the context of prescription drug reform in Quebec. The proximate reason is that these firms were not mentioned in 29 of the 30 cases studies. There was nothing visible for the research team to analyze (although there were ongoing private conversations between representatives of the brand name firms and federal officials on patent law protection and drug prices).

In the case of the large Quebec reform, the Parti Québécois government (1994–2003) included a provision in its 1994 platform that indicated it planned to fix the basic unfairness in the Quebec system of prescription drug insurance. The reforms that occurred in other provinces were connected neither to election platforms nor to a response to reform proposals in the grey literature. The tiny increments to coverage in Alberta (extending palliative coverage and a Child Health Benefit), the counter-consensus benefit reductions in Saskatchewan, and the Ontario Trillium Drug Program were all a response to unique conditions in those provinces as was the absence of reform in Newfoundland and Labrador.

Our research on Quebec's reform found that the major brand-name pharmaceutical firms supported implementation of "the most universal system possible" (chapter 6). At the same time, the companies requested assurance that the government would not attempt to lever its reform to impose new rules that would adversely affect the price structure for their products or market conditions (Pomey, Martin, and Forest 2005, 24). Understandably, the major drug makers wanted as large a market as possible without any new reforms that would constrain price. Then, as now, brand-name firms enjoyed the enhanced protection afforded to their products by amendments to the federal *Patent Act* in 1986 with consumer interests apparently taken into account by the federally appointed Patented Medicines Prices Review Board. Within the scope of its jurisdiction, the Quebec government agreed. For Quebec, mandating universal coverage was one silo. Procurement was seemingly part of a different silo.

Although the main grey literature documents on prescription drugs were published after the reform decisions were taken, they have relevance to our purposes in this chapter. The reports of the government-appointed commissions and task forces saw prescription medicine as "medically necessary." They accordingly called either for universal, first-dollar coverage (in the case of the National Forum on Health 1997b) or, more prudently from a fiscal perspective, for increased public coverage over time as affordable. Given priority were persons with catastrophic expenses, persons receiving drugs for short-term acute or post-acute home care, and persons receiving drugs as part of end-of-life palliative care (Commission on the Future of Health Care 2002, 176-77, 197-98; Standing Senate Committee 2002a, 137-59). On coverage, the drug companies and the grey literature were pointed in the same direction.

Where the difference between the brand-name firms and the grey literature arose was on price. Both the Romanow and Kirby reports called for a National Drug Formulary and a National Drug Agency that would strengthen the ability of publicly administered prescription drug insurance plans to negotiate for lower prices (Commission on the Future of

Health Care 2002, 202-4; Standing Senate Committee 2002a, 143). In the context of ongoing negotiations about fiscal arrangements, there was a brief moment in 2003 when first ministers seemed to buy into the general direction of the Romanow and Kirby recommendations on both coverage and price. They declared that by 2005/06 "Canadians, wherever they live ... [should] have reasonable access to catastrophic drug coverage" (First Ministers' Meeting 2003). We will touch on these developments in chapter 11. The point here is that although the reports of the National Forum, Commission, and Senate Committee became public in the second half of our study period, the ideas were in circulation earlier. Governments took no major initiatives, although some managed procurement more tightly than others. As for the brand-name firms, they might have preferred a system of universal coverage as a way of growing their market. If so, it was not a priority.

The limited visibility of the brand-name firms appears to have been due in part to their comfort with existing arrangements. Business was highly profitable on a global basis (Angell 2004). Big pharmaceutical firms were able to support extensions of coverage seemingly without the concern that there might be a quid pro quo of such an extension in the form of policies that would directly or indirectly exert downward pressure on price. In fact, the public was not privy to the prices that governments paid for their drug purchases from brand-name firms. This was different from provincial expenditures on hospitals and physicians. The tariff that physicians could charge for a specific service was publicly available. The details of hospital funding were accessible. Major foreign-based pharmaceutical firms, however, insisted that their contracts with provincial formularies remain secret. The prices that provincial formularies paid for particular drugs were therefore not accessible to the public. Nor was it possible to obtain that information indirectly because there was no public reporting requirement for Canadian subsidiaries of foreign companies. The silence of the brand-name firms on health reform suggests that they found the status quo to their liking. These firms did not rock their boat unduly.

Nurses and Unionized Hospital Workers. Most of the other associations representing provider groups that showed up in the 30 case studies had less influence on policy reform than hospital associations and were weaker still relative to medical associations and pharmaceutical firms. To the extent that professional associations or unions representing hospital workers attempted to protect the jobs, earnings, and working conditions of their members during the 1990s, they were frequently disappointed. To the extent that they attempted to wield policy influence that put them in opposition to the views of physician and hospital associations, the evidence in the 30 case studies shows no significant impact. Unionized health-care workers in Quebec attempted to steer policy choice in prescription drugs and argued in favour of retaining the regional level when the government proposed to eliminate it. In the drug case, the fact that the ruling Parti Québécois was sometimes perceived as a left-of-centre, social democratic party on some issues and thereby the ideological ally of the unions made no difference. The experience of these provider groups with other social democratic governments was similar. The first Romanow government in Saskatchewan irritated many of its supporters when it closed many hospitals and merged others. Relations between the public service unions and the Rae government were also rocky (Rae 1996, 225-53).

The overarching political goal of these groups was to defend medicare, which was where the general public also stood. These provider groups were part of the great Canadian coalition that successfully protected medicare. They also were part of a large, but less vast, coalition that wished to see medicare expanded but that did not succeed.

Elected Provincial Government Officials. As the authoritative decision makers for all six policy issues analyzed in this volume, provincial government officials, whether elected or appointed, were the target of lobbying efforts by other political actors. In this role, provincial governments served as a sieve or "mediating" variable between the various factors attempting to influence reform decisions. Of course, governing political parties were much more than sieves. To one degree or other, they had core values and interests of their own that they wished to incorporate into the decisions they took. Yet, "elected provincial government officials" were coded as major influences in only seven cases.

This finding was an artifact of our methodology. Fifteen of 22 cases in which elected government officials were major influences were coded under "change in government/leader." Of the remaining seven, four related to for-profit delivery. This issue was almost entirely political. In Alberta and Ontario (Klein and Harris/Eves governments), the political leadership took action to make more space for private enterprise. In Quebec, elected officials decided to do nothing owing to the political sensitivity of this issue. For the same reason, opposition leaders who had a shot at winning government preferred not to campaign on this issue. In Saskatchewan, at the outset of the second Romanow government, legislation was enacted to make for-profit clinics less viable. As for the other three cases, in Newfoundland and Labrador ministers played a key role in introducing regionalization and in opposing needs-based funding. Premier Rae led the prescription drug reform in Ontario.

Provincial Public Servants. The provincial public service is cited as a factor 25 times covering 24 of the 30 cases in annex 2.[18] These influences refer mainly to officials from health ministries but also include finance/treasury officials and other ministers as needed. The breadth of public service influence was in some sense what it should have been. The experience of the various provincial health ministry officials in overseeing if not managing health systems would have afforded them with insights into emerging problems and possible solutions. In most provinces, most of the time, public servants used their knowledge and experience to support the elected government. Where they lacked knowledge and experience was in for-profit delivery. In fact, five of the six cases where public servants were not seen as influential were on this issue.

Three of the four cases where the public service was perceived to be a major independent influence were in Saskatchewan. These cases were regionalization, needs-based funding, and wait times. The first two cases reflected the strong working relationship between the Romanow-led government in Saskatchewan and the public service of that province. The wait-times case occurred more than a decade later, by which time Lloyd Calvert was premier. The fourth case was needs-based funding in Alberta. Both needs-based funding and wait times had a large technical content. (The extent of the distinction that can be made between technical and political issues is discussed in chapter 9.)

On needs-based funding, public servants played comparable roles in Alberta and Saskatchewan despite huge differences in context. In Alberta, Ministry of Health officials effectively advanced and ultimately designed the needs-based funding formula, notwithstanding difficult relations with the premier's office. In Saskatchewan, the influence of public servants on this issue was part of the larger partnership between the government and senior officials in the Health Ministry just mentioned.

It is part of the Canadian political culture that public servants stay silent about their role in advising ministers. Thus, notwithstanding the extensive interviewing done for this book, the above comments might underestimate the influence of public servants. We have no conclusive proof on this question, but two considerations have led us to the view that our assessment is probably close to the mark.

One consideration is that the 30 case studies, taken as a package, showed public servants consistently exerting influence in the direction toward which the ministers were leaning. On its own, this consideration proves nothing since the public servants could have co-opted their ministers. But the policy reform stances of the governments were taken and made public before they became governments in enough cases to make clear that public servants were not the determinative factor in the general policy orientation of elected officials. In this regard, newly elected provincial governments sometimes brought in new deputy ministers when they saw a need to ensure that the public service respected their priorities. For example, within two weeks of assuming office on 1 November 1991, Premier Romanow appointed a former public servant who had been out of government for some time as deputy minister of health. Bob Rae, in his autobiography, discusses the need to bring in fresh blood that he could count on (Rae 1996, 274-84).

The second consideration is based on the only independent analysis that we are aware of that deals with the role of provincial (and federal) health ministry officials over the period that is relevant to our study. Patricia O'Reilly (2001), in her work on the Federal-Provincial-Territorial (FPT) Conference of Health Ministers and the supporting conference of deputy ministers, concluded that health ministers and deputy ministers had reasonable success in dealing with important meso-policy issues like tobacco control, food safety, hazardous products, managing contagious diseases, and perhaps most significantly, developing a new blood transfusion system. It was on these kinds of issues that cooperation between federal and provincial health officials was most effective. But according to O'Reilly, the FPT conferences were much less successful in dealing with macro-policy framework issues.[19] In the O'Reilly analysis, it was not that FPT health ministries did not recognize the need to adapt health-care policy to changing conditions. Rather it was that health spending had become so large and the politics so sensitive that first ministers and finance ministers took the lead on big framework issues and, in so doing, tended to give more attention to financial concerns and constitutional principles than health policy. The dysfunctional FPT relationship was reflected as well in the inability of the different orders of government to work together on big framework issues, as symbolized by Ottawa's decision to establish a National Forum on Health and reject the idea of a provincial co-chair for that process. This led to a provincial/territorial decision to continue with a smaller parallel process and to publish its own ideas in the report *A Renewed Vision for Canada's Health Care System* (Conference of Provincial/Territorial Ministers 1997).

The same reasons that led premiers and prime ministers, and finance ministries and ministers, to appropriate key intergovernmental files from health ministries also applied to a considerable extent in the intraprovincial scene. With provincial health costs increasing to close to 38 percent of provincial program expenditures in 2003 from 33 percent a decade earlier and still growing quickly, it could not have been entirely otherwise (CIHI 2011b, 56). Thus, with premiers and finance ministries in the driver's seat for much of the period covered, the influence of the health ministry public servants was circumscribed. Interestingly, Antonia Maioni (1998) reached similar conclusions in her study of the influence of bureaucrats on the emergence of health insurance. "Bureaucrats involved with the health agenda were clearly constrained," she wrote, referring to public servants in the United States as well as Canada. She also found Canadian public servants to be "less likely to independently initiate reform proposals" than their American counterparts (159). A study of the Ontario Health Services Restructuring Commission suggests that health officials used whatever influence they had to resist reform proposals from sources other than ministers (Sinclair, Rochon, and Leatt 2005, 149). Overall, the evidence suggests that public servants were mainly supportive of ministers instead of being a major reform factor.

Widening our lens beyond health, in a study that compared the paradigms that the Rae and Harris governments brought to public-private partnerships, Neil Bradford (2003) found that both governing parties "curtailed in some measure the lead role of the public service in Ontario policy formulation" and that they "drew on economic ideas circulating outside regular ministerial channels" (1024). Bradford was not writing of health-care policy. Still, he was reflecting on an apparently diminished role for the Ontario public service relative to halcyon days gone by. He asserts that the "Conservatives came to power with their own electoral manifesto, and made it known that the bureaucracy's main policy contributions would be in implementing the party's agenda" (ibid.). Only a few years earlier, Ralph Klein had delivered a comparable message to the Alberta public service.

From the perspective of democratic principles, the wide but not decisive influence of health ministry officials is more than a passing grade. In many circles public servants are expected to provide advice to the elected government, the assumption being that public servants will be only one of several other sources it draws on in its decision process. If our analysis had shown the provincial public service as a major influence in half the cases, then there might be a legitimate criticism that public servants had hijacked the political agenda.

Insider Interest Wrap-Up. Table 8.7 shows how the major insider influences were distributed. Provincial medical associations were found to be a major factor much more often than other insiders, and they were by far the most substantial barrier to reform. Concretely, this reflected the fact that governments did not accept the policy reform proposals of commissions and task forces to shift medical budgets to regions, knowing the political storm that would have arisen in their relations with medical associations. It also reflects opposition of medical associations in some provinces to proposals on wait times and alternative payment plans. With respect to APP, it is arguable that provincial medical associations were *the* main governors of the pace at which APP and primary care reform more generally were introduced.

Hospital interests stood to be affected by all six issues and nurses by most of the six. Yet our analysis shows that neither provider group had much impact on the 30 cases as a package. If we include all variables, and not just major ones, the picture does not change.

The provincial state grew closer both to the hospital sector and to provincial medical associations over the period studied, but the manner in which it did so differed sharply. Provincial governments essentially integrated the hospital sector into the state in most of the five provinces we studied. Rural Newfoundland and Labrador had entered Confederation with state-owned and -operated hospitals. Quebec did the integration in

TABLE 8.7
Distribution of Major Insider Interest Independent Variables on Reform Decisions in 30 Cases

Independent Variable	Phase	Direction				
		Pro-Reform	Middle Territory	Anti-Reform	Counter-Consensus Reform	Total
Medical associations	Governmental/ decision agenda	0	0	6	0	6
	Policy choice	0	4*	0	0	4
	Both	0	4	6	0	10
Hospital interests	Governmental/ decision agenda	1	0	3	0	4
	Policy choice	0	0	0	0	0
	Both	1	0	3	0	4
Elected government officials	Governmental/ decision agenda	2	0	1	2	5
	Policy choice	0	2	0	0	2
	Both	2	2	1	2	7
Public service	Governmental/ decision agenda	0	0	0	0	0
	Policy choice	4	0	0	0	4
	Both	4	0	0	0	4

Notes: *These cases could be added to the governmental/decision agenda phases as well.

the early 1970s. Other provinces studied did so subsequently to varying degrees and at differing rates. Except in Ontario, the task of regionalization was more or less completed in the 1990s. Ontario hospitals, however, retained considerable autonomy during our study years.

Provincial medical associations also became increasingly intertwined with provincial health ministries, but with the opposite effect of that experienced by hospitals. By the 1990s, master agreements set out the relationships in most provinces. These instruments and the structures they created were a means for provincial governments to obtain physician input into planned policy and program changes affecting physicians. Viewed from a physician perspective, these arrangements provided medical associations with privileged access to proposed policy reform.

The health ministry–medical association relationship was in some sense a unique policy subsystem or at least evolving in that direction. Table 8.7 summarizes our findings on insider interests.

CONCLUSIONS

This chapter began with an assessment of the kind and amount of reform experienced for the years 1990 to 2003. The consensus of the reports commissioned by government-appointed commissions, task forces, and advisory councils—the grey literature—was the standard against which provincial performance was assessed. The grey literature favoured the Canadian model for hospital and medical services and aimed at improving its performance rather than replacing it. It also proposed extending the model to cover prescription drugs and home care on a Canada-wide basis in a step-by-step approach as affordability conditions allowed.

One finding was that much of the reform achieved was directionally consistent with the grey literature. Reforms were aimed at strengthening the current model for hospital and medical services, not inventing a new one. On the other hand, despite declarations by First Ministers in 2003 and 2004, there were no first steps toward a countrywide extension of that model. The only big enlargement of program eligibility / benefit generosity was within one province—Quebec's introduction of a mixed public-private model for health insurance. It mandated universal coverage, but not the first dollar coverage that is a fundamental trait of Canada-wide medicare.

As for the amount of policy reform, the evidence showed the results to be meagre.

The greater part of this chapter focused on identifying the categories of independent variables that resulted in meagre reform. To a large degree, influence over and resistance to reform was found in the insider interest category and specifically among provincial medical associations. (Other provider interests were not a significant influence on the 30 cases as a whole.) The second major barrier to reform was public opinion and civil society groups that resisted changes in the existing hospital and medical model. The fact that medical associations and public opinion / civil society groups were the main obstacles to reform does not mean that these actors were always opposed to reform; rather, when they were opposed, reform was difficult to achieve.

Elected government officials had a major influence on seven cases that were "political" as opposed to "technical." None of these cases entailed significant or comprehensive reform. Public servants had a major influence on four cases that were "technical."

Turning to other variable categories, 80 percent of major factors in the four categories of variables that were exogenous—change in government /

leader, fiscal crisis, public opinion / civil society, and media—involved or supported actors who favoured consensus reform. The majority of those actors who did not support consensus reform favoured counter-consensus reform, not the status quo.

The values category included both endogenous and exogenous attachments. Egalitarian values attached to the medicare model and associated with improving and expanding that model commanded significantly more support than the values of personal responsibility, personal choice, and markets that were inspiration for counter-consensus privatization proposals. The values category lent support to reform although mainly within a relatively narrow range of issues, favouring public insurance versus private insurance and Canada-wide programs over provincial programs. Rarely did values stray from this orthodoxy, although the "wellness" agenda of the Saskatchewan NDP of the 1990s did bring a different lens to choice.

Medicare-friendly research communities created many of the proposals for reform. Much of what they produced was focused on the need to improve but not replace the current medicare. Indeed, the "knowledge industry" played a large role in the creation of the grey literature which has served as our standard. It was a voice for large reform although, as we have seen, that voice rarely carried the day. Knowledge played at best a small role in leading reform. Where it was most useful was in crafting solutions when a reform window had been opened by other influences.

This chapter also identified common factors that were associated with the seven cases of large reform. Five of the seven—regionalization in Alberta and Saskatchewan, needs-based funding in the same two provinces, and prescription drug reform in Quebec—involved a newly formed, first-time government that had made commitments during the election campaign or leadership contest that brought it to office. Once in office, the new premier appointed a "policy champion," and the government acted on policy reform within the first half of its mandate. These three governments were re-elected at least once, but all accomplished much more in the first half of their first mandates than in the rest of their years in office. It was also observed that most newly formed, first-time governments did not make health-care reform commitments on a scale that would qualify as "comprehensive" or "significant."

In all five cases, the government reform was helped by fiscal crisis albeit in different ways. The fiscal crisis of the early 1990s helped the governments of Alberta and Saskatchewan to open the reform windows in the regionalization and needs-based cases. Premiers were able to point to recently secured democratic mandates for these reforms and the need for speedy action due to crisis. In the Quebec drug case, the government committed to reform during the election campaign and acted in the first half of its mandate. The decision to act was not supported by fiscal crisis, but the policy choice was heavily shaped by the government's determination to achieve fiscal balance.

Given the paucity of reform, it is not surprising to observe that the most engaged political actors were much more effective in preventing reform than in creating it. Actors who wanted to make a substantial change in the status quo would inevitably bump up against other actors who benefited from the existing arrangements. All interests and institutions played much better defence than offence.

NOTES

1. Deciding whether to publicly fund uninsured services (or to discontinue funding insured services) is classified as "program content."
2. The methodology also understates the extent of regionalization reform in Quebec since it essentially treats two offsetting reforms taken 12 years apart as a single reform.
3. A similar decomposition is provided for the categories of independent variables in Tables 8.3 to 8.7. In some cases a variable may help to explain why a reform occurred while in other cases that same factor may help explain why it did not occur. Indeed, some categories had both pro- and anti-reform elements within a single case, such as when some provider groups supported reform and others opposed it.
4. Changes of governing party: Newfoundland, 1989; Ontario, 1990 and 1995; Saskatchewan, 1991; Quebec, 1994 and 2003. Changes of leadership: Klein (Alberta Conservative), 1992; Daniel Johnson (Quebec Liberal), 1994; Lucien Bouchard and Bernard Landry (Parti Québécois), 1996 and 2001; Brian Tobin and Roger Grimes (Newfoundland and Labrador Liberal), 1996 and 2001; and Lorne Calvert (Saskatchewan NDP), 2001. We have excluded newly formed governments in the second half of 2003 (on the grounds that there was insufficient time to do reforms given our cut-off date of December 2003).
5. The line between policy entrepreneur and policy network is sometimes hazy. For our purposes, policy advisors who interact intensively with government on one issue over a relatively short period may be seen as entrepreneurs. If the relationship covers several issues and is not time-limited, this may be a policy network.
6. The discussion here focuses on hospital interests at the provincial level. While national bodies including the Canadian Hospital Association (until 1995) and the Health Action Lobby (a coalition of 35 national health organizations that represented a broad cross-section of health providers, health regions, hospitals, and other institutions) were active on some issues, their focus was on Canada-wide issues, especially federal government funding.
7. Based on one author's observation while inside government.
8. A study done for the Romanow Commission helps us to understand, indirectly, why this was so (Mendelsohn 2002, 2). The study distinguished among four aspects of public opinion. One was medicare as a symbol of identity. The other three were medicare's core principles, recent performance, and future. It is not a surprise that public opinion about medicare as

a symbol, or about medicare's core principles, did not have a major role in the 15 case studies on regionalization, needs-based funding, and alternative payment plans. Those three policy reform issues had few implications for the idea of medicare as a symbol or for its core principles (i.e., key features of the model). What is more interesting is that these results also applied to the role of public opinion on medicare's recent performance and future prospects.

9. The wait-times issue provides an example of the exceptions. The governments of Alberta under Klein and Saskatchewan under Calvert took fundamentally different decisions based on similar facts. Alberta chose to allow physicians the choice of whether or not to become affiliated with its system of wait-list management. Saskatchewan made its system mandatory.

10. Mendelsohn (2002) cites Daniel Yankelovich, *Coming to Public Judgment: Making Democracy Work in a Complex World* (Syracuse: Syracuse University Press, 1991).

11. Tracking some of these same polls beyond the time period Mendelsohn covered suggests that the public's assessment of the health system reached its low watermark in 2004 and has since recovered significantly (discussed further in chapter 11).

12. Tuohy's (1999) focus was to show how differences in consolidation of power between the United States relative to Canada and the United Kingdom influenced the trajectory of reform. If we were comparing Canadian reform to reform in a country with a weak justice system, then differences in the role of law might explain different reform outcomes.

13. This comparison to earlier periods is discussed in chapters 10 and 12.

14. There is also an argument that the *Canada Health Act* and related provincial health insurance law were important influences in narrowing the range of the possible. This we leave for the last chapter.

15. Hereafter the textual references to medical associations include the two Quebec medical unions.

16. MOHLTC-OMA 2000 Agreement, Appendix A.

17. In Quebec and some other provinces, there were separate agreements for interns.

18. This includes three factors attributed three "public service champions."

19. Her view is shared by both Duane Adams and Duncan Sinclair (Adams 2001a; Sinclair, Rochon, and Leatt 2005, 222-25).

CHAPTER 9

PATTERNS IN THE FACTORS THAT EXPLAIN HEALTH-CARE POLICY REFORM

HARVEY LAZAR AND JOHN CHURCH

We turn next to the question of whether there were patterns in the variables associated with reform. Is it possible to account for differences in the kind and extent of reform across provinces based on differences in the factors identified in chapter 8? For example, why was there more reform in Saskatchewan than Newfoundland? What explained the similarities in the extent of reform between Alberta and Saskatchewan? Were there also differences? What about issues? Were there patterns across issues? Was it easier (or more difficult) to reform some kinds of policy issues than others and, if so, what accounted for the differences?

The section immediately below notes some similarities in the politics and policies of the five provinces studied. We then turn to political and policy differences between four pairs of provinces. The comparisons are instrumental—selected because they reinforce, clarify, or add to the factors identified in chapter 8 as key explanatory variables that helped to account for reform decisions. We compare the two provinces that accomplished the most and the least reform; two social democratic governments; two conservative governments; and a social democratic government and a conservative government.

The third section compares and contrasts the factors associated with our six reform issues. It begins by separating the 30 cases into two groups: the 14 cases of moderate, significant, and comprehensive reform (collectively referred to as "substantial" reform) and the 16 cases of limited or no reform. We did this on the reasonable assumption that the mix of factors associated with cases of substantial reforms might be different than the mix associated with cases of limited or no reform. That turned out to be the case.

We also divided the 14 cases in three ways to determine if there were patterns among these cases. For example, was there a difference among the factors that explained policy reform decisions on issues that touched people directly (seven cases) and those that did not touch the public directly (also seven cases)? Was there a difference in factors associated with counter-consensus reforms (two cases) and consensus reforms (12 cases)? Finally, we also examined whether it was useful to distinguish between "political" and "technical" issues.

SOME SIMILARITIES AMONG PROVINCES

Canada is a country of much diversity. Canada's 10 provinces and three territories vary greatly in history, culture, population size, ethnicity, geographic expanse, economic structure, and socioeconomic well-being. While differences among the 13 jurisdictions are vast,[1] the impact of the diversity lens can sometimes be overstated. Other large countries are diverse.[2] Moreover, much of Canada's diversity is within jurisdictions, not between them. We begin therefore by noting some of the political and policy commonalties among jurisdictions that have special relevance for our purposes.

One similarity was the public's attachment to universal, publicly financed hospital and medical insurance—the medicare legacy. A study of public opinion for the Romanow Commission that examined "thousands of polling questions" found that, with respect to the medicare legacy, "inter-regional similarities far outweigh any minor differences of opinion" (Mendelsohn 2002, 20).

A second similarity was a large and growing concern of provincial governments about the effects of medicare on their finances. This led all five provinces to appoint at least one major commission, task force, or similar body to help point the way forward. The terms of reference for the first-wave reports as well as the reports themselves showed the similarity of conditions. They focused on issues of public finance and cost containment, governance and accountability, as well as delivery issues. Second-wave reports stressed long-term sustainability (as opposed to immediate and short-term cost containment), accountability and transparency, and issues related to access and quality. With relative consistency, reform of primary health care was viewed as a fundamental next step in health-care delivery reforms and the "foundation" of the health-care system (O'Fee 2002a).

Third, in response to concerns about health-care costs, the five provinces more or less froze per capita health-care spending from 1991 to 1996 (a period of "retrenchment and disinvestment" according to CIHI). Oversimplifying, the result was to flat-line the growth of health-care resources while doing little to slow demand. This led to a growing gap between demand and supply that was reflected in longer wait times for some specialists and procedures, pressure on emergency rooms, and demoralized health-care professionals.

Fourth, after the freeze, provincial government expenditure again rose rapidly (CIHI 2012, 3). The longer-term prognostications were for demand to increase in all provinces at a rate that exceeded population growth and inflation (Commission on the Future of Health Care 2002, xvii). New technologies and new drugs promised an improved quality of life for many people, including the growing number with chronic conditions. Partly as a result of these new procedures and medications, population aging was expected to continue with effects on cost. With a better informed public, thanks in part to the Internet, public expectations were also on the rise.

Finally, all provinces shared a desire to recoup the federal dollars, notionally intended for health care, which the 1995 federal budget had removed from their coffers. The federal/provincial numbers war was waged for almost a decade. The provinces argued that the federal government was not paying its "fair share" of provincial program costs. The debate was not so much about what would constitute "fair" but rather how much Ottawa was actually contributing. At the extreme, this included provincial claims that the federal government had cut its financial contribution to provincial health care from the 50/50 cost-sharing principle to just over 10 percent (Provincial and Territorial Ministers of Health 2000, 3). Premiers assessed substantive health-care reform ideas coming from Ottawa mainly in terms of their effects on the bottom lines of provincial and territorial governments. Outside of health care, provincial and territorial governments attacked smaller federal spending initiatives in areas of provincial constitutional competence as "boutique" programs. They argued that these initiatives were being financed out of the money that Ottawa had unreasonably and arbitrarily taken from them in its 1995 budget. The federal government, for its part, insisted that taxes that provinces had been levying for 20 years were still part of the federal contribution (Lazar, St-Hilaire, and Tremblay 2004b).

In some sense the 2004 First Ministers' Health Accord signalled that the provinces had won the war of attrition. The identity of the losers is less clear. While interpretations may vary, it is arguable that Ottawa did not fare badly. Its debt position was many billions of dollars less than it would have been had it acknowledged in 2000 or 2001 what it did accept as a fair result in 2004. More plausibly, the need for health-care reform got the short end of the stick. The valuable time of first ministers, finance ministers, health ministers, and intergovernmental ministers, and some of their most talented public servants was genuinely wasted on a war of numbers.

EXPLAINING DIFFERENCES AMONG PROVINCES

The discussion focuses on differences between four pairs of provinces: the province that did the most reform and the one that did the least; two left-of-centre social democratic governments; a social democratic and a conservative government; and two right-of-centre conservative governments. The governments in each pair are assessed for roughly the same years. One consequence of holding time constant is that some issues are excluded in some of the comparisons. For example, Alberta and Saskatchewan are compared on wait times because the issue reached the governmental agenda of these two provinces at roughly the same time. The same issue is excluded from the Ontario-Saskatchewan comparison because the decisions were taken more than a decade apart and under very different conditions.

The order in which the pairs are presented is from "most different" to "least different."

Saskatchewan and Newfoundland and Labrador: The Most Versus the Least Reform

On four out of six issues we studied (regionalization, needs-based funding, for-profit delivery, and wait times), Saskatchewan's reforms were assessed as "significant" or higher. Newfoundland undertook reform in only one of the six cases. How is this difference explained?

In the decades preceding our study period, these two provinces had much in common. Both were "small provinces" even though Saskatchewan's population was almost double that of Newfoundland and Labrador. Both had experienced stagnant or declining population. The economic well-being of both provinces was linked to commodity prices. Saskatchewan's per capita income was roughly equal to the national average but highly volatile (due in significant measure to the volatility of commodity markets). Newfoundland and Labrador's per capita income was the lowest in the country.

Further, in both provinces in the early 1990s, there was an open reform window. Both provinces had newly formed first-time governments and faced large fiscal crises. In chapter 8, we called the first of these factors "change in government, or leader of a governing party, that committed to reform during the election campaign or leadership contest that first brought the newly formed government to power, and that acted expeditiously on its commitments after assuming office." Hereafter, for simplicity, we refer to this factor as "change in government/ leader." The second factor was referred to as "fiscal crisis/near fiscal crisis" (hereafter "fiscal crisis"). We also distinguished between two stages in the reform process: the governmental and decision phases (combined) and the policy choice phase. We observed that when these two variables were present in the governmental and decision phases, a policy window could open. Whether reform actually took place depended, then, on other factors. This brings us to the differences between the two provinces.

A major difference was in the political priority that the two newly elected governments attached to health care. When the Clyde Wells–led Liberal Party of Newfoundland and Labrador defeated the Progressive Conservatives in 1989, the Liberal Party came to office for the first time since the early 1970s. The province was just beginning to grasp the magnitude of the crisis in the northern cod fishery. Within a few years Ottawa would close the fishery completely, hoping that this might eventually lead to a recovery in the fish stock. The priority for the provincial Liberals was to deal with the massive adjustment process for those who had earned their living in the fishery, especially fishers who lived in isolated outports where there were no local alternative employment prospects. The Wells government made no significant health-related promises during the 1989 or 1993 election campaigns and, in the context of the economic challenges it faced, did not treat health care as a priority once in government.

In contrast, the Saskatchewan NDP had made health care a political priority during its opposition years. As opposition health critic from 1986 to 1991, Louise Simard had attended many of the public meetings of the Saskatchewan Commission on Directions in Health Care (the Murray Commission), which had been appointed by the provincial Conservative government. This kept Simard in touch with both expert and public opinion. The NDP election platform identified the "wellness" concept as a strategic orientation. On winning government, Premier Romanow appointed Simard as his first minister of health and made wellness a fundamental priority. Under her leadership, Saskatchewan Health (1992) laid out key elements of what wellness might mean in *A Saskatchewan Vision for Health: A Framework for Change.* Knowing the direction it wished to travel was no small detail given the fiscal crisis the government inherited. While Premier Romanow would have doubtless preferred to assume office without threats of provincial government bankruptcy, for a government that knew its destination, the fiscal crisis created an opportunity.

The difference in political priority attached to health care was not just a peculiarity of the moment, but can be traced to Newfoundland and Labrador's entry into Confederation in 1949. The leader of the pro-Confederation forces and subsequently the province's first premier, Joey Smallwood, had stressed to the people the social benefits that would accrue to them if they entered Confederation. In health care, this paid off in several ways. In 1961 there was one physician for every 1,991 persons living in Newfoundland and Labrador. The national average at that time was one physician for 857 persons. By 1980 the comparable figures were 674 and 544 (Parliamentary Task Force 1981, 103). In other words, the physician-to-population ratio in Newfoundland and Labrador jumped from 43 percent of the national average to 80 percent of the national average during a period when the national average was itself improving swiftly. The number of physicians in the province more than tripled over those two decades.[3] Much of this improvement was due to the federal government's fiscal support. That support came in three distinct federal programs.

One was the federal government's contribution to the capital cost of creating Newfoundland and Labrador's first and only medical school. Established in the second half of the 1960s, the medical school at Memorial University awarded its first medical degrees in 1973. The federal contribution was made through the Health Resources Fund based on the recommendation of the Royal Commission on Health Services, also known as the Hall Commission, established in 1961. Second were the federal government's cost-sharing arrangements with provinces for hospital and medical expenditures. Regardless of the federal financing formula (whether hospital insurance, medical insurance, Established Programs Financing, or Canada Health and Social Transfer), Ottawa covered a higher percentage of the provincial health-care expenditures of less affluent provinces than wealthier ones. For example, the federal contribution covered 66 percent of Newfoundland and Labrador's eligible hospital expenses at the beginning of the 1960s (Carter 1971, 122). Fifteen years later, just prior to the introduction of Established Programs Financing (EPF), the federal share of Newfoundland and Labrador's hospital and medical insurance program was still 58 percent (Taylor 2009, 426-27). Under EPF, the tax transfer portion of the new transfer program for the provinces was equalized to the national average. This preserved a continued measure of preference for Newfoundland and Labrador and other less wealthy provinces. Third was the federal Equalization program. It transferred large sums annually to Newfoundland and Labrador on an unconditional basis.

The evidence suggests that health care did not receive priority from Newfoundland and Labrador governments for three reasons. First, the province had to manage a massive adjustment challenge associated with the fishery closure. Second, the improvements in health services within the province since the 1960s were large and palpable. Third, the federal "generosity" to Newfoundland and Labrador and other "have not" provinces did not appear through magic. It was the product of intensive and ongoing pressure from the governments of the Atlantic provinces including the government of Newfoundland and Labrador on whatever government was in power in Ottawa (Finance Canada 1996). In this perspective much of whatever priority the government of Newfoundland and Labrador attached to health care was focused on intergovernmental diplomacy rather than "domestic" affairs.

As a result, Newfoundland and Labrador acted on only one issue—regionalization—and not as part of a larger health reform strategy but as a potential money saver. Regionalization was a "one off" measure to integrate services and increase efficiencies. Regionalization was not divisive among the people of the province, although not happily received by most hospitals in St. John's. Needs-based funding and alternative payment plans (APP) for primary care physicians reached the governmental agenda, but the government decided not to undertake reform in either. In the former, the Newfoundland and Labrador Hospital and Nursing Home Association urged reform, but ministers chose to retain the status quo—control of spending in their own hands. In the latter, a group of physicians doing a pilot project encouraged reform, but the government appears to have concluded that this would cost more than the status quo. Other issues did not make it to the governmental agenda (for-profit delivery) or just barely touched it (prescription drugs).

The history and reform outcomes were different in Saskatchewan. The CCF, the predecessor of the Saskatchewan NDP, had been the first government to introduce publicly financed, universal hospital and medical insurance in Canada in part because the people of that province were so conscious of health system failures in the 1930s. The CCF government did so twice without assurances that the federal government would eventually cost share. Once it had introduced a provincially funded program, of course, the Saskatchewan government stood to benefit financially through federal cost sharing.

The Romanow government built on this legacy with a long-term strategy centred on the wellness concept (Saskatchewan Health 1992). The NDP strategy called for regionalization of health services and then restructuring the hospital/institutional system and primary care system. The new regional health authorities (RHAs) would be the driving force to implement these new policy directions. The reality was somewhat "messier" with the sequencing not always following the "textbook." Nonetheless, much was accomplished.

A part of this messiness was that regionalization did not occur in a political vacuum. Even though regionalization was supposed to come first, drug benefits were being cut (contrary to what the NDP platform had signalled) and hospitals were being closed or converted into "wellness centres" as the process of regionalization unfolded. In a nutshell, instead of creating RHAs first and leaving them to do all the "dirty work" of rationalization, the two tracks ran to some degree in parallel. And while the public was consulted, the consultations did not go on for long. Reducing drug benefits and closing or regrouping hospitals were not popular decisions. It was perhaps asking too much to expect people to welcome these changes as the price to be paid for a more effective and efficient medicare system that was some distance into the future.

How, then, did the Saskatchewan government overcome this inevitable resistance? The obvious link between the NDP's historical role in "inventing" medicare and public support for medicare may partially explain why so much reform happened so swiftly. But more important was the fact that the NDP was well prepared and had a narrative to help market its ideas. The fiscal crisis also played a huge role in supplying much-needed political cover for those decisions. Had that spur to swift and decisive action not been present, there is at least a question as to whether the government would have been able to secure the necessary support within its own caucus and among the ranks of its supporters without slowing down and "watering down" its reforms. The crisis forced Premier Romanow out of the starting gate from day one of his mandate. A telling remark in this regard was attributed to the health minister of British Columbia at the time: "You folks have one thing going for you that we don't and I envy you for it.... The fact that people in Saskatchewan know that you're in a desperate financial situation and seem prepared to, you know, make some sacrifices if that had to be done.... In B.C. nobody believes that we're financially strapped" (McIntosh, Ducie, and England 2007, 11).

A new majority government and fiscal crisis in both provinces opened a reform window. But to take advantage of the opening, other factors had to be present. Each of the following was present in Saskatchewan but not in Newfoundland and Labrador. First, prior to the general election that brought it to power, the opposition NDP made health care a priority, included that priority strategy in its election platform, and promoted the strategy during the electoral process.[4] Second, once elected, the "appointment" of a political champion, an excellent partnership between the political executive and senior public servants, and swift action helped to make the pre-election commitments tangible. With a political commitment, a policy champion, and a smoothly functioning relationship between political executive and public service, the government was able to take advantage of the open reform window and make significant reforms before the window closed. These differences are reflected in Table 9.1. The two *P*s in the column "change in government/leader" for the regionalization reflect the above discussion; that is, both factors associated with the change in government/leader category were present for Saskatchewan. This was also the case for needs-based funding in Saskatchewan. The empty cells in this column for Newfoundland and Labrador signify that these same factors were not present there.

The factors that influenced the reform of two other issues—for-profit delivery and wait times—also differed between the two provinces. The Romanow government made itself somewhat unpopular with its own rank and file due to the disruption and hardship associated with reforms during its first term. At the beginning of its second term, the government introduced legislation to make for-profit delivery for hospitals and clinics a financially impractical proposition. The pressure for this originated with political insiders, possibly the premier, as a way of re-establishing the bona fides of the NDP government with its supporters. The fact that this issue was receiving a lot of attention in neighbouring Alberta gave the issue some profile. There was no comparable action in Newfoundland and Labrador. Being a small province with relatively low income, there were no commercial firms looking to open for-profit hospitals in that

TABLE 9.1
Influence of Major Factors on Reform by Category
Saskatchewan (1991–2003) vs. Newfoundland and Labrador (1989–2003)

		EXOGENOUS				EXOGENOUS/ENDOGENOUS			ENDOGENOUS
		Change in Govt/ Leader	*Fiscal Crisis*	*Public Opinion/ Civil Society*	*Media*	*Values*	*Knowledge*	*Institutions*	*Insider Interests*
SK	**1991–2003**								
1	Significant	PP	P			P			A
2	Significant	PP	P			P	P	P	P
3	Limited	P	P	M					PA
4	Significant					P			P
5	Significant			PP	P	P	PP	P	P
6	Counter-consensus limited		C						
NL	**1989–2003**								
1	Moderate								PA
2	None							A	AA
3	None		A						
4	None								
5	None								AA
6	None		A						

Notes:

The six issues/case studies are as follows:

1 = regionalization
2 = needs-based funding
3 = alternative payment plans
4 = for-profit delivery
5 = wait-times management
6 = drug coverage

The letters indicate the direction of reform. Two reform letters in a cell mean that there were two major reform independent variables in the same category. If an issue is not known to have reached the governmental agenda, cells are empty.

P = pro-reform
A = anti-reform
M = mediating between pro- and anti-reform factors
C = favoured counter-consensus reform

province. The table thus shows a *P* under "insider interests" for that issue in Saskatchewan. The comparable cell is empty for Newfoundland and Labrador.

The issue of wait times was on the governmental agenda in most provinces by the late 1990s or early 2000s. In Saskatchewan, public opinion and civil society pressures put it on the governmental agenda. There was no comparable public pressure in Newfoundland and Labrador. The outcome in Saskatchewan involved much technical policy work, which is reflected under the knowledge and institutions (policy community) columns. In Newfoundland and Labrador cardiac surgeons began to coordinate on a voluntary basis, a relatively easy task since they were few in number and lived in St. John's, the only place where such procedures were undertaken in the province.

Saskatchewan and Ontario: Comparing Two Social Democratic Governments

The point of comparison here is between the Ontario NDP government of Bob Rae (1990–1995) and the first NDP Romanow government in Saskatchewan (1991–1995). Both shared a social democratic left-of-centre philosophy. Both came to office in very difficult fiscal conditions. But the Ontario government decided on only one issue—drug coverage—whereas the Saskatchewan government decided on five.

The Rae government modestly expanded drug coverage with the creation of the Ontario Trillium Drug Program. This decision was taken in the months leading up to the 1995 general election under strong pressure from civil society groups. In contrast, the Saskatchewan NDP cut its drug program substantially in a series of decisions between 1991 and 1993. Perhaps the main factor that explains the difference in direction was timing. The worst of the fiscal crisis in Ontario was over when Rae acted, whereas the Romanow government was "forced" to act when the Saskatchewan crisis was at or near its peak. There were also institutional considerations at work in Saskatchewan. It was easier to cut prescription drug benefits than hospital or medical budgets. Federal hospital and medical transfers required provinces to cover first-dollar expenditures (no deductibles), and there was no such constraint on drug expenditures. Moreover, there were insider interests that would have to be dealt with if hospital budgets or medical tariffs were cut. There was no comparable lobby for consumers of prescription drugs.

On all the other issues except wait times (which did not become a pressing concern in Saskatchewan until the second half of the 1990s), the Saskatchewan NDP accomplished significantly more reform than the social democrats in Ontario. The Romanow government acted swiftly on regionalization with the goal of making the system better coordinated and more efficient. The fiscal crisis spurred the government to close or merge hospitals, whereas in Ontario the fiscal crisis was perceived as an obstacle. The Saskatchewan NDP was able to use the fiscal crisis as cover for tough political decisions because the party had a coherent, long-term strategy on winning office. The Ontario NDP did not. The NDP in Saskatchewan faced a decimated and weak opposition. The NDP in Ontario did not.

The Ontario NDP made an explicit decision not to regionalize. In so doing, it effectively precluded the idea of needs-based funding since such funding was premised on some form of geographic division in the administration of health services. Neither issue had a champion within the government at the political or civil service level. The Ontario Hospital Association and Ontario Medical Association were opposed. The Rae government reached the view that regionalization would be particularly difficult in a context of deficit reduction. One reason was that needs-based funding would be a natural corollary of regionalization. Given the fiscal circumstances, needs-based funding would have had to be a zero-sum game. In turn, that game would have meant politically difficult, absolute cuts to some regions.

The Saskatchewan Medical Association (SMA) did not challenge the early decisions of the Romanow government. Where it did draw the line was in the government's plans to eliminate fee-for-service (FFS) for primary care physicians as a necessary precondition for primary care reform. By the time the government was ready to tackle this issue, its first mandate was no longer fresh. The threat of provincial bankruptcy had also receded. Both factors meant that the reform window of 1991 was almost shut. The timing was no longer right for taking on the doctors in a political battle. The province had become health-care weary. The government had established an Alternative Payment Unit that undertook pilot projects, but it lacked traction with the SMA. Well before the 1995 general election, the government had concluded that any changes in the method of compensating primary care physicians would have to be voluntary. [5]

In Ontario, the question of APPs for primary care physicians was part of an ongoing dialogue between the Ontario Medical Association (OMA) and the governments of the era: the Peterson Liberals, the NDP under Rae, and then the Mike Harris–led Progressive Conservatives. Some voluntary initiatives flowed from the dialogue, but the issue of APPs was not a focal point of decision-making while the Rae government was in power. It negotiated a five-year contract agreement with the OMA in 1991 that included provision for a Joint Management Committee of ministry officials and OMA representatives to oversee the contract and manage the relationship. Despite the agreement, the ongoing relationship was adversely influenced by the fiscal context, including on physician remuneration. In 1994, the government received a report commissioned by the Conference of Federal-Provincial-Territorial Ministers of Health recommending the elimination of fee-for-service (Gafni, Birch, and

O'Brien 1994). Our research does not indicate whether it was discussed in cabinet, but we do know that the OMA was pressing for improvement in the fee-for-service schedule.

To account for these differences in reform, we need only replicate the factors that were present in Saskatchewan but not in Newfoundland and Labrador: these same factors were also absent in Ontario. First, prior to the general election that brought it to power, the opposition Saskatchewan NDP had made health care a priority, included its strategy in its election platform, and then promoted the strategy during the electoral process. Second, once elected, the appointment of a political champion, the strong relationship between ministers and the public service, and speed from the starting line made quick decision-making possible.

While it may at first glance seem unusual that a social democratic government in relatively affluent Ontario would have more in common with a Liberal government in relatively low-income Newfoundland and Labrador than with another social democratic government, there were at least four reasons for these differences between the Saskatchewan NDP and its Ontario cousins. First, the Saskatchewan NDP knew well in advance of the 1991 election call that it would likely win office, thanks to the self-destruction of the Progressive Conservative government led by Grant Devine and the very weak third-party status of the Liberals. The Ontario NDP had no expectation of forming a government when the 1990 general election was called (Rae 1996, 144 and 244). Second, there was a big difference in experience. From the time that Tommy Douglas led the social democratic CCF to victory in 1944 until the general election of 1991, the CCF and then the NDP (the successor to the CCF) had been the governing party in Saskatchewan two-thirds of the time. Romanow's first government marked the ninth time the CCF/NDP had succeeded at the polls. The Rae government was Ontario's first social democratic government, and it was sorely lacking hands-on experience in governing. The third difference was in some ways an extension of the second. The Romanow government had an excellent relationship with senior officials in Saskatchewan Health. Where the relationships were lacking, the government knew from previous experience how to fill gaps swiftly. Romanow appointed a deputy minister of health from outside the public service within weeks of achieving power. The Rae government found it difficult to create a comparable partnership with the Ontario Public Service (Rae 1996, 151-54). Rae gradually brought in fresh resources, but that took time. It was nine months after winning office that Rae appointed a new deputy minister of health from outside the public service. The interaction of these three factors was reflected in many of the political difficulties the Ontario government encountered in its first year in office and beyond.

Fourth, the Romanow government used the grey literature. It borrowed from the Murray report (Saskatchewan Commission on Directions in

Health Care 1990) that had been commissioned by the Devine government and massaged it to its needs. It brought in researchers from outside the province where such expertise was available. This was notably the case with needs-based funding. For these and other reasons, the Saskatchewan NDP had a vision of where it was headed and something of a road map about how to get there. The Rae government ignored the grey literature. Although much of that literature had its origins in Ontario academe, for whatever reasons it did not catch the eye of the government. Reports that originated in the Peterson years were not taken up by the NDP. The three building blocks in the Saskatchewan strategy—regionalization, needs-based funding, and a focus on alternative payment plans for primary care physicians—were not adopted by the Ontario NDP. These issues had no internal champions. They were someone else's agenda.

By the middle of his term, Rae was caught up in negotiations with public service unions that ended in an impasse. The Ontario legislature enacted the terms of the "Social Contract" without union agreement. By that time, too, it was clear that Ontario had one further item in common with Newfoundland and Labrador. The economy was the priority, and wrestling with the deficit was part of what needed to be done. What the Rae government then wanted from the Ministry of Health was much better control of spending, which in fact it did deliver.

The differences in reform and the explanations for the differences are summarized in Table 9.2. More than any other factor, the numerous empty cells for Ontario reflect the differences in the governmental agendas of the two governments.

Saskatchewan and Alberta: Comparing Social Democratic and Conservative Regimes

Of the five provinces studied, Alberta had the second most reform. Whereas social democracy had deep roots in Saskatchewan soil, economic and social conservatism had equally deep roots in Alberta, maybe deeper. Yet some of the reforms the two governments adopted were very similar. Both assigned to regional health authorities the task of coordination and delivery of hospital and other institutional services. Both adopted a new method of funding the regions (and hence hospitals and other institutions) that was broadly alike. Neither accepted the idea of eliminating fee-for-service (FFS), and both made a place for APPs as a mode of payment that individual physicians might choose. On APPs, the Alberta Medical Association was a policy entrepreneur with the government eventually following, while in Saskatchewan the Romanow government led the reform but eventually backed off because of strong opposition from the SMA.

TABLE 9.2
Influence of Major Factors on Reform by Category
Saskatchewan (1991–1995) vs. Ontario (1990–1995)

		EXOGENOUS				EXOGENOUS/ENDOGENOUS			ENDOGENOUS
		Change in Govt/Leader	Fiscal Crisis	Public Opinion/ Civil Society	Media	Values	Knowledge	Institutions	Insider Interests
SK	**1991–1995**								
1	Significant	PP	P			P			A
2	Significant	PP	P			P	P		P
3	Limited	P	P	M					PA
4	Significant					P			P
6	Counter-consensus limited		C						
ON	**1990–1995**								
1	None		A						
2	None								
3	None								M
4	None					P			
6	Moderate		A	P		P			M

Notes:
The issues/case studies are as follows:
1 = regionalization
2 = needs-based funding
3 = alternative payment plans
4 = for-profit delivery
6 = drug coverage
The table excludes wait times as this issue was dealt with in Ontario just prior to the NDP winning office, and it did not become a big issue in Saskatchewan until the second half of the 1990s.

The letters indicate the direction of reform. Two reform letters in a cell mean that there were two major reform independent variables in the same category. If an issue is not known to have reached the governmental agenda, cells are empty.
P = pro-reform
A = anti-reform
M = mediating between pro- and anti-reform factors
C = favoured counter-consensus reform

Although these three reforms were similar, there were some differences in motivation. Premier Klein came to power espousing a policy of rapid deficit elimination and debt reduction. Alberta announced huge cuts in health spending including in physician remuneration and then took policy decisions to give substance to the deficit targets. These decisions included regionalization and population-based funding. As outlined in chapter 3, the government determined fiscal targets and then introduced legislation for the disestablishment of 200 local hospital, public health, and continuing care boards with provision to replace them with 17 new regional health authorities (RHAs) and two provincewide health authorities. The new RHAs, appointed by the government, were required to achieve efficiencies by rationalizing existing institutions. The new funding model was left to the experts. The cut in physician pay was arbitrary, not designed to change incentive structures or pave the way to primary care reform. Klein was focused on the bottom line first and foremost.

Much of the Klein government's enthusiasm for fiscal restraint terminated with the rebound in oil prices in the second half of the 1990s. The Alberta government had cut health-care spending more sharply than other provinces. With its coffers replenished, the Alberta government increased its expenditures as oil prices took off (CIHI 2012, Table B.4.2). Thereafter, apart from Klein's passion for more private for-profit delivery, the political will to support further significant policy changes in health care evaporated. Thus, as already noted, it was the Alberta Medical Association (AMA) that proposed to the government that physicians in Alberta should have a choice about mode of payment and not be confined to fee-for-service. Although the government resisted, the AMA proposal remained on the table and eventually led to APPs on a pilot project basis.

Romanow left office in 2001 and was replaced by Lorne Calvert. Calvert won a fresh mandate in 2003 and was defeated in 2007. In 2008, Klein resigned. Of the six issues we have studied, the pattern was set on three issues—regionalization, needs-based funding, and APPs—during the first elected terms of the Klein and Romanow governments. Their accomplishments were also roughly comparable.

In the above comparisons between Saskatchewan and Newfoundland and Labrador, and between Saskatchewan and Ontario, a number of key factors found in Saskatchewan were not present in the other two provinces. Klein's government, however, had most of them: quickly restoring the fiscal balance was a priority, and this could not be done without a plan for health care. During the 1993 election campaign, Klein promised health reforms. Once elected, his government immediately organized roundtables to discuss and lay out a health-care strategy. Klein himself was a policy entrepreneur when it came to selling expenditure cuts and the need for restructuring. Like Romanow, he too went through the starting gate quickly. The sole area where Alberta lagged Saskatchewan was in relations with the public service. Where the Romanow government developed a strong relationship with Saskatchewan Health, Klein was actively trying to do away with much of the Ministry of Health. Yet, our case studies suggest that the Klein government was effectively served by its public service.

The difference in ideology showed in the other three issues: prescription drugs, for-profit delivery, and wait times. The government of Saskatchewan cut prescription drug benefits while the government of Alberta expanded its drug program. But the timing of the Saskatchewan decision dictated its outcome. The Alberta decision was taken well after oil prices had bounced back and the government was running a budgetary surplus. The Alberta decision to make two minimal reforms in prescription drugs reflected its attachment to the idea of the residual state. The beneficiaries of these small changes—families with children that were making the transition from welfare to work, and end-of-life patients in palliative care settings—suggest that the government was not trying to save the treasury from further claims but to emphasize the importance of self-reliance.

With respect to for-profit delivery, Klein pressed hard to create more room for private for-profit delivery with modest results at best. Romanow brought in legislation early in his second term to make it practically impossible for private for-profit hospitals and clinics to start up in Saskatchewan. Romanow took his anti-for-profit delivery legislation further than Klein did his for-profit delivery policies.

Both governments worked hard to achieve a workable way of tracking wait times. Alberta introduced a voluntary, publicly accessible, Internet-based wait-list registry in 2003. The intention was to provide all stakeholders, including patients, with accurate and understandable information so that they could make smart choices about where and how to access the necessary services. The voluntary aspect of the registry ensured that individual physicians were not coerced to surrender control over local information about wait times. Saskatchewan chose to create a centralized and mandatory management instrument for surgical care. Romanow's government came very close to meeting the grey literature definition of "comprehensive" reform on wait times whereas the Klein government chose a limited reform that fit with its culture.

The similarities and differences are shown in Table 9.3.

Alberta and Ontario: Comparing Two Conservative Regimes

The Progressive Conservative Party of Alberta had been in power for 30 years when Ralph Klein became premier. It was a one-party province at the provincial level and equally conservative in federal elections. Although the Progressive Conservative (PC) Party of Ontario had held office without interruption for over 40 years—from 1943 until 1985—by

TABLE 9.3
Influence of Major Factors on Reform by Category
Saskatchewan (1991–2003) vs. Alberta (1992–2003)

		EXOGENOUS				EXOGENOUS/ENDOGENOUS			ENDOGENOUS
		Change in Govt/ Leader	Fiscal Crisis	Public Opinion/ Civil Society	Media	Values	Knowledge	Institutions	Insider Interests
SK	**1991–2003**								
1	Significant	PP	P			P			A
2	Significant	PP	P			P	P	P	P
3	Limited	P	P	M					PA
4	Significant					P			P
5	Significant			PP	P	P	PP	P	P
6	Counter-consensus limited		C						
AB	**1992–2003**								
1	Significant	PP	P						
2	Significant	PP	P			P	P	P	P
3	Moderate		P					P	M
4	Counter-consensus limited			P		PC		P	C
5	Limited			P	P	C	P		M
6	Limited					C		P	

Notes:

The six issues/case studies are as follows:

1 = regionalization
2 = needs-based funding
3 = alternative payment plans
4 = for-profit delivery
5 = wait-times management
6 = drug coverage

The letters indicate the direction of reform. Two reform letters in a cell mean that there were two major reform independent variables in the same category. If an issue is not known to have reached the governmental agenda, cells are empty.

P = pro-reform
A = anti-reform
M = mediating between pro- and anti-reform factors
C = favoured counter-consensus reform

the time Mike Harris and the PCs were back in power, provincial politics in Ontario had become highly competitive. Indeed, in voting behaviour both provincially and federally, Ontario was a less conservative province than it had once been and less conservative than Alberta.

While the Alberta polity was more conservative than Ontario's, in the mid-1990s the Progressive Conservative parties of both provinces were close to one another in ideology: both endorsed lower taxes and smaller government as central to their purpose and vision. Neither party, in its first or second term of office, had in place all of the elements of a broad strategy for health care. Klein's first campaign had focused on things that needed doing in health care as a necessary corollary of fixing the fiscal balance. After the 1993 general election, a committee of the legislative assembly consulted publicly and provided Klein with a report (Alberta Health Planning Secretariat 1993) that emphasized that service delivery should concentrate on patient choice, integration of health services under unified governance and administrative structures, and greater opportunities for not-for-profit associations and private for-profit delivery. The report may have given the Klein government a sense of direction although not a road map.

Like the Alberta platform in 1993, the Harris government's Common Sense Revolution, which served as its platform in the 1995 general election, promised less spending on lower-priority items, cuts to welfare, and lower taxes. Unlike Alberta, however, it did not promise to cut health-care spending. Nor did it do so, although certain categories of expenditure were reduced.

During the nine years that the Ontario Progressive Conservatives were in power, the government undertook reforms in two of the six issues and acted on a third issue in a unique way that merits discussion. First is APP. Soon after taking office, the Harris government attacked the master agreement that the NDP had signed with the Ontario Medical Association (OMA) including its provision for joint management. The government initially attempted to negotiate separate arrangements with different groups of doctors rather than dealing with all the physicians in one contract through the OMA. It took about 18 months for relations between the Harris government and the OMA to settle. While these issues were being worked through, the government was considering alternative approaches to primary care as a result of several reports recommending reforms. In July 1996 the Ontario minister of health and the chair of the OMA Committee on Health Reform jointly announced pilot projects for capitation and reformed fee-for-service (FFS) as a basis for primary care reform. Two years later the minister of health and OMA president announced the launch of five pilot projects to evaluate the effectiveness of primary care networks. In 2000, the Ontario government and the OMA reached a new master agreement. It included two points of note in our context. First, it created incentives for family practitioners to join group practices that provided around-the-clock care seven days a week. Second, and equally significant, the money for the APP budget was taken from the FFS budget. This signalled in some sense that the new arrangements were becoming permanent. Once the FFS budget was tapped to pay for alternative payment arrangements, it would not be realistic politically to return the funds to the FFS budget.

In Alberta, in the context of dealing with large planned cuts in physician compensation, it was the medical association that proposed the idea of allowing individual physicians to have alternatives to the standard fee-for-service method of remuneration. The government was not enthused, but agreed to explore alternative payment plans after the AMA went public on the issue. The fact that a general election was on the horizon helps to explain the change in government position.

Key points in common between the Ontario and Alberta PCs in respect of APPs included the following: both governments had a rocky start in relations with their provincial medical associations; relations improved over time; the medical associations used forthcoming elections to improve their bargaining positions on issues relating to compensation including APPs; and in both cases the agreements were voluntary. The main difference was that Ontario developed its stance as an offshoot of a long-term plan to encourage primary care reform. In Alberta, the agreement was not linked in the same way. It was seemingly an end in itself.

In the health-care sphere the most controversial item tackled by both governments was for-profit delivery. Their successes and failures were roughly comparable as seen in Table 8.1, where the reforms are described as "counter-consensus moderate." The Ontario Progressive Conservatives chose to encourage private for-profit investments in diagnostic imaging to overcome shortfalls in the availability of MRIs and CT scanners in the province. In Alberta, the focus was on medical services and allowing private for-profit clinics. Both governments had a philosophic disposition to provide more opportunity to private for-profit enterprise. They also saw for-profit enterprise as a way to improve delivery without making a major call on their strained finances. The opportunity in both cases was due to technological changes. Services that had previously been delivered in hospitals, where they were covered by the *Canada Health Act*, could be provided "in free-standing clinics in the community, where physicians' services continued to be covered under medical care insurance but where patients were being charged additionally to cover operating and capital costs" (Gildiner 2006, 30).

Despite ideological similarity, the governments took different approaches to the task. Premier Klein, seemingly at times well ahead of his cabinet and caucus, took on for-profit delivery as a personal cause. This effectively meant that it was on the decision agenda from the time that Klein won his first majority in 1993. In conjunction with Klein's "in your face" style, the result was to guarantee that all opponents of for-profit delivery (mainly extra-legislative and led by the grassroots Friends of Medicare) were alerted and mobilized. The struggle forced Klein to withdraw policy proposals and legislation on more than one occasion. Finally, in 2000, the *Health Protection Act* (usually known as Bill 11) passed. It created a framework for some for-profit delivery of surgical services, a considerably narrower measure than his initial hopes.

In contrast, the Harris and Eves governments proceeded in a way that was less visible. They inherited the *Independent Health Facilities Act, 1989* (*IHFA*), a statute that regulated the growing number of free-standing clinics performing diagnostic services and, to a lesser extent, day surgeries in the province. The Progressive Conservative government introduced two sets of amendments to the statute—one in 1996 and the second in 2002. Both were embedded within much bigger legislative changes, which likely made the public less aware than it otherwise might have been. In 2002, seven years after the PCs assumed power, the government announced the names of the bidders that had been selected to provide new scanners. By that time Ernie Eves had replaced Mike Harris as premier.

Ontario's handling of this file was in contrast to its open and seemingly "no holds barred" approach to many other big files such as the forced amalgamations of cities, a tough approach to social assistance reform, and reductions in environmental regulation. In a nutshell, the Harris government was relatively cautious in its approach to for-profit delivery in view of the public's ongoing attachment to medicare and its readiness to pounce on any "faux pas." Ontario politics were more competitive than Alberta's, and this seems to have influenced its strategy.

The Harris PCs showed no public interest in regionalization, but they did believe that Ontario's hospital "system" was inefficient. It needed to be rationalized by closing uneconomic hospitals, merging others, and breaking down silos between delivery institutions that remained. Such actions, however, would create lots of "losers." While other provinces, including Alberta, established arm's-length regional health authorities, at least in part, to deflect political blame, Ontario chose a different path. Premier Harris appointed a Health Services Restructuring Commission, which differed from other provincial commissions and task forces in having the authority to restructure hospitals—to "direct" hospitals—and its directives were binding. The commission also recommended other changes in health care. By the end of its four-year term, the commission had made a difference. Many acute care hospitals in urban municipalities were consolidated. Following the commission's recommendations, the government invested in the "expansion of home-care services and the creation of more nursing-home places to accommodate hospitalized patients categorized as ... alternative level of care" (Sinclair, Rochon, and Leatt 2005, 2). The point of interest here is that the outcomes in some ways paralleled the restructuring (especially of acute care) in Alberta despite the difference in mechanism.

In sum, on the two (or three if hospital restructuring is included) items that both the Klein and Harris/Eves governments tackled, the extent of reform was roughly comparable (see Table 9.4). On APP, they were heavily influenced by their medical associations and ended up with broadly similar reforms. They used different mechanisms to rationalize the hospital sector, but again, the results were not markedly different. The results on for-profit delivery were also comparable.

The Klein government elected in 1993 had much more detailed plans for the health sector than the governments led by Harris and Eves. But once oil prices rebounded, the Alberta government eased up on its plans except for the premier's for-profit delivery dreams. As a government that preferred a small state, it appears to have been more than satisfied to manage issues one at a time once its fiscal crisis had passed. Its approach to drug reform was, we saw above, a reflection of its philosophy. In Ontario, the PC's 1995 election platform—the Common Sense Revolution—signalled a different approach to government than the Peterson and Rae governments that had preceded it. With its mandate, the Harris government was bold and determined in many areas of policy including social assistance and municipal government. But the Common Sense Revolution document said little about health care other than identifying it as a priority service. The PC government under Harris worked on health-care files one at a time without a seemingly clear destination. In this respect Ontario's approach was similar to Alberta's after oil and gas prices had improved. Both governments knew that there were limits to what they could do to move their health systems toward markets or market-like mechanisms for delivery. Even in provinces where there were right-of-centre governments, the commitment to the medicare legacy was powerful enough to limit a determined premier.

Discussion

These comparisons and earlier analyses suggest a few observations. First is that there was no simple gradient of most or least reform based on the wealth or size of a province. The poorest province (Newfoundland and Labrador) did the least reform, but a middle-income province (Saskatchewan) did the most. The two largest provinces (Ontario and Quebec) did less reform than two provinces that were smaller (Alberta and Saskatchewan) but more than the smallest (Newfoundland and Labrador).

Second, happenstance mattered. The political dynamics of a province influenced the time when issues reached, or did not reach, the governmental agenda (prescription drugs in Saskatchewan relative to Alberta) and influenced the substantive policy choices that were made.

TABLE 9.4
Influence of Major Factors on Reform by Category
Alberta (1991–2003) vs. Ontario (1995–2003)

		EXOGENOUS			EXOGENOUS/ENDOGENOUS			ENDOGENOUS
		Change in Govt/ Leader	*Fiscal Crisis*	*Public Opinion/ Civil Society*	*Media*	*Values*	*Knowledge*	*Institutions*	*Insider Interests*
AB	**1991–2003**								
1	Significant	PP	P						
2	Significant	PP	P			P	P	P	P
3	Moderate		P					P	M
4	Significant					P			C
5	Limited			P		C	P		M
6	Limited					C		P	
ON	**1995–2003**								
1	None								
2	None								
3	Moderate						PP	P	M
4	Moderate			P		PC			C
5	Moderate			P	P	P			
6	Moderate		A						

Notes:

The six issues/case studies are as follows:

1 = regionalization
2 = needs-based funding
3 = alternative payment plans
4 = for-profit delivery
5 = wait-times management
6 = drug coverage

The letters indicate the direction of reform. Two reform letters in a cell mean that there were two major reform independent variables in the same category. If an issue is not known to have reached the governmental agenda, cells are empty.
P = pro-reform
A = anti-reform
M = mediating between pro- and anti-reform factors
C = favoured counter-consensus reform

Third, other things equal, provincial governments that committed to reform and had a plan for reaching their objectives (Saskatchewan and Alberta in the first half of the 1990s) were more likely to achieve reforms than provinces that did not (Ontario and Newfoundland and Labrador in the same period).

Fourth, broad differences in governmental ideology mattered little to health policy reform outcomes on some issues (such as regionalization) but mattered more on others (such as for-profit delivery and wait times). Provincial governments with right-of-centre conservative orientations (Klein's second and third governments in Alberta and Ontario under Harris and Eves) had greater similarity of policy reform outcomes than provincial governments with left-of-centre social democratic orientations (Romanow's first government in Saskatchewan and Ontario under Rae).[6]

EXPLAINING DIFFERENCES AMONG ISSUES

Chapter 8 provided an aggregate analysis based on the assumption that the five provinces covered constituted a reasonable proxy for all of Canada and that the six issues were a representative sample of the challenges facing Canadian health care. The main question examined here is what kinds of factors were associated with different *kinds* of reform. The kinds of reform compared include

- those that touched Canadians directly (program content and delivery) and those that did not (governance and financial arrangements);
- counter-consensus (for-profit delivery) and consensus (the other five issues); and
- political (regionalization, APP, for-profit delivery, and drug coverage) and technical (needs-based funding and wait times).

Comparing Reforms That Touched Canadians Directly and Those That Did Not

When we began our research, we selected six issues for study with at least one in each of the four policy domains using the taxonomy outlined in chapter 2. At that time we did not make any assumptions about the patterns that might emerge from the analysis.

One intriguing finding emerged when we divided the 30 cases between the 14 cases of comprehensive, significant, and moderate reforms and the 16 cases of limited and no reform. For the latter group, the factors explaining the extent of reform were broadly similar. Endogenous variables, including insider interests, were paramount. Perhaps most surprising was the association between "major reports" and little or no reform. It was noted earlier that such reports often were written by persons with inside experience (former ministers and deputy ministers, for example), usually with research support from those with technical knowledge. It appears that many major reports gathered dust.

When we examined the factors associated with the 14 cases of comprehensive, significant, and moderate reform (hereafter "substantial" reform), a quite different picture was observed. As shown in Table 9.5, seven of these 14 cases fell within the governance or financial arrangements domains and the other seven fell under the delivery or program content domains. Note that the order in which the variables are shown differs from the order for tables in chapter 8. Exogenous variables are displayed in the top two rows and the bottom three rows. The main endogenous factor, insider interests, is in the third row. The other variable categories in the middle rows include influences that are both endogenous and exogenous.

TABLE 9.5
Categories of Variables That Substantially Influenced Extent of Reform:
14 Cases Assessed as Moderate, Significant, or Comprehensive Reform

	Governance and Financial Arrangements 7 Cases			Delivery Arrangements and Program Content 7 Cases		
	Regionalization AB SK NL	*Needs-Based Funding* AB SK	*APP* AB ON	*Wait Times* SK ON	*For-Profit Delivery* AB SK ON	*Drug Coverage* ON QC
Change in government/leader committed to reform	xxxx	xxxx				xx
Fiscal crisis	xx	xx	x			xx
Insider interests	xxxx	xx	xx	x	xxx	xxx
Institutional arrangements		xx	xx	xx		
Knowledge		xx	xx	xx		x
Values	x	xx		xx	xxx	xx
Public opinion/ civil society				xxx	x	x
Media				xx		x
Technological change						xx

Notes:
x = number of major observations
AB = Alberta
NL = Newfoundland and Labrador
ON = Ontario
QC = Quebec
SK = Saskatchewan

The principal insight from the table arises from the broad pattern it shows, not the case-by-case details. There are striking differences in the incidence and distribution of independent variables across the governance and financial arrangements domains and the delivery and program content domains. In the discussion that follows, we therefore group these four domains into two clusters: the governance and financial arrangements cluster, and the delivery and program content cluster.

The bottom three rows summarize the incidence and distribution of public opinion/civil society, media, and technological change for each of the six issues. The nine cells on the left side of the table are empty. For the same three rows on the right side, there are 10 observations located in six of the nine cells under the delivery and program content domains. The plain message is that public opinion/civil society, media, and technological change were associated with the three issues in the delivery and program content domains but not with the three issues in the governance and financial arrangements domains.

Moving from the bottom to the middle of the table, we see that 10 of 17 observations in the values and knowledge rows were associated with the delivery and program content grouping and seven with the governance and financial arrangements grouping.

For the top two rows of variables, we see a pattern that is almost the opposite of that in the bottom three rows. There we find 13 observations in the change in government/leader and fiscal crisis categories in five of the six cells for the issues under the governance and financial arrangements domains. There are only four observations in two of the cells in the delivery and program content domains.

The absence of public opinion/civil society, media and technological change variables from the three issues under the governance and financial arrangements cluster suggests that the issues in these domains were decided mainly, if not entirely, by "elites." The presence of those same three variable categories under the delivery and program content cluster suggests that the three issues in this cluster can be thought of as "people" issues. That is, the issues in the delivery and program content grouping touch people directly. In contrast, the public is not touched directly by the elite-driven issues on the left side of the table under the governance and financial arrangements cluster.

One other point worth noting is that values played a far greater role in the people cluster than they did in the elite cluster.

Comparing Counter-Consensus and Consensus Reforms

Two of the seven cases of substantial reform in the delivery and program content cluster ran counter to the consensus found in the grey literature.

Both cases involved for-profit delivery—one in Alberta and the other in Ontario. The questions we consider here are whether and to what extent these decisions involved a substantially different mix of variables than the other seven cases in the delivery and program content domains.

Referring back to Table 9.5, three points merit attention. First, the political leadership in these cases is captured in the third row under "insider interests," not in the first row under "change in government/ leader committed to reform." In other words, neither Premier Klein nor Premier Harris made firm electoral commitments on this issue. Neither could claim a mandate from the electorate.

Second, there was in fact strong grassroots opposition to for-profit delivery in both provinces. There was no comparable grassroots opposition to proposed policy direction in the other five cases in the delivery and program content domains. To the contrary, there were calls from the public for more reform, not opposition to the reform direction, in respect of some of the wait times and drug coverage cases.

Third, the basis of the arguments of each side (those favouring and those opposed to for-profit delivery) was rooted in values, not knowledge (Table 9.5).

With respect to values, the views espoused by the conservative governments led by Premier Klein in Alberta and Premiers Harris and Eves in Ontario were out-of-step with mainstream Canada. But they were not new to the Canadian polity. Even before the 1945–1946 Dominion-Provincial Conference on Reconstruction, there were competing views about the way in which health care should be funded and delivered in Canada. In the Reconstruction debates, the premiers of Ontario, Quebec, and Alberta were among the strongest opponents of the proposals for public health insurance that were tabled by the Liberal government led by Mackenzie King. The three premiers were vehemently opposed to the state's displacing private arrangements for insurance and delivery and also to the Dominion government's meddling in a sphere of provincial legislative competency under the Constitution (Dominion-Provincial Conference 1945, 7-19, 36-45, 339-52). The positions taken by both the Klein and Harris/Eves governments were a contemporary version of that competition.

Premier Klein won the first of four majorities in 1993. In the Westminster system, the party that controls the legislature controls the executive. Yet reform achievements were moderate, and arguably barely so. The opposition to the Alberta government's policy solutions came from organizations at different levels in society. In response to a question about whether the government "should allow the private sector to provide some health care services to those people who can afford to pay for them," one-third of Albertans agreed, the same share as for all of Canada (Mendelsohn 2002, 29 Figure 10). The most active opposition came from grassroots civil society organizations, especially the Friends of Medicare (the provincial affiliate of the Canadian Health Coalition), which included unions representing health-care workers and other groups of the political left. They could not directly block government policy reforms in the legislature, but they could rally support against the re-election of Progressive Conservative members. Opposition also came from the federal government. Ottawa's opposition not only made it politically harder for the provincial government to act. It also gave heart to the grassroots that they were not alone in resisting the premier's policy on this issue. The effectiveness of the opposition was remarkable in the face of a popular premier with a majority in the legislature and a clear sense of strategic direction, if not the details.

The ultimate compromise took seven years to emerge. It came in the form of legislation to create a regulatory framework that allowed the government to deal through a single policy instrument with several unresolved policy issues relating to for-profit delivery and the need for increased accountability in the health-care system (Church and Smith 2006).

The Ontario Progressive Conservative Party won a majority in the 1995 general election, ousting the NDP government. The style adopted by the Ontario PCs on for-profit delivery of health care was low key relative to what transpired in Alberta. The election brought to office a government and premier that believed in the need for an empowered private sector. Harris's Common Sense Revolution declared that "many of the things that government does can be done cheaper, faster and better if the private sector is involved" (Ontario Progressive Conservative Party 1995, 16). The platform neither explicitly included nor excluded health care. However, when a survey by the Fraser Institute drew attention to a relative shortage of medical imaging capacity, the government was afforded an opportunity to advance for-profit delivery by encouraging commercial suppliers to help fill the gap.

At the grassroots level, the Ontario Health Coalition organized 22 rallies across the province to protest for-profit delivery as a solution to long wait times. Indeed, polling data showed that fewer Ontarians favoured a for-profit, private delivery solution as a response to perceived increases in wait times than was the case for residents in all other provinces (Mendelsohn 2002, 29, Figure 10). This strong public attachment to medicare explains why the government moved with caution down the for-profit delivery track.

The evidence of this book suggests that first-term governments are more likely to take on large reforms than governments that have been in power for several terms. A first-term government that can point to a campaign commitment that gives it a mandate for action is also more likely to succeed in its reform objectives than a newly elected government without a mandate on an issue. Neither the Alberta nor the Ontario PCs had such a mandate coming out of their first election campaigns in 1993 and 1995, respectively. It was toward the end of their second mandate that they implemented their reforms. In Alberta, Klein was rebuffed by his own caucus at least twice before securing his 2000 package. The Harris government was hardly shy in its election platforms, but it was timid when it came to for-profit delivery of health care.

For those who wished to see alternative approaches to delivery tested fully, the civil society resistance to market-driven reforms would have been yet another example of rigidity in Canadian health care. For opponents of for-profit delivery, it may have been reassuring that an activist citizenry could slow a legislative majority that did not share its views. The "moderate" outcomes suggest that the resistance to more for-profit enterprise was not much weaker or stronger than the resistance to other reform proposals, but the sources of opposition were different.

Comparing "Technical" and "Political" Cases

The literature suggests that there is a distinction between cases that are essentially grounded in technical knowledge and those that are more grounded in the political aspects of decision-making. Having said this, Bozeman and Panday (2004) note that rarely is a decision purely political or purely technical, and sometimes distinguishing between one and the other is difficult. With this caveat in mind, we tested this hypothesis by using some basic criteria developed in the literature to analyze our 22 cases where some degree of reform occurred. Table 9.6 summarizes these criteria.

Four criteria in Table 9.6 were taken from the US literature: technical requirements of the reform, goal consensus, time span of the decision, and role of technical experts. The remaining two criteria, change in government/leader and fiscal crisis, were derived from our analysis of the cases described in chapter 8 (exogenous factors). Cases that were political in nature were sensitive to these last two factors; cases that were exclusively technical in nature were not.

Table 9.7 depicts the cases according to political attributes versus technical attributes. Each *x* in the table refers to one of the 22 cases in which there was reform. For example, the three *x* markings in the far right cell of the last row indicate that technical participants were key decision-makers in the three provinces—Alberta, Quebec, and Saskatchewan—that undertook reform in the needs-based funding case.

At the government agenda stage, all cases were mainly influenced by political considerations. Technical knowledge played a limited role. At the policy choice stage, the result was somewhat different. For those decisions requiring a high degree of technical knowledge, politicians were sometimes willing to cede their chairs to officials with essential technical knowledge. In other cases, while technical knowledge was an ingredient in the decision, political considerations trumped technical knowledge.

TABLE 9.6
Criteria for Distinguishing Decisions That Are Mainly Political from Decisions That Also Involve Technical Expertise

Mainly Political	Political and Technical
Decisions were not based on high levels of technical knowledge and did not require high levels of scientific understanding	Decisions were based on technical knowledge and/or required high levels of scientific understanding
Low goal consensus	High goal consensus
Decisions were taken in relatively short time span	Decisions were taken over longer time span
Technical experts had little or no role in the policy choice	Technical experts played a central role in the development of a policy choice
Decisions were linked to "change in government/ leader" associated with elections	Decisions were not linked to "change in government/ leader" associated with elections
Decisions were directly related to fiscal crisis	Decisions were not directly related to a fiscal crisis

The analysis indicates that reforms related to alternative payment plans, for-profit delivery, regionalization, and prescription drugs were heavily influenced by political factors through to the policy choice stage.

Alternative payment plans were introduced in Quebec, Saskatchewan, and Alberta. Despite a substantive body of evidence supporting an end to fee-for-service as a precursor to primary care reforms, none of the provinces achieved either comprehensive or significant levels of reform. Reluctance to "force" reform on doctors and low goal consensus trumped best available evidence.

The decision on for-profit delivery in all provinces, whether the reform was categorized as being "consensus-based" (meaning opposition to for-profit delivery) or "counter-consensus" (favouring for-profit delivery), was heavily driven by values. None of the decisions required any degree of scientific or technical knowledge in order to arrive at the policy choice stage.

Regionalization was heavily driven by the fiscal crisis and not incidentally the escalation in health-care costs that played a role in creating that crisis. Only Quebec had regionalized before the 1990s. Further changes made to these structures in Quebec during the time period of our study were political and motivated for reasons similar to other provinces—a perceived need for better service integration and more efficiency. In the other four provinces, there was a change in government/leader just before

TABLE 9.7
Categorization of Health Reform Case Studies as Mainly Political or Technical/Political Based on Six Criteria

		Alternative Payment Plans	For-Profit Delivery	Regionalization	Prescription Drug Coverage	Wait Times	Needs-Based Funding
Political Criteria	Low goal consensus	xxxx	xx		x	xxx	
	Short decision times	xx	xx	xxx	xxxx	x	
	Not based on technical feasibility	xxxx	xxx	xxxx	xxxx		
	Fiscal crisis	xx	xx	xxxx	xx		
	Change in government/leader	xxxx	xx	xxxx	xxx		x
	No technical participants	xxxx	xxx	xxxx	xxxx		
Technical Criteria	High goal consensus		x	xxxx	xxx	x	xxx
	Long decision times	xx	x	x		xxx	xxx
	Based on technical feasibility					xxxx	xxx
	Not related to fiscal crisis	xx	x		xx	xxxx	xxx
	Not linked to change in government/ leader		x		x	xxxx	xx
	Technical participants					xxxx	xxx

Note: x = number of major observations.

or shortly after the turn of the decade. That change, in conjunction with the fiscal conditions and goal consensus, led to relatively quick decisions by mainly political actors. In Ontario there was much political opposition to regionalization and no champion for the cause, and the decision not to regionalize was taken swiftly. In Alberta and Newfoundland and Labrador, regionalization was seen as part of a broader effort to improve efficiencies within health-care delivery and thereby reduce costs or at least contain expenditure growth. This was also the case in Saskatchewan, but in that province regionalization was also seen as a precondition to a broader wellness agenda. Premiers Romanow and Klein acted in their first electoral mandates. The regionalization decision in Newfoundland and Labrador was taken after decades of study in the second mandate of Premier Wells. In Saskatchewan, Alberta, and Newfoundland and Labrador, determining the borders of regions was more a by-product of political pressures than technical considerations.

Finally, drug reform also proved to be highly political. The case studies in all instances were driven by a combination of cost considerations and dynamics related to change in government/leader and the electoral cycle.

Moving along to the more technical side of the spectrum, the issue of wait times as seen in Table 9.7 tells a compelling story about the interplay between technical and political reform. Wait times is a reform that relied heavily (and still does) on a technical knowledge base and high goal consensus. Yet even technical decision-making took place within a context that was influenced by political concerns. While the actual mechanics of effectively tracking wait times (collecting data, determining appropriate wait times, and prioritizing treatments) were highly technical, engaging physicians without invading their professional autonomy was highly political. The issue of providing choice for both physicians and patients was also political. Once a decision had been taken to do reforms, the decision process became highly technical. Once complete, it gave rise to normative political questions about how to use wait lists: as a tracking device for the information of government and physicians only, as a management tool, or as public information that would allow people to make informed choices.

Needs-based funding was the most technical reform of the six. It initially involved a political decision about whether to depart from the historically based funding models. Once consensus was reached in principle, there were many technical decisions that had to be considered in developing a funding formula.

In Saskatchewan, the move to develop a needs-based funding formula was driven primarily by the civil service in conjunction with technical experts. Similarly, in Alberta, public servants were seen to be proponents of population-based funding. Once politicians endorsed the concept, public servants were left to their own devices to work out the technical details through expert committee input. In Quebec, the government deliberately avoided implementing its needs-based formula in a fashion that might have created regional inequities with political consequences.

In general, the analysis of the case studies reveals that issues can almost never be defined as being exclusively political or exclusively technical. However, the analysis does suggest a spectrum in the mix of technical and political elements that drive the decision-making process. Our case analysis suggested that certain conditions—low goal consensus, short decision times, fiscal crisis, change in government/leader, lack of technical feasibility, lack of technical participants—helped to facilitate reforms that were highly political in nature, while other conditions led to more technical reforms that involved high levels of participation from subject matter experts.

Although the sample size does not enable us to develop hard-and-fast rules about the two categories, the analysis does suggest that all (or at least a large majority of) issues must have some "political" characteristics to find a place on the government agenda. The politics of the electoral cycle create the opportunity to advance health-care reforms that are not heavily related to scientific or technical feasibility. Crisis has the same effect. When both conditions are present, the opportunity for reform for politically driven issues increases. Conversely, the most successful technical reforms are much less reliant on the dynamics of the electoral cycle at the policy choice stage. Reforms that are technical in nature are more likely to be successful when decisions are made over time, under the guidance of subject matter experts where there is limited political opposition.

Conclusions

In 16 of 30 cases, there was limited or no reform. Eight of the 16 cases were in the governance and financial arrangements grouping and eight in the delivery and program content grouping. Simply put, existing interests benefited from the status quo and they were good at protecting their turf. Most of these interests were insiders—provider groups (especially medical associations) and governments (except newly elected first-time governments). But it was not just insiders that were attracted to the status quo. Canadian public opinion and civil society groups wished to retain the benefits they enjoyed from the status quo. Public opinion was very protective of medicare as an icon and committed to the principles on which it rested. On the whole, there was not much difference between the two groupings in the categories of factors that led actors to resist reform.

For the 14 cases of substantial reform, the pattern of factors associated with reform was much different than for the 16 cases. Among the 14, there was a big difference between the mix of variables that shaped policy reform decisions in the two clusters. For issues in the governance and financial arrangements cluster, there was no gradient among provinces in the direction or amount of reform based on traditional left/right values. Rather, the extent of reform was a function of the political priorities of provincial governments, their political and administrative preparedness, and accidents of timing. Reform decisions were shaped heavily by elites focused on efficiency/cost-containment and effectiveness, or by technical considerations in needs-based funding. An open reform window was a necessary but not sufficient condition for reform. Political actors had to be ready and able to take advantage of the opening. On political priorities and preparedness, other things equal, newly elected first-time provincial governments that had committed to reform and that had a plan for reaching their objectives (Saskatchewan and Alberta in the first half of the 1990s) were more likely to achieve reforms than provinces that did not (Ontario and Newfoundland and Labrador).

By contrast, the issues that made up the delivery and program content grouping were influenced by whether a government was left-of-centre, centre, or right-of-centre. The left/right division was most evident in the for-profit delivery issue (Romanow in Saskatchewan vs. Klein in Alberta and Harris/Eves in Ontario). But it was reflected as well by differences between the Saskatchewan (Calvert) and Alberta (Klein) governments on whether to mandate surgeons to participate in a wait-list management system (Calvert) or leave them the choice of participating in a voluntary tracking system (Klein).

For left-of-centre social democratic governments, a common philosophic orientation was not associated with similar reform decisions (Romanow and Rae governments). Right-of-centre conservative governments (Klein and Harris/Eves governments) were more similar in their reform decisions. There were, nonetheless, significant differences between them (e.g., needs-based funding was brought into force in Alberta and ignored in Ontario). Conservative governments were also constrained by the power of the medicare legacy.

The range of factors that caused items to reach the governmental agenda in the delivery and program content grouping was broader than for the governance and financial arrangements cluster: public opinion and civil society groups supported reforms on wait times and prescription drugs, and opposed for-profit delivery; elected government officials were instrumental in for-profit delivery reaching the governmental agenda in four of the five provinces. Competing values were influential at the governmental agenda stage (e.g., for profit-delivery) and even more so in policy choice (e.g., the difference in policy choice between Alberta and Saskatchewan on wait times). Knowledge was important in policy choice for wait times.

No political party or contestant for party leadership ran for office committed to for-profit delivery. Even the parties that had a disposition toward a greater role for the for-profit sector did not campaign on this issue. This made it difficult to claim a mandate from the people and ultimately constrained the magnitude of the counter-consensus reform that was achieved.

Finally, it was concluded that different reform issues displayed different intrinsic properties. Some reforms were characterized by a very high measure of political sensitivity at all stages in the decision process through to completion of the policy choice. Other issues became increasingly technical as they moved through to the policy choice stage.

Chapter 12 will suggest some implications of this analysis. Before we get there, however, two further steps are needed. One is to compare the conclusions based on our methodology to alternative ways of assessing the extent of reform. The other is to assess whether our results would be altered by updating the analysis to 2011. These two steps are the subject of chapters 10 and 11.

NOTES

1. For example, the population of Ontario is about 150 times larger than that of the smallest province, and the geographic expanse of Quebec is more than 10 times the size of the three Maritime provinces together.
2. For example, the United States, Russia, India, Brazil, and China.
3. Hospital beds also increased. But the number of beds per population in Newfoundland and Labrador in the 1950s was comparable with the national average, and therefore the increase was less rapid than physician growth (Taylor 2009, 235).
4. This does not mean that health care was *the* priority for the NDP. In fact, much of the NDP's election campaign was focused on the maladministration of the government. But the NDP was on record with commitments to undertake substantial health reform.
5. The Saskatchewan government's reliance on a voluntary approach did not change during our study period. Fast-forwarding to the mid-2000s, despite the NDP's ability to secure re-election in 1995 and 1999 (under Romanow) and 2003 (under Calvert), little progress occurred on the APP file under its watch.
6. To the extent that the PQ of the 1994–2003 era under Parizeau, Bouchard, and Landry can be thought of as a social democratic party, its reform record was unlike that of the second and third Saskatchewan NDP governments (1995–2003) led by Romanow and Calvert.

CHAPTER 10

VERIFYING THE RELIABILITY OF RESEARCH RESULTS

HARVEY LAZAR AND JOHN CHURCH

This chapter has two purposes. First is to test the sensitivity of our results. Did the choice of time period for study or the choice of issues bias the results in any way? Second, are the results of the research and analysis broadly consistent with existing literature or are they an outlier?

SENSITIVITY OF RESULTS

In this section we set out an alternative to the case study methodology for answering the initial research question regarding the nature and extent of reform. Second, within the case study methodology, we consider whether the issues selected for study might have unintentionally biased the results.

Alternative Methodology: Comparing Reform in 1990–2003 to Reform in Earlier Decades (1944–1989)

The discussion below compares the nature and extent of the 1990–2003 reforms to reforms in earlier periods in post–Second World War Canada. To that end, we divided the years from 1944 to 1989 into four periods (referred to as T1, T2, T3, and T4 for ease of exposition) and examined the record of reform in each period with a focus on the macro-policy framework and larger meso-level reforms. We then compared these findings to our base case (1990–2003). As the circumstances of each period were different, so too were the priorities for reform. How did the reforms in each period compare with the priorities? To answer this question, it was necessary to take a view about the priorities of each period. This we did by examining statements by governments, actions by governments, and public opinion. The exercise was part science and part art.

The periods selected are similar (but not identical) to those used by Malcolm Taylor in his book on the history of Canadian health insurance (Taylor 2009).[1] The first period begins with events in Ottawa and Saskatchewan in 1944 and ends with events between 1953 and 1955, before the Canada-wide hospital insurance plan was adopted. In 1944, Ottawa was preparing draft legislation (more than one model) for a national health insurance system through interaction among federal political leaders, federal public servants, researchers from academe, and representatives of the Canadian Medical Association. That same year in Saskatchewan, a general election brought the Co-operative Commonwealth Federation (CCF) to office for the first time anywhere in Canada. During the campaign, the CCF renewed its commitment to bring universal publicly financed health care to Saskatchewan (it was on record before then as favouring such a reform). In 1945, at the Dominion-Provincial Conference on Reconstruction, Ottawa proposed a shared-cost system of universal publicly financed health care. When the proposal did not garner sufficient provincial support to move forward, the Saskatchewan government acted swiftly and on its own, introducing legislation in March 1946. The Saskatchewan government program of universal publicly financed hospital insurance began in January 1947.

The second and third periods (T2 and T3) coincide with the introduction of Canada-wide public hospital insurance (1953/1955–1961) and medical insurance (1961–1971/72), respectively. The fourth period (T4) begins in 1972. By that time all jurisdictions had begun delivering medical services in a manner consistent with the framework set out in the federal *Medical Care Act*. With the national hospital and medical insurance systems up and running, much of what the federal government had proposed in 1945 had been achieved. For Ottawa, the question was what should come next. Early on in this period, the federal minister of national health and welfare, Marc Lalonde, published *A New Perspective on the Health of Canadians* (Lalonde 1974). The Lalonde report was received as a call for society to recognize that much more than health care determined the health status of the population. Less noticed, however, was that it also was an effort to consult the public on what Ottawa's role in health-related matters should be going forward (Forest, forthcoming).

T4 marked the beginning of a quarter century of annual fiscal deficits in Ottawa. At the beginning of T4, close to one-quarter of federal expenditures involved the transfer of cash grants to the provinces. Two-thirds of that amount involved matching grants (Bird 1979, 57). The more the provinces spent, the more it cost Ottawa. This led Ottawa to sever the link between its contributions for health care and provincial spending on health-care services. Under the *Established Programs Financing Act, 1977,* federal matching grants to the provinces were replaced by a combination of block grants and a transfer of federal tax room to the provinces.

This change in intergovernmental fiscal arrangements led to two challenges. First, in the 1980s, the growth rate in provincial revenues associated with Established Programs Financing (EPF)—tax points and cash combined—did not keep pace with the growth rate in provincial health expenditures. Since health care was the largest expenditure "envelope" in all provinces and growing rapidly, provinces inevitably began a search for ways to make health-care delivery more efficient. They also began to consider the kinds of structural modifications that would improve health services without adding to costs.

The second challenge was the growth in extra-billing by physicians and to a lesser degree user charges by hospitals (facility fees). EPF did not make clear what conditions Ottawa would require in exchange for the new block transfers. Nor did it specify the manner in which the federal authorities would enforce those conditions. This situation might have, over time, impaired access to medical and hospital services and eroded key principles of medicare. The result was the *Canada Health Act*.

The 1990–2003 base period studied began with the onset of recession and a per capita freeze (more or less) on health-care spending by each province. It ended with the Romanow and Kirby reports, both released in 2002, and the First Ministers' Health Accord reached in 2003. The priorities of the base period have been analyzed in this book. But we have focused on six issues only. It is clear that cost containment was a major priority in the first part of this period. Other issues that could be considered as priorities are discussed later in this chapter.

T1: 1944 to 1953–1955

At the outset of T1, there were three overriding health policy objectives: first, to make health insurance universally available, preferably through a social insurance program or other mechanism that shifted the burden of uncertain health costs from the level of individual or family to the widest possible base (Dominion-Provincial Conference 1946, 84-95). The second and linked priority was to build the supply side of health services including for Canadians living in rural areas. There was an expectation that demand for services would grow with the provision of publicly funded insurance. A third priority was to improve the health of the people of Canada (Dominion-Provincial Conference 1946, 85-95; Taylor 2009; 5-6). For example, for infant mortality rates, the Dominion Bureau of Statistics data ranked Canada 17th "among developed nations in 1937" (cited in Taylor 2009, 5) and 21st in "maternal mortality" (cited in Canadian Public Health Association 2012, 4.3). In 1941 the Dominion Council of Health[2] observed that the "maternal mortality rate in Canada is high, and when compared to other countries with a similar standard of living, may be considered excessively so" (cited in Taylor 2009, 5).

The Canadian Public Health Association (2012, 5.4) reported that during the Second World War 40 to 50 percent (depending on the year) of new recruits for military service were rejected because of poor health. Similar priorities applied in T2 and T3.

The first priority required a wide measure of buy-in from provincial governments. Above and beyond a general concern about revenues that was shared by all provinces,[3] it was further recognized that to secure the participation of the lower-income provinces in a national health scheme, including the Maritimes (and Newfoundland after it entered Confederation in 1949), it would be necessary politically to find a funding formula for health insurance that would be affordable to the treasuries of those provinces.

As events unfolded, the federal-provincial fiscal arrangements included both a formal Equalization program (beginning in 1957 although the differing needs of each province had been recognized in various ways since the 1867 Constitution) and what the fiscal federalism experts of the era sometimes referred to as "implicit equalization." The latter involved funding formulas under which the federal government paid for a higher share of the health-care programs of lower-income provinces than the more affluent ones. To achieve agreement in this complex intergovern-mental bargaining process was in some sense a fourth priority for our purposes. The process was led by first ministers and finance ministers with assistance from health ministers.[4]

What was achieved in T1? At the provincial level, Saskatchewan and British Columbia introduced universal publicly financed hospital insurance programs. Newfoundland maintained the cottage hospital program that had been available to persons living in rural and remote areas (covering around 47 percent of the population of the province) when it entered Confederation in 1949. Alberta implemented a program of subsidies for its numerous municipally sponsored hospital insurance plans. Second, across the country, due in part to National Health Grants, there was an expansion of the supply side. For example, the number of hospital beds grew from 109,000 in 1944 to 168,000 in 1955 (Dominion Bureau of Statistics, "Rated Bed Capacity"). The population per nurse ratio improved in parallel, dropping from 389 to 305 (Dominion Bureau of Statistics, "Number of Physicians"). At the same time the population per physician ratio was flat in part because public expenditure was con-centrated on hospitals and other health infrastructure (ibid.). Whether achieved or not, the Dominion's 1945 commitments were a beacon of light. Canadians did not forget. But there was no national program.

Third, the health status of Canadians improved. The available data do not correspond precisely with T1. But from 1941 to 1956, the life expect-ancy at birth rose from 67.6 to 72.7 years for females and from 63.0 to 66.3 years for males (Dominion Bureau of Statistics, "Life Expectancy"). While this improvement was partly due to higher living standards, the continued migration of Canadians from rural areas to urban centres, and new drugs, public policy also played a role. In 1948, the federal government began making annual grants to provinces to combat certain illnesses (such as tuberculosis, cancer, mental illness, and venereal disease), to help with the treatment of children with disabilities (referred to then as "crippled" children), and to fund training of public health personnel.

T2: 1953–1955 to 1961

In T2, the priorities remained what they were in T1 except the insurance focus was narrowed to hospital insurance. Advancing publicly funded hospital insurance became more difficult to achieve by political changes "on the ground." Commercial insurance companies and private not-for-profit insurance firms owned or supported by physician groups were selling medical insurance policies in all provinces; these companies were also selling hospital insurance in all of Canada, except in the two provinces (Saskatchewan and British Columbia) with universal coverage (Taylor 2009, 170-73). This was a market these insurance companies were reluctant to give up. The Canadian Medical Association and its provincial divisions were also opposed, fearing that if pan-Canadian hospital insurance were brought into force, Canada-wide medical insurance might soon follow (Maioni 1998, 97; Taylor 2009, 189-92).[5]

Nonetheless, the achievements were large: broad federal-provincial fiscal arrangements were settled through five-year agreements in 1952 and again in 1957.[6] Canada-wide, universal, publicly financed hospital insurance was implemented. The details of the funding formula (which on the whole favoured less affluent provinces) made participation attractive to less wealthy provinces. The supply grew substantially. In short, "the combination of hospital construction grants and voluntary insurance followed by the universal hospital insurance program enabled Canada to increase enormously its hospital resources" (Taylor 2009, 234-35).

Life expectancy at birth between 1956 and 1961 continued to grow (Dominion Bureau of Statistics, "Life Expectancy"). Improved living standards and the continued migration from country to city played a role in this improvement. But so too did the attention of governments to disease prevention and health promotion. Issues like food safety, potable water quality, and air contaminants received enhanced attention as did promotion of healthy diets.

T3: 1961 to 1971–1972

The T3 priorities were to achieve Canada-wide medical insurance and to increase the supply of physicians and other health professionals. Saskatchewan led the way again. In 1961 it introduced its universal publicly financed medical insurance plan. Ottawa followed a few years later with a Canada-wide plan. This priority was even more heavily contested than hospital insurance. Unlike T2, there was strong opposition to a federal government–led initiative from most provinces including the four largest provinces. There was also a well-organized medical and insurance lobby that strongly resisted the federal proposal. This lobby connected with some of the provinces that were against the federal plan. Indeed, the governments of Alberta, British Columba, and Ontario were ready to proceed with medicare systems of their own based mainly on private for-profit insurance (Maioni 1998, 131; Taylor 2009, 368). Quebec declared it would have its own medical insurance program, which substantively turned out to be consistent with the federal medicare law (Maioni 1998, 131; Taylor 2009, 365-66).

Yet the federal *Medical Care Act* was passed in 1966, and by the end of T3 it was operating in all provinces and territories. By 1971 Canadians had a system of publicly financed medical insurance coverage that was universal and portable between provinces. The supply side had grown as well. With federal government financial support through the Health Resources Fund, four new medical schools were established and the 12 existing schools expanded or upgraded. The number of medical school graduates increased from 881 in 1966 to 1,796 in 1983 (Taylor 2009, 418-19). The population per physician dropped from 857 in 1961 to 659 in 1971. For nurses the comparable numbers were 182 and 140. Life expectancy continued to grow.

The T3 decade also saw an explosion of social programs aimed broadly at improving social security (e.g., improving retirement and disability pensions and widening the scope of unemployment insurance), enhancing equality of opportunity (expanding post-secondary education and skills development), and providing more and better support for those most in need (through social services and social assistance). Although not presented to the public as motivated by a desire to improve population health, these initiatives were consistent with health promotion.

T4: 1972 to 1989

The priorities of T4 reflected collateral side effects of what had been achieved in T1–T3 inclusive. Due to the costs associated with the health, post-secondary education, and social programs created or expanded in T2 and T3, public sector expenditures grew throughout T4. The rate of economic growth fell (first stagflation, then recession followed by slow growth) with adverse effects on federal and provincial government revenues. Annual deficits became the "new normal," first at the federal level and then in the provinces. Public debt rose.

One knock-on result was Ottawa's decision to download the risks of greater than expected cost increases for publicly financed health care and post-secondary education to the provinces. In 1977, it replaced its three matching grant programs with a new transfer program under the *Established Programs Financing Act*. The new program had both cash and tax components. Under these arrangements, the federal government transferred cash to the provinces equal to roughly one-half of the amount that would have been payable under the matching grants programs. This new block transfer was to escalate thereafter at a rate of growth linked to gross national product and not the rate of growth in health-care spending. The remainder of the federal contribution was paid for by federal legislation that reduced Ottawa's take from the income tax base. This left room for provinces to increase their income tax revenues and fill the gap without adding to taxpayer burden. This so-called tax transfer was designed to cover the other half of what Ottawa had been paying to the provinces under matching grants.

As events unfolded, the EPF transfer, including cash and tax components, grew more slowly than the rate of increase in provincial health-care programs. Due to ongoing budgetary pressures, during the 1980s Ottawa cut its planned rate of increase in the cash transfer several times. At the same time, income tax yields grew more slowly than had been anticipated in 1977, reducing the value of the tax transfer. Ottawa's "notional" share of provincial health-care expenditures thus dropped. More of the financial burden of health care was borne by provincial treasuries.

Whether EPF and its amendments are viewed as a major reform of health care, de-linking Ottawa's contribution from provincial health-care spending, or as a major reform to public finances with downstream implications for the affordability of provincial programs, provincial budgets were squeezed. In some provinces, this squeeze contributed to the introduction of user fees at point of delivery by some physicians. The federal Liberal government objected. Controversy erupted leading to venomous relations between some provincial medical associations / provincial governments on the one side, and the federal government and its many friends on the other. A solution was required. Politically, this was the priority issue in Canada during T4. But economically and financially, the priority was for provinces to make efficiency gains and undertake structural reforms to help offset the fast-rising costs of the health-care programs that they were funding.

With regard to user charges at point of delivery, arguably this priority was met in that the *Canada Health Act* came to be accepted by provincial governments, provincial medical associations, and the general public. Had Ottawa chosen not to intervene, some provinces would have almost certainly taken this as a signal that the principles that had applied prior to EPF (i.e., under the *Hospital Insurance and Diagnostic Services Act* and the *Medical Care Act*) were no longer a condition of Ottawa's ongoing EPF block transfer. Such provinces would have likely tolerated, if not encouraged, hospitals and physicians to charge user fees at point of service

(Evans 2000, 893-96). Polling data indicate that a substantial majority of Canadians were "satisfied" with way in which the federal government handled health care during the second half of 1980s (Mendelsohn 2002, 34).

Governments were not successful in dealing with the second priority: improving efficiency or making the kinds of structural changes that would contain costs without impairing service. This observation is inferred not by the rate of increase in provincial health-care spending in T4 (there was no "right" number) but by the appointment of numerous commissions and task forces through the second half of the 1980s and into the 1990s. The terms of reference indicated that provincial governments were worried about cost control and that reform was needed in a number of areas including primary care, physician remuneration, regionalization, hospital funding, and hospital rationalization (annex 1; O'Fee 2002a). The failure to contain cost growth would be seen in the retrenchment that began in 1991–92. T4 thus left a legacy of unsolved problems relating to the delivery and cost of health care.

For Ottawa, the question was what should come after the creation of countrywide hospital and medical insurance. One possible answer was reflected in a "working document" released in 1974 by the federal minister of national health and welfare, Marc Lalonde. The Lalonde report, *A New Perspective on the Health of Canadians,* was received as a call for society to recognize that much more than health care determined the health status of the population. It was a way to consult the public on the federal government's future role in health care (Forest, forthcoming). The report may have influenced the way in which researchers and public servants thought about issues of population health; however, policy decisions in the 1980s suggested that, on the whole, the determinants of health philosophy was not a major factor in policy reform agendas.

T1 to T3 had been mainly concerned with establishing universal, Canada-wide, publicly financed health insurance and increasing the supply of health-care professionals and hospital beds. The success of those years created many vested interests, including patients and their families; organizations representing physicians, nurses, and other unionized health workers; local dignitaries attached to hospitals in small towns as well as big; political parties (that claimed political paternity for these achievements); and public servants who helped to manage the health systems. As this book has underlined, the presence of these many interests, some more than others, made reform politically difficult.

Base Case: 1990 to 2003

This brings us to the base case. What about the years from 1990 to 2003? What were the priorities, and how were they addressed? The underlying objectives at the start of the period can be inferred from the first wave of grey literature reports: cost containment, cost-effectiveness, and efficiency (O'Fee 2002a). These objectives led to a focus on decentralization, regionalization, and hospital rationalization. In other words, it was held that "organizational change is facilitated first and foremost by structural change" (ibid., 2). Moreover, throughout the 1990s not only did provincial governments continue to appoint commissions and task forces, the federal government appointed its National Forum on Health in 1994 and then a Commission on the Future of Health Care in Canada in 2001. These actions indicated that federal political leaders were also concerned with health system performance. These second-wave reports focused on matters such as governance, information systems, transparency, and accountability.

The priorities are somewhat ambiguous compared to the four previous periods. Arguably, however, cost considerations came first at least in the first half of the period. The Canadian Institute for Health Information used the terms "retrenchment" and "disinvestment" to describe the years 1992 to 1996. Since demand for services continued to grow during these years, a supply-demand gap opened up. Canadians began to experience difficulty in accessing specialists and certain diagnostic services. Emergency rooms became overcrowded even as the fiscal situation improved.

The 1995 federal budget, which included a very large reduction in cash transfers to provinces, ensured that fiscal issues would also play a large role in the second half of the period. The provincial governments gave priority to "forcing" the federal government to restore transfers to the levels they would have been without the 1995 federal budget.

As the 1990s unfolded, there were also proposals to extend the coverage of the *Canada Health Act* to prescription drugs and home care. The prescription drug issue had become more salient with the arrival of expensive new breakthrough drugs. Home care had grown in importance because of increased reliance on ambulatory care and the aging of the population. The argument for acting was strong. The *Canada Health Act* was not amended, however. Premiers were generally uninterested in such reforms unless and until federal cash transfers were restored. In Ottawa, the Prime Minister's Office and the Department of Finance held sway, and they ceded ground on transfers too slowly for premiers to make new commitments.

Perhaps the largest reforms of the period involved regionalization. Regionalization, particularly because of how it altered provincial governments' core bargains with hospitals in some if not most provinces, occurred more or less in parallel with retrenchment. It was hoped that the regional structure would serve as a platform from which it would be possible to achieve efficiency and effectiveness gains. Some decision-makers viewed regionalization as the key to many desired reforms—hospital budgeting, hospital rationalization and better integration of services, and potentially primary care reform—that would help reduce the pressure on provincial health budgets when retrenchment had passed. To one degree or other, all provinces except Ontario decided to create regional systems. At the beginning of the 1990s, Quebec had already had a system of regional administration for close to two decades. Nonetheless, Quebec made two major reforms to its system in 1991 and 2003.

Regionalization did facilitate reform of hospital budgeting in two of the provinces we studied (Saskatchewan and Alberta). Hospital rationalization preceded regionalization in Alberta and to a degree in Saskatchewan, and was done independently of regionalization in Ontario. Primary care reform was not significantly advanced in most provinces and was not correlated with regionalization. (Indeed Ontario, which did not regionalize its services, accomplished more primary care reform than Saskatchewan, which did regionalize.) Integration of services was talked about more than done. Regionalization was, in many quarters, also intended to be an exercise in democratization with regional boards at least partly elected and, in some instances, with provider interests included. The democratization aspect of regional boards was not a major component by the end of the base case.

At the meso-policy level, there were some important achievements that were linked in part to the social determinants of health perspective such as federal-provincial child tax benefit agreements, and agreements on early childhood development. Other achievements are better thought of under the rubric of public health including the fix of the blood system and the anti-smoking campaign. But the broader picture was less encouraging. In a paper prepared for a workshop on Intersectoral Action and Health, Michael Rachlis wrote: "Health status is stagnating and some of the determinants of health are deteriorating. Canada's official infant mortality rates have continued to decline but the rate of low birthweight remains around 6 percent and the rate of premature birth has increased by almost 10 percent in the past decade" (1999, 4). It was not a lack of knowledge that led to these conditions. Only a few months before the 1995 federal budget, the federal/provincial/territorial ministers of health had released the report *Strategies for Population Health: Investing in the Health of Canadians*, prepared by an advisory committee on public health. The report stated,

> A framework based on the broad determinants of health presented in this paper, as the foundation for planning and action to improve population health will significantly enhance our chances for success. The health sector cannot act alone, because most of the determinants of health fall partly or wholly outside its purview. (Federal/Provincial/Territorial Advisory Committee 1994, 38)

What was the relationship between the First Ministers' Meetings of 1999, 2000, 2003, and 2004 and the above reform agenda? In short, most of the items were endorsed at these meetings. Actual reforms were slow in coming, however, as the main agenda for provincial premiers was restoration of transfers.

In 2003 the health-care share of provincial budgets was higher than it had been in 1990. Regionalization was proving to be a "hit and miss" affair in the sense that provinces appeared unable to decide how much real authority to assign to regional bodies. Home care and pharmaceuticals were still outside the coverage of the *Canada Health Act*. Concerns about wait times for certain specialists and procedures had begun to attract attention (in the form of methodological advances and data development), but improvements on the ground were not noticeable. There was no shortage of pilot projects for primary care reform. Yet, once again, real change was barely noticeable. Public opinion was critical of performance. In sum, relative to priorities, achievement was at best meagre. Table 10.1 summarizes the discussion of the five periods.

Whether one agrees with the details or not, it is hard to find a basis for rating achievements in 1990–2003 as equal to any of the first three periods. Less clearly, the achievements of T4 strike us as somewhat larger than the base case although the difference was not great. What is of equal note is that the societal consensus that determined the priorities of T1–T3 was less firm in the latter two periods. This may be a variation of the idea that, for some issues or items, it is easier to start from scratch than reconstruct the building while operating it. The accomplishments of T1 through T3 had created vested interests that were reluctant to open up the arrangements from which they benefited.

In sum, there were many calls for substantial reform from 1990 to 2003 at the macro-policy and higher meso-policy levels. Some reforms, of course, did occur. In the governance domain, most provinces regionalized services although they shied away from including medical budgets in this reform. In the delivery sphere there was hospital rationalization and integration, and the displacement of some expensive acute care services by less expensive ambulatory care. While these were important achievements, the macro-policy framework remained unchanged. The incentive structure for physicians was largely intact. Two of the provinces we studied reformed hospital funding substantially, but three did not. Calls for reforms at the meso-policy level were acknowledged but, apart from a few exceptions, changes were incremental and slow, especially in the funding sphere. "Incremental and slow" is not a bad thing when a health-care system is firing on all cylinders. That was not the case in Canada between 1990 and 2003.

TABLE 10.1
Comparing Health Reform across Five Periods, 1944–2003

Period	Priorities: Explicit or Inferred	Reforms	Reform Achievements Relative to Priorities
T1 1944–1953/1955	1. Canada-wide, universal, publicly financed health insurance administered by provinces 2. Expansion of supply 3. Public health, especially in rural areas 4. Equalization to enable less wealthy provinces to participate (in Canada-wide insurance)	1. Saskatchewan and BC introduce universal publicly financed hospital insurance 2. National Health Grants for hospital construction and training of health personnel begin 1948 3. National Health Grants also used for combatting specific diseases. Federal government begins to acquire data on health status of the population. 4. No progress	1. None Canada-wide; major within two provinces 2. Considerable; substantial 3. Considerable (probably). Hard to attribute most improvements to specific reforms 4. None
T2 1953/1955–1961	1. Canada-wide, universal, publicly financed hospital insurance 2. Expansion of supply 3. Public health 4. Equalization to enable less wealthy provinces to participate	1. Canada-wide hospital insurance 2. Strong supply growth 3. No major achievements since supply was focus of expenditures 4. Substantial element of equalization in cost-sharing formula	1. Major 2. Major 3. Variable 4. Major. Atlantic provinces participated in Canada-wide plan
T3 1961–1971/1972	1. Canada-wide, universal, publicly financed medical insurance 2. Expansion of supply 3. Public health 4. Equalization to enable less wealthy provinces to participate (a lesser priority than it was for hospital insurance)	1. Canada-wide medical insurance 2. Health Resources Fund: strong supply growth—4 new medical schools and increased intake in existing 12 schools. Comparable growth in professional nurses 3. Huge growth in social services, post-secondary education, skills training, and retirement incomes 4. Equalization less strong than hospital insurance but sufficient for all provinces to participate	1. Major 2. Major 3. Major 4. Major

T4 1972–1989	1. Clarification of principles that undergird Canada-wide health-care system 2. Cost-containment/efficiency while maintaining quality of service 3. Determinants of health mindset (Lalonde)	1. *Canada Health Act* and amendments to provincial health insurance law where needed 2(a). Provinces not successful in controlling costs 2(b). High level of public satisfaction with services 3. Little evidence of this mindset influencing policy outcomes	1. Major 2(a). Considerable 2(b). Major 3. Little
Base case 1990–2003	1. Cost-containment/efficiency 2. Cost-effectiveness through structural change 3. Scope of insurance coverage 4. Social determinants of health	1. Five-year period of retrenchment (1992–1996) followed by sharp escalation in costs 2. Regionalization, some funding changes, some hospital rationalization; little progress in primary care reform 3. Absence of changes in insurance to respond to growth of ambulatory care; Quebec drug coverage improved; other provinces variable on drug and home care coverage 4. Some achievements: anti-smoking campaign; some setbacks with growth of income inequality	1. Considerable in short run but not sustained 2. Modest 3. Substantial in Quebec; modest and variable elsewhere 4. Variable at best

Note:
Scale: major, considerable, modest, variable, little, none. These adjectives differ from the terms used in the case-by-case analysis to avoid confusing the analyses. The case-by-case analysis involved detailed examination of specific programs, whereas here we focus on higher-level trends.

Reconsidering the Case Selection

The aspect of the methodology considered here is the choice of issues for study. Chapter 2 set out our method for selecting cases relying on a decomposition of health-care policy reform into four domains (Lavis et al. 2002). We refined this methodology into a comprehensive taxonomy that serves as a one-stop shop for research evidence about health systems (www.healthsystemsevidence.org).

The specific question posed here is whether, with the benefit of hindsight, any of the six cases selected have somehow turned out to be inappropriate, perhaps by being too small in the context of the overall health-care reform issue, insufficiently representative of the reform challenges, or not readily researchable. Is there an inadvertent bias in our case selection that has led to either an overstatement or an understatement of the extent of reform or its direction? It will be recalled (chapter 2) that before making the choices, we consulted with 10 key informants—two from each of the five provinces—with one being a senior government official and one a member of the research community.

With regard to the governance domain, regionalization was our choice. The first wave of provincial grey literature reports focused on regionalization more than any other single governance issue (O'Fee 2002a). Regionalization was also the biggest governance issue on provincial agendas, at least in the first half of the 1990s. In some provinces, regionalization was seen as a precondition to the reform of hospital funding and improvements in health services. For these reasons, it seemed an obvious choice and a fundamental challenge to the core bargain with hospitals in some provinces.

In the second half of the 1990s, in the aftermath of the unilateral federal government cuts in cash transfers to the provinces associated with the introduction of the Canada Health and Social Transfer (CHST), provincial priorities changed. The rules of the game concerning the interpretation and enforcement of the *Canada Health Act*, and the link between the CHA and the CHST, became an overriding concern of provincial premiers, finance ministers, and health ministers (Conference of Provincial/ Territorial Ministers of Health 1997, 9). Thus the governance of the CHA/ CHST—who gets to make decisions about what health-care services are publicly insured, and under what terms—might have been an alternative to regionalization as our case study (although that would have entailed intergovernmental governance). Had the CHA/CHST been substituted for the regionalization case, the result would have entailed less reform: during our study period, the provinces made only minor inroads on this issue in their negotiations with Ottawa.

Needs-based funding and alternative payment plans (APPs) were the two cases selected in the financial arrangements domain. Hospitals were the largest recipients of provincial health-care funding throughout the 1990–2003 era. Physicians were the second-largest recipients in 1990 and remained so until 1997 when provincial spending on drugs eclipsed spending on doctors. For the remainder of the period, physicians were the third-largest recipients. Given the slow progress on financial reform, the grey literature through to the Kirby and Romanow reports continued to highlight the necessity of altering the incentive structure for hospital funding. As for physician compensation, APP was not only an important issue in its own right, but generally was seen as a precondition to implementing primary care reform. These case choices thus remain as suitable selections. But had pharmaceutical financing been chosen, the results would not have been more reform.

Wait-times management and for-profit delivery were selected as the case studies in the delivery domain. Wait times was a way of focusing on issues of accessibility. By the second half of the period, the wait-times issue was in the process of becoming perhaps the largest single challenge to the delivery system. This was reflected in the September 2000 First Ministers' "Action Plan for Health Delivery," which stressed that "both the timely access to and quality of health services" were "the highest priority to Canadians" (Canadian Intergovernmental Conference Secretariat 2000, 2). This priority was reaffirmed in the 2003 and 2004 First Ministers' Accords (First Ministers' Meeting 2003, 2004).

To achieve a fair sample of reform issues, it was appropriate to assess how effective strongly market-oriented governments were in advancing their reform agendas. For-profit delivery was a way of capturing this alternative paradigm.

Both issues grew in relative importance over the period covered, but with limited to moderate effects only. There were certainly other substantive cases that might have been selected in their stead. An argument can be made, for example, that had the project included a case focused exclusively on hospital rationalization (which was linked to regionalization), the result might have increased the amount of reform since Ontario's rationalization of hospitals was carried out without regionalizing services. A second alternative would have been to develop a case around electronic health records. This too was potentially a large delivery issue, but one characterized by little progress despite significant public investment. A 2009 Commonwealth Fund International Survey of 11 industrialized countries showed that Canada ranked *last*, and by a large margin, in terms of "health information practice capacity" (cited in CMA 2010, 23). Had it been selected, the result in all probability would have decreased the overall amount of reform in our sample. In short, in the delivery category there were other possible cases of similar magnitude but not obviously more representative than the ones selected.

As for the program content domain, there were two major proposals for enhanced universal insurance coverage during the period: prescription drugs and home care. The drug case was the larger of the two in terms of potential cost and the one where more progress was made. Had home care been selected, the result likely would have shown less reform.

In sum, the cases selected were large in their own right, covering a substantial proportion of the health-care reform agenda. Some were also preconditions to other reforms. The cases were reasonably representative of the challenges in health-care reform.

RELATING RESEARCH RESULTS TO PUBLIC POLICY AND HEALTH LITERATURE

This section first considers our research results relative to the Kingdon framework. To what extent did the framework help us to illuminate the decision process? Kingdon developed his framework on the basis of case studies of decision-making in two sectors, one of which was health care. How did our results on health-care reform in Canada compare to his findings in the United States? Next, we discuss our findings relative to the wider public policy and health policy literature.

Kingdon's Framework

A decision to root an empirical research project in one or more theories or models of decision-making is made with the expectation that applying the theory will illuminate and clarify what are often very complex processes. The research for this book takes into account many schools of thought, but we relied mainly on two theories in structuring the research program. One was John Kingdon's "agenda-setting" model. We hoped it would help us understand the early and middle phases of the decision process.

Kingdon's (2003) book rests on an empirical base that included 23 case studies in two broad areas of public policy—health care and transportation—in the United States. The fact that Kingdon had tested his ideas about agenda-setting in the health-care sphere added to our interest in his theory. Nonetheless, there were important differences between his purposes and the work that underpins this book. Kingdon used questions about health care and transport to shed light on the decision process in general. His goal was to observe policy change on a wide enough range of issues to be able to offer hypotheses about decision-making in the United States, especially during the agenda-setting phase. In the preface to the second edition of *Agendas, Alternatives and Public Policies,* Kingdon wrote that he had become "convinced that scholars had learned quite a bit about such authoritative decisions in government as legislators' roll call votes and presidents' final decisions," but much less about how issues "got to be issues in the first place" (2003, xvii). He studied two policy areas to "insure that generalizations about policy processes would not be due to idiosyncrasies of one case or policy area" (231).

In contrast, our purpose was specific to health-care policy and why it was so hard to reform this sector despite widespread calls for such reforms. We wondered whether there were idiosyncrasies in Canadian health care, and how substantial they might be in shaping the record of reform. In effect, we were testing the applicability of Kingdon's insights to a different jurisdiction. We found that much of what Kingdon wrote did in fact have application for our purposes. However, we set out below some further differences and similarities between the two research projects, and their results, so that readers can form their own assessments.

In addition to different purposes, there are other differences worth noting. Kingdon's major project was carried out in the 1970s in the United States and focused on issues that were current then. Ours was carried out in the mid-2000s in Canada and investigated decisions that had already been taken. His work had all the benefits of observation in real time. Ours had the benefit of some historical perspective. Since Kingdon was most interested in what made an issue, his focus on current activity or inactivity made considerable sense. Since our purpose was to account for policy outcomes, it followed that we could do our work only after decisions had been taken or had failed to reach the governmental agenda within our period of study.

Kingdon was interested in decision-making at the federal level. We did not seek to exclude the federal authority in Canada but, as things turned out, health-care reform in the years we studied involved mainly provincial governments. In effect, we tested the explanatory value of his theory in five provincial jurisdictions.

Perhaps the biggest difference between the two projects was the institutional setting. Due to the fusion of decision-making processes in the Canadian Westminster model—that is, the integration of executive and legislative powers—and the strong discipline in Canadian political parties, decision-making in Canada was highly integrated. This was true for decision-making in both the federal and the provincial orders of government. Researchers in Canada can learn much about a decision if they find the "right" person to interview, as that person might well know most of the history of the issue from its earliest stages through to the policy choice stage. And that interviewee will often be able to point to the few other people who can fill in the blanks. This is less true in the United States since the executive and legislature are separate. Adding to the difference is the bicameral nature of the legislature in the United States with substantive power found in both the House of Representatives and the Senate. Provincial legislatures in Canada are unicameral, and the Canadian Parliament has a weak upper house.

One difference in our results relative to Kingdon's project is in the role of the policy entrepreneur. Kingdon reported that in "our 23 case studies, we coded entrepreneurs as very or somewhat important in 15, and found them unimportant in only three" (180). In our 30 case studies, the role of policy entrepreneurs was cited in eight cases and only two of these were major influences. While the difference may be research-related, it is also plausible that there is a greater need for policy entrepreneurs in the more fragmented American system of government than is the case in Canada, where the executive usually has a majority in the legislature.

All these institutional factors suggest that decision-making in Canada should be more researcher-friendly. But it was not, mainly because governance in the United States is more transparent than in Canada. Members of Congress may talk publicly about an issue long before it hits the administration's radar screen. The frequent use of congressional committee hearings may help the researcher to follow the pathway of an issue. Relatively weak caucus discipline in the United States reinforces the transparency, because legislators are not breaching the "rules of the game" if they take a public stand that does not jibe with the majority in their caucus. These processes are more publicly visible in the American system than in the Canadian system.

Yet there were also strong similarities between the two research projects. For example, Kingdon focused on proposals to encourage health maintenance organizations as a way of increasing competition and controlling health-care costs. Our project studied proposals to encourage for-profit delivery for similar reasons. Kingdon analyzed proposals to expand Medicare and Medicaid insurance coverage, while we studied decisions to extend publicly financed insurance for prescription pharmaceuticals. Kingdon was interested in economic regulation of various modes of transport from the perspective of the user or consumer. Our interest in wait times and in regional and hospital funding had both a consumer (patient) and fairness perspective.

On the role of interest groups, Kingdon wrote,

> Actually, much interest group activity in these processes consists not of positive promotion, but rather of negative blocking.... Interest groups often seek to preserve prerogatives and benefits they currently are enjoying, blocking initiatives that they believe would reduce those benefits.... While it is not possible to estimate quantitatively..., it is clear that a substantial portion of interest group effort is devoted to negative, blocking activities. (2003, 49)

We report in almost identical terms in chapters 8 and 9.

Kingdon distinguished between "predictable windows" and "unpredictable windows" for reform. Predictable windows, he wrote, can be linked to the budget cycle, statutory requirements (such as requirements for periodic legislative review or sunset provisions), and election cycles.

On the election cycle he observed that "basically, a window opens because of change in the political stream (e.g., a change of administration, a shift in the partisan or ideological distribution of seats in Congress)" (2003, 186). Our research found that a change in government/leader that had committed to reform in the election campaign or leadership contest and that acted swiftly on its commitment once in office constituted one of two key factors that led to large reforms.

With respect to "unpredictable windows," Kingdon (2003, 187-90) observed that the problem, policy, and political streams usually run in parallel with one another. But occasionally random events bring these streams together. While they flow together, there is an opportunity for policy reform (the open window). This opportunity is generally short lived, however, and for reform to occur the policy stream must have a solution that fits the problem and politics. Kingdon observed that crisis can play a role in opening a window. This paralleled our findings on the role of fiscal crises linked to recession. Political change sets the broad direction for policy change, but it is rare, in Kingdon's research (or it was rare until he updated his book), for the new administration to have concrete ideas on which it is ready to act. In Kingdon's model, this is where the policy stream comes into play. Similarly, in six of the seven largest Canadian reforms identified in Table 8.1, the policy community supplied all or much of the policy design.

Kingdon's research was first made public a quarter century prior to Barak Obama's becoming the president of the United States. Under Obama's leadership, Congress passed legislation that involved the first large reform in health care in decades. This led Kingdon to update his book to ascertain whether his framework could account for Obama's success. The update is in the form of an epilogue. In it Kingdon examines the factors that enabled President Obama to achieve health-care reform where President Clinton had failed during his years in office (2010, 231-47). Kingdon reminds readers about the sheer complexity of the health-care system and the numerous veto points within it that make reform inherently difficult. What, then, made the difference for Obama?

Kingdon begins his epilogue by focusing on the "problem stream" that not only contributed to putting health care on the governmental agenda but also helped move it swiftly to a decision. The growing cost of health care, and to a lesser extent the gaps in insurance coverage, were the well-known basic problems. They had been present in the Clinton era but had worsened since then. Second, the "greatest recession since the Great Depression of the 1930s ... threw into sharp relief the downside of employer-based health.... If one were to lose one's job, not only did one lose the income and status of employment, but one also lost the health insurance for both the employee and his or her family" (2010, 234). Kingdon cites White House chief of staff Rahm Emmanuel that "you never want a serious crisis to go to waste" (235). The Clinton years did not "benefit" (our word) from such a crisis. Third, the ongoing process of globalization was creating a problem for American firms in trade-sensitive industries. Firms that were sponsoring or contributing to employee health insurance were increasingly at a disadvantage in competition with foreign firms that did not bear the financial burden of contributing to the health insurance of their employees. This situation was not new but had worsened since Clinton had occupied the White House. It meant that some business leaders were prepared to rethink their self-interest.

The "policy streams" affecting the two administrations were also different. Kingdon (2010, 238) observes that there was "disarray among health policy specialists before President Clinton took office." In contrast, when Obama took office in January 2009, "most of the prominent advocates had settled on one basic approach.... The current system of private insurance would be left in place, as would the current government programs and employer-based insurance policies" (ibid.). The centrepiece of the approach is the "individual mandate" under which individuals are required to obtain health insurance privately to the extent that they are not covered to a minimum standard under a public plan.

As for the "political stream," there were similarities in the situations that faced the Obama and Clinton administrations (Democrats in the White House and Democrat majorities in both houses of Congress) as well as differences ("the filibuster-free majority of sixty in the Senate" enjoyed by Obama). Importantly, the Obama administration and its allies were "keenly aware" that the reform window would not stay open for long, and they acted accordingly. In sum, Obama had run for office committed to reform, was organized to take advantage of the consensus within the policy community, and acted swiftly on it. Members of the Obama administration were able to meet and negotiate with interests that had opposed reform in the past because they knew their basic direction. This had not been the case under Clinton.

Although on a different scale, the Obama-Clinton comparison is qualitatively similar to the cross-province comparison between premiers Romanow and Rae (chapter 9). Presidents Obama and Clinton were members of the same political party and shared a roughly comparable centre to centre-left worldview. Premiers Romanow and Rae also shared a common worldview, and one that was similar in the Canadian context to the Obama and Clinton stance in the American context. Neither Rae nor Clinton achieved substantial reform. Rae's party had not committed to health reform, so that outcome was not a surprise. Clinton had committed to reform but had not prepared for it. He did not have a clear vision of his destination and an effective strategy to overcome his opposition, or at least to negotiate a compromise that was a stepping stone to something larger. His outcome was roughly comparable to Rae's (meagre) achievements (at least in respect of our six issues). Political commitment was a necessary ingredient for reform but not a sufficient one. Both Obama and Romanow were politically committed to reform. Both were prepared from a policy perspective—not the details but the fundamentals. Both were organized to act immediately on taking office, and did so. Neither, it must be added, secured all of what they originally intended. Of course there were differences: Romanow acted a quarter century earlier than Obama. The institutional settings—the Westminster system relative to separation of powers in the presidential system—were large. The political opposition was weak in Saskatchewan but fierce in Washington. What is noteworthy about the Obama-Romanow comparison is that the commonality of the factors that bred success outweighed the differences between the two cases.

In a nutshell, the Kingdon framework proved illuminating in a Canadian setting as well as in the United States. Put more generally, these comparisons point to the convergence of the three streams—problems, policies, and politics—in both countries. The integration of executive and legislature in the Westminster system and the usual four-year life of Canadian legislative bodies may enable more frequent and longer lasting open windows in Canada than in the United States. The Canadian system of government does not require general elections every second year as does the House of Representatives in the United States (so political honeymoons may last longer in Canada). There may even be more policy capacity (of a certain kind) within government ministries in Canada because the top levels of the public service usually do not change whenever a government changes as is the case in Washington. Probably the public service in Canada, relative to its US counterparts, is better informed about the mix of policies that represent the status quo and what kinds of nips and tucks are needed to make it better. Experience teaches Canadian officials that big reforms are not necessarily better, and are very difficult to make happen. In the United States, changes of administration do bring new ideas because the new team is not wedded to what is. They are the winds of change, yet that they rarely succeed is also part of the legacy.

The more salient message is that despite big differences in institutions and big differences in political culture, until "Obamacare" the records of reform in the two countries were not vastly different. The last major reform in Canada was in the 1960s in favour of universal health care; at about the same time, Lyndon Johnson presided over the creation of Medicare and Medicaid. These reforms marked a parting "at the crossroads," to borrow Maioni's (1998) evocative phrase. The roads have diverged, but achieving reform of any magnitude in either country remains a huge challenge.

Comparing Our Results to Those of Other Researchers

In this subsection, we compare our conclusion of meagre reform with the conclusions of other researchers. We then compare our explanations for the reform outcomes as set out in chapters 8 and 9 with what other researchers have found on this question.

On the Extent of Reform

The literature on the *extent* of reform from 1990 to 2003 is limited. Researchers apparently took for granted that little reform had occurred; possibly they looked at the action and lack of action at the Canada-wide level and concluded that there was little need to explain the obvious. In the discussion here, we begin with the literature that deals with reform at the Canada-wide level. Next, we consider what other researchers have had to say about the extent of reform on the six issues we studied.

At the Canada-wide level, reform of the *Canada Health Act* was not on the agenda of the Mulroney Conservative government nor seemingly was any other aspect of health-care policy.[7] In a letter to provincial ministers of health, the federal minister of health Jake Epp (1985) committed to "honour and respect provincial jurisdiction and authority in matters pertaining to health and the provision of health-care services."[8]

The rhetoric of the Chrétien Liberals (1993–2003) was much different from that of the Tories, and so was the federal/provincial/territorial dynamic. Yet when all was said and done—notwithstanding the work of the National Forum on Health, the Social Union Framework Agreement, and the apparent agreements among governments at the First Ministers' Conferences in 1999, 2000, and 2003 (the latter two involving health agreements, whether called "accords" or not)—policy reforms at the Canada-wide level were few and of modest consequence. Commitments entered into by provinces and territories with the federal government were neither legally binding nor for the most part politically enforceable.

What, then, did researchers have to say about the extent of reform? Carolyn Tuohy noted Canada's resilience to health policy change (1999, 89-90):

> In the three decades after the establishments of the federal Medicare programme (which was fully in place by 1971), the Canadian health care system showed a remarkable structural and institutional stability. No major policy change on the order of the NHS internal markets reform occurred, nor was there even an unsuccessful attempt at major change as occurred in the United States.[9]

Tuohy's comparators were the United Kingdom and the United States. Other researchers have come to similar conclusions but took the dearth of reform as evidence of rigidity, not stability (Evans 2000, 889; Pink and Leatt 2003, 1-2). In arguing the case for a renewal of national health goals and objectives, Duane Adams observed that the "difficulty inherent in achieving intergovernmental consensus seems to be so great that principal stakeholders are at times unwilling to modernize, amend, or update an intergovernmental agreement for fear of unraveling the original consensus that formed the 'national' foundation for the programme" (2001a, 60). Adams had been deputy minister in the early Romanow years and brought the perspective of an insider. With some reason, he saw national health policy "as a pawn on a much larger federal/provincial/territorial ... game board" (2001b, 271). Redden (2002, 69-70) used the word "stasis" to describe health care in Canada. Stasis, she argued, was made up of three factors: federal-provincial deadlock, resistance to delisting, and stability in the face of evidence of the need for change.

At the subsector/issue level, regionalization was where we found the most reform. Indeed, in the early 1990s, four of the five provinces we studied undertook reforms on this issue—qualifying as "significant" in Alberta and Saskatchewan, and "moderate" in Newfoundland and Labrador. Quebec furthered its regional system of governance in 1991 and then reversed some of those decisions in 2003. The "net" result in Quebec was a limited counter-consensus reform. Among the provinces we studied, there was less reform on needs-based funding than on regionalization and less still on the alternative payment plans (APP) issue.

As for the literature on regionalization, Naylor (1999) wrote favourably that nine provinces and one northern territory had moved toward some form of regionalized governance of health care during the 1990s, and he saw hospital rationalization as one positive linked outcome. He lamented the fact that "two provinces have created regional boards but have not actually devolved budgets to them" (14). Two years later, Steven Lewis and colleagues argued (Lewis et al. 2001, 929),

> With the introduction of regionalization, the 1990s saw dramatic organizational changes in health services, but the main elements of the reforms recommended in a series of extensive reviews in the 1980s have yet to be adopted. Fee-for-service remains the dominant payment method for doctors, despite widespread and longstanding recognition of its perverse incentives.

These authors reached the conclusion that considerable reform was achieved on the issue of regionalization, as does this book. Their worry was that it was not generating the reform results that had been expected.

Population needs-based funding was implemented to a significant degree in Saskatchewan and Alberta once the provincial governments had their regional authorities in place. A smaller reform (in the sense of covering a small part of hospital budgets) was introduced in Quebec. Within the health policy research literature, how hospitals were funded, as opposed to how they should be funded, was not controversial (Federal/Provincial/Territorial Advisory Committee on Health Services 1995).

On APP, and primary health-care reform more generally, other researchers agree that reform was slow in coming. Hutchison and co-authors set out their conclusions on primary care reform in the title of their paper, "Primary Care in Canada: So Much Innovation, So Little Change" (Hutchison, Abelson, and Lavis 2001). Their take was: "Despite their wide variety and substantial numbers, innovations in the organization, funding, and delivery of primary care in Canada have been at the margins of primary care rather than at its core" (122).

For-profit delivery was the only one of our six issues that examined a reform proposal that was not consistent with the consensus of the grey literature. Our research showed two cases of moderate counter-consensus reform (Alberta under Klein and Ontario under Harris/Eves), two cases of no reform (Quebec and Newfoundland), and one significant reform, Saskatchewan (remembering that "reform" in this context means supporting the grey literature opposition to for-profit delivery). What is particularly noteworthy is that the premiers of Alberta and Ontario, despite their personal commitment and effort, were not able to achieve significant counter-consensus reforms.

As for wait times, the research community agreed on the need for substantial reform. By the early 2000s, there was a veritable "industry" of individuals and organizations doing research on wait times and wait-list management. Much of what the country's leading researchers on health policy thought about these issues was captured at a colloquium, The Taming of the Queue, held in 2004.[10] Over 80 participants discussed what "needs to happen next in Canada to move towards better measurement, monitoring and management of wait times" (Canadian Policy Research Networks 2004). Participants were surveyed about the seriousness of the wait-times issue, and 55 percent agreed that "there is excessive wait times for many treatments and services across all jurisdictions" (ibid., Appendix C). When asked whether "access to timely services has worsened, improved, or stayed about the same over the past few years," 55 percent thought it had worsened, 5 percent thought it had improved, and the rest either did not know or thought it had remained the same. In 1999, Naylor wrote that "waiting lists for many procedures remain lengthy and inconsistently managed.... The true extent of under-servicing and implicit rationing is still unknown, in part because systematic audits have not been carried out" (22).

On prescription drug coverage, our cross-provincial analysis mirrored the perception of other researchers that equity was lacking. We found one case of limited counter-consensus reform (Saskatchewan), one of no reform (Newfoundland and Labrador), one of limited reform (Alberta), one of moderate reform (Ontario), and one of comprehensive reform (Quebec). Demers and colleagues "found that eligibility criteria and cost-sharing details of the publicly funded prescription drug plans differed markedly across Canada, as did the personal financial burden due to prescription drug costs" (Demers et al. 2008, 405). Taking account of both publicly and privately financed drug insurance plans, 96 percent of Canadians had some coverage (Kapur and Basu 2005, 181-93). Eighty-four percent of the population had "conventional" (i.e., non-catastrophic) coverage; in three provinces, conventional coverage was in the 67–69 percent range. Quebec alone had universal coverage (ibid.).

In sum, the basic conclusion of meagre reform during the 1990–2003 period is consistent with literature at both the overarching and the sectoral/issue levels.

On the Factors That Account for Reform Performance

We have accounted for these meagre reforms in chapters 8 and 9. How do our explanations for the paucity of reform compare with the explanations put forward by other researchers who have studied these issues? In answering this question we begin by referring to the general literature on public policy, then very briefly on health policy in other countries and comparative health policy, and finally on Canadian health policy.

The literature on public policy places considerable emphasis on the role of political *institutions* (one of the three I's) and the way they evolve. The argument is that previously enacted public policies structure the behaviour of policy actors, creating constraints and opportunities for policy change. In focusing on the politics of welfare states, for example, Paul Pierson (2000) noted that postwar social welfare programs had created powerful vested *interests* (another of the I's). Once created, and given time to sink roots, these actors had the resources to punish political leaders who threatened the structural arrangements from which they benefited. In reviewing the literature on policy-making, Howlett and Ramesh (2003, 217) note that "path dependency" describes "the situation whereby once a system's trajectory is in place, it tends to perpetuate itself by limiting the range of choices or the ability of forces both outside … and inside … the system to alter that trajectory." When policy change is called for, and happens, the change is almost always incremental and within the framework of the existing model.

Decisions to protect the existing framework—the status quo—or modify it at the margin are not, however, neutral. Some existing interests benefit more than others. Decades ago Bachrach and Baratz (1970, 44) referred to such decisions as a "mobilization of bias, [which is] a set of predominant values, beliefs, rituals and institutional procedures (rules of the game) that operate systematically and consistently" to the benefit of certain interests. In a similar vein, Sabatier (1988) noted that via a set of reinforcing *ideas* (the third "I") and institutions, certain interests were privileged over others through a symbiotic relationship with government. Relative stability within the policy community was maintained unless some external shock, such as a major change in socioeconomic conditions or an entirely new technology, arose to alter "the causal assumptions of present policies" (Sabatier 1988, 131). These "policy regimes" are seen by scholars as an attempt "to capture how policy institutions, actors, and ideas tend to congeal into relatively long-term, institutionalized patterns of interaction that combine to keep public policy contents and processes more or less constant over time" (Howlett, Ramesh, and Perl 2009, 86). These regimes limited the opportunities for significant reforms to occur because of the path dependency and policy legacies that were created (Doern 1998; Pierson 2000).

With respect to the literature on health care, American scholars pointed to the central power position of physician interests in shaping health-care policy in the United States (Alford 1975; Mechanic 1991). They observed that health policy was determined through an ongoing process of negotiation among major governments, medical interests, and non-medical interests. Alford suggested that the interests of some groups such as organized medicine and the pharmaceutical industry were "dominant" in the health field, although he wrote before the growth of managed care in the United States and the ascension of private insurers. In comparing European jurisdictions, Freddi and Bjorkman (1989) concluded that the close and formal relationship between organized medicine and governments embedded and enhanced the power of physicians. Bluntly, physician interests were more likely to co-op governments than the other way around.

As identified by a number of Canadian scholars, some examining health care in Canada through a comparative lens (Maioni 1998; Tuohy 1999) and others through a mainly Canadian prism (Lavis 2004; Naylor 1986; Taylor 2009), past policies in Canada created core bargains between provincial governments and medical associations. These legacies served to reinforce and institutionalize the central power position of medical associations. For example, the case studies of alternative payment plans undertaken for this book found that over time provincial medical associations and provincial governments were developing increasingly closer and more formalized governance relations through joint-management committees.

Naylor (1986), Lomas and Barer (1986), Tuohy (1988), and Lavis (2004) observed that organized medicine in Canada has been successful in protecting its core clinical and economic interests as defined through the core bargain between provincial governments and provincial medical associations and medical unions. Lavis added that medical associations did not always have to demand something in order to get what they wanted: "Reform proposals may never make it past the consideration stage because provincial officials anticipate opposition from political elites ... and do not feel they have the necessary political resources to take on this opposition" (2004, 270). At the same time, medical associations used their considerable resources to protect and enhance the private delivery aspect of their core bargains with provincial governments and what they saw as its corollary—the right to fee-for-service.

In their study of health reform in Quebec, Contandriopoulos and Brousselle (2010, 6) noted that "the unimplemented elements were always those that entailed significant transformations for powerful interest groups (i.e., doctors, hospital associations, teaching hospitals and faculties of medicine). On the other hand, the implemented elements were mostly modifications to the system's administration."

Medical associations were not the only voices that were heard. Both Maioni (1998, 173) and Tuohy (1999, 102) noted that once medicare benefits were created, the Canadian public became very attached to them. For some, medicare was the stuff of Canada's DNA. Governments, both federal and provincial, were reluctant to be seen as taking any action that would leave them vulnerable to the charge of being an enemy of medicare. Lavis (2004) observed that the federal government drew on its financial and political resources to create and entrench the public payment side of the core bargain. He suggested that provinces were loath to challenge it because, for the most part, they believed that public opinion would be on Ottawa's side. We return to this important theme in chapter 12.

Where do our findings fit with the literature discussed above? First, like other researchers, we have found government reform agendas to be incremental. No government approached health care in a way that might be described as a "big bang." Second, the largest of the reforms found in our 30 cases had their origins outside the heath sector, driven by newly elected governments with commitment to reform and helped by fiscal crises that could be used to provide cover for such reform. By the same token, we found insider interests generally opposed to reforms that touched their interests.

Third, on the influence of medical associations, our findings are broadly similar to the results of other researchers. Only one of the seven cases assessed as "significant" or higher involved physician interests (Saskatchewan wait times), and it was developed with physician experts playing a lead role. We found that medical associations were the most influential when reform proposals that affected the interests of their members reached or were about to reach the governmental agenda. On such issues, medical associations were able to shape the nature and pace of reform. Their influence on such matters far exceeded that of associations representing other health-care professionals such as nurses. It also outstripped organizations representing hospital interests. (We did not do sufficient cases to express views on the influence of pharmaceutical producers and distributors.)

Fourth, we noted that public opinion and civil society advocacy groups were also very protective of the medicare legacy. We described formal coalitions at both the Canada-wide and provincial levels dedicated to that

very purpose. Although their views were barely perceptible on governance and financial issues, public opinion and civil society groups carried
considerable weight on policy reform issues within the delivery and
policy content domains. They were more influential in protecting existing
arrangements within these policy domains, however, than in extending
them. In general, public opinion and civil society groups vigorously opposed any opening up of the medicare legacy unless it was to extend its
scope. For example, Tuohy (1999, 114) argued that public opinion was
neither a necessary nor a sufficient condition to open reform windows.
Our findings are similar. It is noteworthy that public opinion and civil
society groups gave greater priority to protecting existing benefits than
they did to extending them.

Thus the evidence points to physicians and public opinion—to doctors
and patients—as the main bases for the stability, or rigidity, depending
on the reader's view, of Canada's medicare arrangements. The third
principal partner in this political triangle was elected government. With
the important exception of the "change in government/leader" cases,
government was generally content to preside over what existed rather
than to challenge it.

Finally, we noted the effect of Canadian federalism. Tuohy (1999, 246)
argued that strong institutional arrangements were required to implement
national macro-policy reforms: a centralized decision-making body and a
high level of support from political actors were essential factors to initiate
substantive change. In this view, Canada's non-centralized system, with a
relatively weak federal constitutional authority, was a barrier to Canada-
wide reforms during our study period.

Our analysis also pointed to the conduct of federal-provincial relations
as an obstacle to reform on matters within the jurisdiction of individual
provinces. Each province had the constitutional authority to undertake
reforms in the six representative issues we researched. That they did
not do much was linked to disparate opposing factors, most of which
were noted in previous chapters. One factor that we have not discussed
in great detail was the state of federal-provincial fiscal relations. We are
not referring here to the conditional nature of federal health transfers to
provinces (which created a barrier to certain kinds of reforms, especially
those that might have involved user charges at the point of delivery).
Rather, we observe that the dysfunctional nature of federal-provincial
dynamics (Marchildon 2004) arising from the 1995 federal budget became in itself a reform barrier. Premiers were reluctant to undertake any
reform that might undercut their claims that Ottawa was shortchanging
the provinces on the federal contribution to health care. This theme is
picked up again in chapter 12.

CONCLUSIONS

The first purpose of this chapter was to test the sensitivity of our findings. To do so, we compared the nature and extent of reforms in our study period to reforms in four earlier periods. This historical approach generated similar results to the case study method—meagre reform. We also found that altering the mix of issues within the case study method would not likely have changed the results.

We then compared our research results to John Kingdon's findings in his analysis of agenda-setting in the United States. The results were remarkably similar. This does not mean that reform in Canada was similar to reform in the United States, but that the methodology Kingdon developed to understand policy change in the US could be constructively applied in the Canadian setting.

Finally, we demonstrated that our explanations for meagre reform were broadly consistent with the explanations of other researchers.

Taken together, the arguments in this chapter point to the robustness of the methodology we employed. The study period ended in 2003, however. Has the nature or extent of reform changed since then? Have the various factors that shaped reform outcomes between 1990 and 2003 changed? If so, in what ways? These are the questions addressed in chapter 11.

NOTES

1. The first three periods overlap because of overlapping events and the related difficulty in selecting a single moment when one era ended and another began. For example, it can be argued that the events that precipitated the federal government's willingness to proceed with a long-postponed promise to introduce federal-provincial shared-cost hospital insurance began at a First Ministers' Meeting in the spring of 1955. At that meeting, Ontario premier Leslie Frost reversed his previous public stand and pressed federal prime minister Louis St. Laurent to include health care on the agenda of a First Ministers' Conference to be held in the autumn of that year. Alternatively, the events that triggered Frost's change of heart could be the starting point. They dated back to the 1953 general election when federal Liberal backbenchers persuaded a reluctant St. Laurent to include, in the Liberal party's election platform, a commitment to proceed with a federal-provincial shared-cost hospital insurance program when a majority of provinces were willing to participate (Martin 1985, 218-47; Taylor 2009, 108).

2. The Dominion Council of Health was created under Section 6 of the federal *Department of Health Act* of 1919 and reaffirmed under the *Department of National Health and Welfare Act* of 1944. It advised the minister of national health and welfare on matters relating to the health of Canadians. The council focused on coordination of federal-provincial health programs and liaison between the two levels of government. The council was composed of a chair (the deputy minister of national health), the chief executive officer of each

provincial department or board of health, and five members representing various segments of the Canadian population. It ceased functioning in the 1970s.

3. During the war years, the provinces had agreed to temporarily "rent" their constitutional right to levy taxes on personal income and corporate income to the dominion government. The Constitution allowed the dominion government to tax personal and corporate income as well and there was a concern that tax competition between the orders of government would weaken the ability of Canada to prosecute the war. In return for these rental arrangements, Ottawa made grants to the provinces. The rental arrangements were to end a year after wartime hostilities had terminated. But there was no agreement on what would replace them when the war did come to an end. Provincial governments did not know, therefore, what their revenue would be when peace returned.

4. With regard to the dominion government's health insurance proposals to the provinces at the Dominion-Provincial Conference on Reconstruction, Taylor (2009, 66-67) cites the dominion government's minister of national health and welfare to the effect that "at times it was made to appear as the gasoline tax alone stood in the way of an agreement" on health insurance.

5. The CMA had shown support for the "principle of health insurance" (cited in Taylor 2009, 27).

6. Neither Quebec nor Ontario reached a postwar rental agreement in 1947 with the federal government regarding personal or corporate income tax-sharing or collection. Quebec chose not to do so again in 1952 and 1957 and has not done so to this day (2013). Ontario reached an agreement with the federal government in 1952. Nonetheless, the word "settled" is used here to reflect informal understandings among governments that enabled Ottawa and Quebec City to informally coordinate their approach to income tax law and administration.

7. The Progressive Conservative government introduced amendments to the *Patent Act* that modified and strengthened the protection that patent holders enjoyed. Enacted by Parliament in 1987, its purpose was to encourage investment in the pharmaceutical industry. A Patented Medicine Prices Review Board (2012) was subsequently created with a mandate to ensure that the "prices of patented medicines sold in Canada are not excessive."

8. It has been standard practice to include this letter as an annex in the annual report on the operations of the *Canada Health Act*.

9. The NHS reference is to the National Health Service in the United Kingdom.

10. Held on 31 March–1 April 2004, the colloquium was funded by the Canadian Medical Association, the Association of Canadian Academic Healthcare Organizations, the Institute of Health Services and Policy Research, the Canadian Institutes of Health Research, and the Canadian Institute for Health Information. Health Canada contributed indirectly. The colloquium was facilitated by the Health Network at Canadian Policy Research Networks.

Chapter 11

Health-Care Reform: Where Things Stand

Harvey Lazar

Introduction

This chapter extends the analysis of the 1990–2003 period to the end of 2011 for two reasons. One is curiosity. The research team was interested in how reform had evolved in the years since the end of the study period. The other relates to three changes in the external political environment that enabled us to test the robustness of some our conclusions in chapters 8 and 9.

The first of these changes was the substantial turnover of governments that began just as our study period was ending. Earlier chapters showed the association between newly created, first-time governments committed to reform and the achievement of larger reforms. We also found an association between an absence of reform commitments and lesser degrees of reform. We were naturally curious as to whether these findings held true during a period of widespread governmental turnover.

The political complexion of governments also changed. In a majority of the provincial jurisdictions that we studied, centre and centre-left political parties were in office for much of the time from 1990 to 2003 (hereafter referred to as period 1 or "P1"). From 2004 to the end of 2011 (hereafter "P2"), centre and centre-right political parties were dominant in provincial governments. Chapter 9 found that political ideology (right/left) was not a major factor in explaining reform decisions in the governance and financial arrangements grouping but that it was important in accounting for reform decisions in the delivery arrangements and program content grouping. Did this finding for the study period also apply in the years that followed?

A third change was at the federal level. We wondered about the effects of federal/provincial/territorial relations on health-care reform during P1 and since then. The 2006 federal election brought the Conservatives to power in Ottawa under the leadership of Stephen Harper. The Harper Conservatives had a different view of the appropriate role for the federal government in the federation than the Liberal governments that had preceded them. Where the federal Liberals were centralizing, sometimes in their actions and more often in their rhetoric, Harper was a non-centralist in matters of health-care reform. This provides us with an opportunity to consider whether the non-centralist view has made a difference.

To these ends, this chapter has two purposes. It considers what happened to the reform momentum for each of the 30 cases during P2 relative to what it had been at the end of P1. Was there a change in reform direction or not? Was the magnitude of reform larger, smaller, or about the same?

We then consider what happened during P2 to some key independent variables identified in P1. We also note a few variables that were not a part of the P1 analysis.

THE 30 CASES: 2004–2011

Developments in the 30 Cases, 2004–2011

Table 11.1 provides an update on each of the cases. It summarizes whether and to what extent the reform momentum that was signalled by the original P1 assessments, updated to the end of P1, had noticeably altered by the end of P2.

It will be recalled that our reform assessments for the 30 cases were based on the proximity of the reform to the consensus of the proposals in the grey literature produced from the late 1980s through P1. Where reform met the consensus position, it was considered to be "comprehensive" (annex 1 provides details). Those definitions of comprehensive reform are referred to below as "reform goals," and since these apply to the period from 1990 to 2003, they are "P1 goals."

For each case, the following sets out the possibilities for P2:

- momentum in respect of P1 goals was unchanged
- momentum accelerated or a new momentum started toward consensus P1 goals
- momentum decelerated or reversed direction away from P1 goals

Movement away from P1 goals may refer to a shift back to an earlier status quo or toward a much different end point, a counter-consensus reform.

Table 11.1 shows the results. Note that the table does not compare the extent of reform among provinces. Rather, for each case where there has been reform since 2003, it indicates the direction and extent of the change. An empty cell signifies no change in momentum. For example, on the needs-based funding issue, the cells are empty for three provinces. This

TABLE 11.1
Direction and Extent of Momentum Change in 30 Cases in 2004–2011 Relative to 1990–2003 Assessment

Province	*Four Domains and Six Policy Issues*						*General Comments by Province*
	Governance	*Financial Arrangements*		*Delivery*		*Program Content*	
	Regionalization	*Needs-Based Funding*	*Alternative Payment Plans*	*For-Profit Delivery*	*Wait Times and Wait-List Management*	*Prescription Drug Coverage*	
Alberta	B+	b	A				Centralizing delivery big change
Saskatchewan	b	b		b		a	Trend cautiously toward for-profit delivery within frame of publicly financed system
Ontario	a		A	A+	A	a	Reforms large and privilege medicare model
Quebec	b		a	B	A		Statutory guarantees of maximum waits for specified services
Newfoundland and Labrador					a		Lags despite oil wealth

Notes:
Letter "A" indicates *substantial* shift toward P1 goals.
Letter "B" indicates *substantial* shift away from P1 goals.
A lower case "a" or "b" indicates shift is *modest*.
An upper case "A" or "B" with a plus sign indicates the shift is *big* (comparable to significant as defined in chapter 8 or higher).

signifies that there was no momentum change relative to the reform situation in 2003 for each of those provinces, not that there was no reform or that previous reform was scuttled.

This table leads to several observations. First, as in P1, there was no "big bang" in P2. Second, the pace of reform in P2 was moderately faster than in P1. Reforms or momentum shifts occurred in 17 of the 30 cases over the eight-year span of P2, more than two shifts per year. There were 22 reforms over the 14 years of P1, just over 1.5 per year. (Note that two reforms during P2 reversed the P1 reform direction—regionalization in Alberta and for-profit delivery in Ontario.) Third, during P1, the reform direction in 18 of the 22 cases where there was reform (over 80 percent) was consistent with the consensus of the grey literature. In P2, 10 of the 17 cases of reform (less than two-thirds) involved additional substantial momentum or moderate momentum or entirely new momentum toward P1 goals.

The combination of a modestly higher rate of reform (momentum shift) in P2 than in P1, but with a smaller proportion of those reforms aimed at P1 goals, is open to more than one interpretation. One is that, in a big picture perspective, not much changed in P2 relative to P1. An overlapping interpretation is that some P1 goals had become stale by P2 (e.g., the desirability and political feasibility of *quickly* eliminating fee-for-service). The perception that regionalization would, willy-nilly, generate benefits that outweighed costs, was also more in doubt. A third interpretation focuses on the similarities and differences in momentum shifts across issues. For some reform issues, progress was made in P2 relative to the consensus of the grey literature in P1. For others the momentum shift was away from that consensus. A fourth interpretation relates to the differences among governments. In particular, Ontario, the sole centre or centre-left government, did much more reform than the other governments.

All four interpretations fit with reality to one degree or other. It will require the further passage of time—greater historical perspective— to be able to weigh them. In what follows, we focus on the last two interpretations.

Casting an eye on Table 11.1, we see that Ontario went from its status as a tortoise in P1 to the province with the greatest shifts in momentum during P2. During its first year in office, the newly formed Liberal government under the leadership of Dalton McGuinty, and with an activist health minister George Smitherman, moved quickly to undo the Conservative push toward for-profit delivery. With a majority in the legislature, the Liberals enacted legislation to reverse the policy path that its predecessor Progressive Conservative government had pursued on for-profit delivery.

On other issues as well, Ontario moved in the direction of P1 goals (grey literature consensus). Although not a part of its 2003 election platform, in 2004 the government created its unique approach to regionalization through Local Health Integration Networks (LHINs). Reform momentum accelerated on both alternative payment plans and wait-list issues. The proportion of primary care physicians being paid exclusively on a fee-for-service basis fell substantially while the proportion remunerated "through blends of fee-for-service, capitation, salary, or payments per session ... and targeted payments designed to encourage or reward the provision of priority services" (Hutchison et al. 2011, 267) grew. APP was not only an issue on its own but also a window into primary care reform. The province moved forward on wait times with the appointment of a prominent physician, Dr. Alan Hudson, the former chief executive officer of Toronto's University Health Network, to lead the charge. Hudson had the necessary knowledge and standing in the physician and hospital communities to persuade hospital administrators to sign "accountability agreements" in return for incremental funding for high priority wait-time cases (MOHLTC 2007, 3). Expanding the scope of provincial prescription drug insurance was not a priority, but by reforming the manner in which drugs were purchased and reducing the prices, coverage was presumably made more sustainable (for both generic and brand-name drugs).[1] Much of this overall reform effort was aided by the appointment of a Health Results Team made up of public servants and experts from outside the public service. Its annual reports on results, in relation to targets, were made public (MOHLTC 2005).

The 2003 general election in Quebec saw the Quebec Liberal Party returned to office after nine years in opposition with Jean Charest as leader. We have already noted new momentum in primary care reform, including APP, in Quebec (Hutchison et al. 2011, 267). The government also introduced a new legislative framework for clinics and patient access to services. For patients it included a "guaranteed-access mechanism" under which Quebecers would have alternatives to the existing delivery system if access was not provided within predetermined time limits (Ministère de la Santé et des Services sociaux 2006, 54). According to one commentator, the Quebec policy entails two distinct access mechanisms. One is a public guarantee that applies to tertiary cardiology and radiation oncology services—areas "where a patient's safety could be in serious jeopardy" (Prémont 2006, 7). Other selected services are covered by a "public-private" arrangement that is "associated both with duplicate private insurance and provision of services by private, for-profit institutions" (ibid., 8). The public-private guarantee was initially introduced for a small group of elective surgeries (hip and knee replacements and cataract surgery) and was to be gradually expanded over time. The same legislation also authorized the sale of private insurance by commercial insurers for those elective surgeries. To help ensure that time limits were met, the framework contemplated the "idea of affiliated clinics," which would allow the government to certify medical and surgical centres that were "managed by the private sector (firm, cooperative, etc.)" (Ministère de la Santé et des Services sociaux 2006, 49).

Alberta made a substantial shift toward P1 goals on the APP issue, but reversed the trend on regionalization. Alberta centralized its delivery system without forewarning or explanation, thus bringing to an end a 15-year period of regional delivery.

P2 has seen what could be the beginning of a trend. In both Quebec and Saskatchewan, for-profit delivery mechanisms were introduced or given clearer status as part of a strategy to meet wait-time targets. Both provinces created regulatory frameworks that set out specific ways in which certain categories of for-profit firms could be used to help deal with long wait times.[2]

It is also noteworthy that despite its much-enhanced fiscal situation, owing to the development of offshore hydro-carbon resources, the government of Newfoundland and Labrador did not prioritize health-care reform.

These findings suggest that the fourth interpretation—differences among governments—largely explains the differences in reform momentum between P1 and P2. The government that was most identified with the political centre or centre-left—with values closest to the grey literature consensus—made the strongest reform commitments during P2 and achieved the largest momentum shifts (Ontario). The government that promised the least also accomplished the least (Newfoundland and Labrador). At the same time, the four centre-right provincial governments did not win office promising to undo publicly financed medicare. They were parsimonious in their electoral commitments and cautious in their actions. They tried to make medicare work better—not to overtly roll it back.

The third interpretation—differences in momentum shifts across issues—can also be seen in Table 11.1 although it does not jump out to the degree that the cross-provincial comparison does. There were only two issues—APP and wait times—in which large momentum shifts occurred in more than one province. Both required the cooperation of the medical profession. We return to this point below.

EVOLUTION OF FACTORS IMPACTING REFORM

Earlier chapters have analyzed the factors that hindered or helped reform in each of our 30 cases. That analysis ended in 2003. What has happened to those factors since then? This part traces their evolution since 2003. By considering not only the magnitude of reform in P2 but also the trend in factors that helped to determine the magnitude, we shall have a base for looking forward. The discussion is selective, focusing on those factors where we observed differences in P2 relative to P1. For the convenience of readers, Table 11.2 compares the list of P2 independent variables discussed in this chapter to the more comprehensive list for P1 found in annex 1.

Note that some of the P2 variables or variable categories are discussed jointly with others and not as stand-alone categories.

Change in Government/Leader

During P1, "change in government/leader" was one of two categories of exogenous variables associated with large reforms. This category was made up of two variables—public commitment to reform prior to or during the election campaign or leadership contest that resulted in the formation of a new government, and evidence that the commitment retained its priority status with the newly formed government post-election.

There were six changes of government among the five provinces in P2.[3] The rate of change in government in P2 (six changes in eight years) was a little slower than in P1 (13 changes in 14 years). More significant was the direction of change. Whereas there had been a right-to-left shift in P1, the trend was reversed in P2. The shift began in Newfoundland and Labrador (Liberal to Progressive Conservative) and Quebec (PQ to Liberal) in 2003. In 2007, the right-of-centre conservatives won office in Saskatchewan (NDP to Saskatchewan Party). The one jurisdiction that did not change its formal complexion was Alberta, while Ontario bucked the trend and shifted back to the centre and beyond to a centre-left stance in 2003 (Progressive Conservative to Liberal). A further round of elections in 2011 was characterized by the re-election of sitting governments regardless of political stripe (although the Ontario Liberals slipped to minority status).[4] As for the federal level, the Conservative Party defeated the Liberals in 2006 and formed a minority government. In the general election of 2008, the Conservatives won a second and stronger minority. In 2011, Prime Minister Harper's conservatives were returned to power with a majority.

On the whole, the conservative opposition parties that won power in P2 were either silent or vague about health-care priorities, or focused on program details during the elections that brought them to office. They did not offer a vision of a different kind of health-care system or a more innovative way of fulfilling the existing vision. The platform of the incoming Progressive Conservative government in St. John's in 2003 made no promises on health. Nor did the incumbent Stelmach Progressive Conservatives in Alberta make significant reform commitments in 2008. There was not a hint of the major "de-regionalization" reform it was to announce within a few short months of its election. In 2007, the incoming Saskatchewan Party declared its opposition to the NDP government's promise to introduce universal coverage of prescription drugs. It also promised a "Patient First Review of the health care system to determine how best to ... reduce surgical wait times and ensure patients get more timely access to the care they need" (Saskatchewan Party 2007, 11). On the whole, this promise has played out as a commitment to make health-care delivery more efficient.

The Quebec Liberal Party made health care a key issue in its 2003 general election campaign while remaining vague about what it would do. Thus, it both declared its support for the single-payer system and hinted at making more use of the for-profit sector in delivery, with the issue of "sustainability" a subtext to this last point. The single-payer system and for-profit delivery are not inconsistent with one another. They may, however, send different signals making it difficult for the electorate to discern the broad strategy of the party. In an election context, that ambiguity may well have been purposeful.

In chapter 8 we saw that there was a close association between change in government/leader and large reforms during P1. Table 11.1 shows seven cases where there was a "substantial" shift in momentum: three in Ontario, two in Quebec, and two in Alberta. Were these shifts in reform associated with newly formed governments that had committed to reform publicly during the election campaigns or leadership contests that preceded their assuming office? Did these newly formed governments take policy reform action in the first half of their first mandates?

The answer is "yes" to both questions for the three substantial momentum shifts in Ontario. During the 2003 general election, the Ontario Liberal Party campaigned to "end the Harris-Eves era of creeping privatization" (3). The platform contained 21 pages of health-related promises. The party had less reason to be cautious about medicare, as its egalitarian values fit well with medicare values. In its first year in office, the new government passed the *Commitment to Medicare Act*.

> On wait times the Ontario Liberal Party promised it would work with experts to set and meet maximum needs-based waiting times for care. These standards will be made public, so you know you will get treated within a safe time period. We will begin by setting and meeting standards for cardiac care, cancer care, total joint replacements and MRI/CT scans. We will meet these standards by making the smart investments described in this plan and by building on successes like the Cardiac Care Network. (Ontario Liberal Party 2003, 6)

This reform was up and running in its first year in office (MOHLTC 2005).

The Ontario Liberal Party also committed to establishing "at least 150 family medicine teams" and, in that regard, undertook to "create incentives for doctors to practice in teams" (2003, 8). This shift, with its implications for alternative payment plans, was also launched in its first year (MOHLTC 2005).

In Alberta, the answer to our questions is "no." Reform decisions in Alberta were associated with change in government/leader but not foreshadowed by commitments to reform made during an election

TABLE 11.2
Comparing Independent Variables Discussed in 2004–2011 (P2) to 1990–2003 (P1)

Independent Variable	2004–2011 (P2)	1990–2003 (P1)	Comments
Exogenous			
Change in government/ leader	x	x	
Values	x	x	
Fiscal crisis	x	x	Not a major factor in P2
Public opinion and civil society	x	x	Interacted with government/leader
Media		x	
Justice system	x		Chaoulli judgment; not present in P1
Exogenous or endogenous			
Knowledge		x	
Institutions	x	x	P2 focus on federal-provincial relations and master agreements
Endogenous			
Insider interests	x	x	P1 broad discussion whereas P2 only Canadian Medical Association

campaign or leadership contest. The decision to de-regionalize (or create one super-board) was not telegraphed by Premier Stelmach either in his 2006 campaign for party leadership or in the 2008 general election that saw him win a mandate. On APP, the accelerated momentum appears to have been linked not to an election commitment but to ongoing interaction between the Alberta Medical Association, the provincial health ministry, and Alberta's regional health authorities that led to a 2005 agreement among these three bodies (Hutchison et al. 2011, 264).

It is harder to answer these questions for the two substantial momentum shifts in Quebec. This is in part because when the Quebec Liberal Party ran for office in 2003, it made health care a high priority but did not make commitments as precise as the Ontario Liberals did. In Ontario the government's platform was left-oriented, whereas Quebec's was more nuanced. The 2004 Quebec budget restated the Liberal Party's 2003 election pledge "to make health care the No.1 priority of our government.

We promised to fix the health-care system" (Quebec 2004, 4). The Quebec Liberals subsequently published a consultation document and then passed legislation that included statutory guarantees of maximum waits for specified services. The new legislative framework also allowed for the regulation of for-profit clinics. In so doing, the Quebec Liberal Party was seeking to rebalance the role of government, the commercial sector (in the provision of health services), and citizens.

Thus, an overall assessment of the seven substantial shifts in momentum suggests that three fully met our criteria (Ontario), two did not (Alberta), and two met some of the criteria (Quebec's commitments were imprecise, but the government did act quickly once in office).

Values

During P1, the egalitarian values associated with Canadian medicare (universal publicly financed hospital and medical services with priority of access based on medical need and not size of bank account) were politically stronger than competing values based on personal responsibility, personal choice, and a greater role for markets and market-like instruments. In P2 the shift to the right was broad and reflected at least in part a concern about government costing too much and the need to stop or reverse government growth as a share of the economy. This shift was reflected in provinces as diverse as Quebec and Saskatchewan. During the election campaigns that brought them into power, the Quebec Liberal Party (2003) and the Saskatchewan Party (2007) both campaigned with an eye on making governing more affordable and sustainable. But they were cautious not to do this by attacking publicly financed health care. Both parties continued to support medicare. They may have been ready to make small adjustments, but the values that were built into medicare seemingly remained sacrosanct. They and other conservative parties were wary about extending their overall approach to government and governing to include health-care services. In contrast, as noted earlier, the government that was most at ease with medicare values was the centre-left McGuinty Liberals in Ontario. The P2 goals fit well with Ontario's values and its strong attachment to the directions embedded in those goals.

Fiscal Conditions

In P2, the instability in the financial markets that began in late 2008 roiled the international financial system. As 2012 drew to a close the fallout from these events was still being felt worldwide. Canada was not and still is not immune to these pressures (e.g., a higher than anticipated unemployment rate and higher budgetary deficits). The knock-on effects of the recent turmoil have nonetheless been less severe in Canada than in many other countries. Prior to the turmoil, Canada's public finances were in good shape compared to the public finances of many other countries. Canada's financial institutions were more conservatively managed and more tightly regulated, and they weathered the storm better than most. Thus, while the existential threat of permanent global economic and financial damage was greater in 2008 and its aftermath than was the case in the recession of the early 1990s, the effects on Canadian governments' expenditures, including health-care spending, were less severe in the more recent period than in the early 1990s. Provincial health-care spending grew substantially in 2008, 2009, and 2010. Although the growth rate slowed in 2011 and 2012 (CIHI 2012, 3), the financial events since 2008 did not provide the same kind of political cover for health-care reform as they did in the early 1990s.

Accordingly, for four of five provinces, much was missing in P2 that had aided P1 reforms. These governments had not made strong commitments before arriving in office, and they did not "enjoy the benefits" of fiscal crisis to help them undertake difficult reform decisions.

Public Opinion/Civil Society Groups

Chapter 8 referred to two studies prepared for the Romanow Commission in 2002 that inquired about the state of public opinion concerning medicare (Maxwell et al. 2002; Mendelsohn 2002). Together, those studies serve as our baseline for the role of public opinion in P2.[5] Both studies remarked on Canadians' continuing attachment to the medicare model. They also observed a growing concern about the quality of its management, the need for improved accountability, and a greater willingness among Canadians to consider, given certain conditions or qualifications, an enhanced role for the private for-profit sector in both delivery and payment (and for some out-of-pocket payments). One of the studies was updated in 2007 in work commissioned for the Health Council of Canada and the Canadian Health Services Research Foundation (Soroka 2007), and again in 2011 (Soroka 2011).

There are six points to note about the state of public opinion during P2. First is that "support for the Canadian health care system, it seems, is as strong as ever" (Soroka 2007, 5). In a further 2011 update, it was concluded that most Canadians still have "a very clear preference for a strong single-tier public system" (Soroka 2011, 4). At the conclusion of an extensive public dialogue that involved town hall meetings in six cities and towns and an extensive online dialogue in 2011, the president of the Canadian Medical Association declared (CMA 2011b), "The message that came through most strongly from the public was the need to preserve and strengthen the current principles underpinning the *Canada Health Act* to ensure continued support for a universally accessible, publicly funded healthcare system."

Second, Canadians' assessment of the quality of health care fell during the 1990s and early 2000s before rebounding modestly in P2. In 1991, 85 percent of Canadians thought that "Canada's health-care system and the quality of medical services ... was excellent, very good, or good" (Ipsos Reid as reported by Mendelsohn 2002, Figure 3). In 2001, Ipsos Reid posed a slightly modified question about the "overall health of services available to you and your family" and asked respondents for a letter grade. The low watermark occurred in 2004, when only 59 percent of respondents gave the system an "A" or a "B." By 2011, 70 percent gave the system more than a passing grade (Ipsos Reid 2011, 22). Other data sets showed lower levels of public satisfaction with quality but similar trends (Soroka 2011, 6-7).

The third point relates to the political salience of health care. Ipsos Reid asked the same question periodically between 1988 and 2000: "Thinking of the issues presently confronting Canada, which one do you feel should receive the greatest attention from Canada's leaders?" In 1988, no respondents ranked health care as issue number one. In 1996 and 1997, from 12 to 15 percent of respondents did so. By 2000, 51 percent put it on top (Mendelsohn 2002, Figure 14). Health care has since been ranked at or near the top of the issue list every year. In 2010, it was by far the largest concern at 34 percent, three times as large as the second item, "the economy/recession" (Ipsos Reid 2010, 17). The Commonwealth Fund International Survey also captured this significant shift in public attitudes (Nanos Research, cited in Spencer 2010; Soroka 2007, Figure 3).[6] These views were summarized as follows (Soroka 2011, 4):

> Healthcare is, without question, one of the most salient domestic policy issues in Canada. The issue regularly tops the "most important problem" survey list; indeed, it has done so for most of the last decade. It has in recent years been a major focus of election campaigns, a federal Royal Commission and Senate committees. Healthcare policy is, in short, a regular preoccupation for Canadian policy-makers, the public and mass media.

Fourth, the public held both federal and provincial governments responsible for the things that went wrong. At the beginning of P1, public opinion polls showed that a sizeable majority of Canadians credited both federal and provincial governments with doing a good job in improving health care. By the end of P1, a similar majority thought governments were doing a poor job (Mendelsohn 2002, Figures 20, 21, and 22 from two pollsters). Toward the end of P2, governments had regained some ground but a small majority continued to grade government performance poorly (Ipsos Reid 2011, 30; Soroka 2011, Figures 21–24 citing data from three different pollsters).

Fifth, in 2007 more than twice as many Canadians pointed to inefficient management as the main cause of problems in the system rather than insufficient funding (Soroka 2011, 19). This continued a trend that had been noted in 2002 in the Maxwell and Mendelsohn studies.

Lastly, the discussion of how to fix health care's ailments led inexorably to questions about the role of for-profit firms in delivery. Data in Soroka's 2011 study suggested that the public had moved decisively on the idea of a larger role for private for-profit clinics and hospitals *within* a publicly financed system provided that the private entities were paid no more than the public sector and did not charge patients facility fees (Soroka 2011, Figures 35–37).

On health insurance, when asked whether more health care should be privately or publicly financed, only 12 percent answered "more private," whereas 55 percent favoured "more public" (Soroka 2011, Figures 27 and 33). Moreover, when asked about Canada-wide public financing of coverage for prescription drugs and home care, a strong majority supported such coverage (ibid., Figures 27 and 28). Yet more than one-half agreed that "individuals should be given the right to buy private health care within Canada if they do not receive timely access to services in the public system" (ibid., Figure 30). These data could be interpreted as indicating ambivalence about the role for private insurance. An alternative view is that a substantial majority of Canadians continued to prefer the single-payer system but had become more flexible about some additional role for private insurance or out-of-pocket payment in specific situations.

There was not, however, any ambivalence on the part of health-care coalitions, trade unions, and other civil society groups that pay close attention to health issues. Whether the issue was delivery or insurance, they consistently voiced their opposition to an enhanced role for private for-profit businesses. On delivery, their goal may have been to protect union jobs. In some cases, the union stance reflected its interpretation of an employer-employee collective agreement.[7] Where collective agreements were not involved, unions argued that privatizing jobs would lead to inferior service and jeopardize lives. They pointed to studies that compared publicly owned and privately owned nursing homes and hospitals, which documented the better performance of the publicly owned facilities (Canadian Health Coalition 2001; McGregor and Ronald 2011). More generally, these groups remained vigilant in protecting medicare. They encouraged members to quiz candidates for public office on their positions on health care.[8] They kept an eye open for organizational changes that had the potential to affect not only their members, but the public as well.[9] Wherever they detected what they considered to be an infraction of the *Canada Health Act*, they informed their membership and attempted to pressure government to disallow the activity or transaction.

The position of civil society groups did not change between P1 and P2. Public opinion was also similar between the two periods when issues were expressed mainly in terms of values. When expressed in practical terms, however, public opinion had evolved. For example, whereas in P1 a majority of people saw additional health-care spending as a solution to some problems, by the later P2 years many citizens saw improved management as the best way of mending the ailments of the health-care system. The public continued to see governments as stewards of the health-care system. Well before the end of P2, public opinion had become more open to delivery through private for-profit enterprises as contractors to the public system. The preference was to maintain the single-payer system, but the public was willing to consider exceptions under specified conditions.

Supreme Court Judgment: *Chaoulli v. Quebec (Attorney General)*

The justice system did not show up as a factor in our 30 case studies during P1. But it did appear in P2 owing to the 2005 judgment of the Supreme Court of Canada in the *Chaoulli* case. At issue was whether the health-care regime in Quebec infringed the constitutional rights to life, liberty, and security of person of a Quebecer, George Zeliotis, under the Quebec Charter of Rights and Freedoms. The case arose when Mr. Zeliotis had to wait a long time to receive a hip replacement. Jacques Chaoulli was Mr. Zeliotis's physician, and he wanted to establish his own private medical practice. They joined together and took their case to court.

Quebec health insurance and hospital insurance statutes did not allow for the sale of private insurance for health and hospital services that were insured publicly. Due to the length of time Mr. Zeliotis had to wait, the Court ruled in a controversial (Flood and Sullivan 2005) majority decision (4-3) that the prohibition on the sale of private insurance was a violation of Quebecers' rights to life and security of the person under the Quebec Charter of Rights and Freedoms. The ruling had a direct effect only in Quebec as the case did not deal with the health-care systems of other provinces. (Three of the seven judges also found that the laws violated provisions of the Canadian Charter of Rights and Freedoms.) The earlier discussion about Quebec's new regulatory framework and its guaranteed access mechanism was in part a response to the court judgment.

The Supreme Court judgment in some sense also put other provinces and territories on notice. They too might be vulnerable in a similar type of case under the Canadian Charter. Based on the information available to us, however, the *Chaoulli* decision appears not to have been a major influence in P2 outside Quebec.

Federal/Provincial/Territorial Relations

Chapter 8 distinguished between the direct and indirect effects of federal-provincial relations and federalism during P1. It was noted that in P1 federal-provincial relations and federalism were cited infrequently as a factor in the 30 health-care reform cases. It was suggested, however, that federal-provincial relations had some indirect effects that our case study analysis had not picked up. One such indirect effect was linked to the federal Liberal government's focus on politically divisive issues. Examples included the federal government's interpretation and enforcement of the *Canada Health Act*, its opposition to the idea of having a provincial premier as co-chair of the National Forum on Health, and a communications strategy that promoted medicare as a national icon and attacked those who were seen as its political adversaries. The latter included not only the Reform Party of Canada (1987–2003) and then the Canadian Alliance (2000–2003) at the federal level but also right-of-centre provincial governments (Klein in Alberta and Harris/Eves in Ontario) that occasionally gave Ottawa the opportunity to question their support for medicare. We argued that, unintentionally, Ottawa may have lessened the time and attention that civil society groups, the public, and the media gave to the actual reform agenda (the kinds of issues that this book has examined such as regionalization, needs-based funding, and drug coverage).

A second indirect effect was the fallout from the federal government's 1995 budget. Despite the frequency of federal-provincial meetings on matters of health-care reform, the priority of provincial governments was to force the federal authorities to restore cash transfers to the level they would have been had the federal government not enacted the large cuts in transfer payments to the provinces in its 1995 budget. This led to an intergovernmental fiscal struggle and to highly dysfunctional federal/provincial/territorial (FPT) relations, especially from 1998 to 2004 (Boychuk 2003, 321; Lazar et al. 2004a, chapter 4; Marchildon 2004, 4-8; Standing Senate Committee 2002b, section 1.2). From the viewpoint of this book, the question is whether that deterioration in FPT relations resulted in a feedback loop with implications for health-care reform.

When the federal *Medical Care Act* was passed in 1966, the Liberal government in Ottawa had used the inducement of federal cost sharing to pressure recalcitrant provinces to sign on. Again, in 1984, the federal Liberals relied on the popularity of medicare to persuade reluctant provincial governments to amend their health insurance legislation to comply with the *Canada Health Act*. In both cases public opinion provided important political support to the federal Liberal government in making these huge health-care reform decisions. By the late 1990s and early 2000s, the shoe was on the other foot. Provinces held that the federal cutbacks to the provinces were responsible for the deterioration in health-care services (Premiers' Council 2002; Provincial and Territorial Ministers of Health 2002). This position was contested by Ottawa (Dion 2005, 153-71).

It took several years, but the provinces eventually gained enough support from public opinion to "persuade" the Liberal governments of Jean Chrétien and Paul Martin to restore Ottawa's funding to a more appropriate level.[10] In the vocabulary of this book, the *dependent* variable had become fiscal fairness in relations between the federal government and provincial/territorial governments; health care was an independent variable that provincial/territorial governments invoked to help dictate the outcome. As for the health-care reform commitments that Ottawa was able to "buy" when restoring funding, some were not implemented, some were implemented but would have been in the absence of federal dollars, and a few were incremental. On the whole, the purchases were a fig leaf to provide political cover for the fact that the provincial/territorial undertakings were neither legally binding nor politically enforceable (as subsequent events were to show). In releasing its 2012 review of the 2004 Health Accord, the Standing Senate Committee on Social Affairs, Science and Technology observed that "real systematic transformation of health care systems across the country had not yet occurred, despite more than a decade of government commitments and increasing investments." In its review of the accord, the Health Council of Canada (2012) repeated an earlier message that there is "much to celebrate and yet much that falls short of what could—and should—have been achieved by this time" (1).

The fig leaf was not without influence on events, however. By pointing to the 2003 and 2004 FPT Health Accords, the Liberals were able to claim some high ground in health-care reform at the federal level. In so doing, they attempted to insert medicare as a wedge between their policies (friendly to medicare) and those of the Conservative Party (with its alleged secret plan to weaken medicare). In the 2004 general election campaign, for example, the Paul Martin–led Liberals promised a health-care "fix for a generation" as the centrepiece of its electoral platform (Liberal Party 2004, 16-23). To counter the Liberal strategy, the 2004 Conservative platform endorsed the 2003 First Ministers' Health Accord (Conservative Party 2004, 25-27).

Soon after the election, Martin negotiated the 10-year 2004 Health Accord with provincial/territorial first ministers—his fix for a generation. During the 2006 election campaign, the Conservatives endorsed the 2004 Accord. Harper promised to work with the provinces to develop a Patient Wait Times Guarantee to ensure that all Canadians would receive essential medical treatment within clinically acceptable waiting times, or could be treated in another jurisdiction, as required by the Supreme Court of Canada's *Chaoulli* decision and the Canadian Charter of Rights and Freedoms (Conservative Party 2006, 30). Wait times had become the leading political health concern in the country. Harper subsequently characterized this promise as one of the five most important in his party's platform. The key point is that Mr. Harper and his party were not willing to cede the political high ground to the Liberals. The FPT Accords thus helped shape the position of the Conservative Party. If there was a "secret plan" to do away with medicare, it remained secret.

Over the next five years, the Conservatives honoured the transfer commitments of the 2004 Accord, and sporadically lent support to the Patient Wait Times Guarantee. But on other matters that were part of the 2004 Accord—from a pharmaceutical strategy to primary care reform and from health human resources to home care—the Harper government did not act. The Conservatives apparently viewed these issues as beyond the writ of the federal government, notwithstanding that the commitments entailed the involvement of federal as well as provincial governments.

In its 2011 election platform, the Conservative Party promised to "work collaboratively with the provinces and territories to renew the Health Accord and to continue reducing wait times." The party platform also emphasized the importance of "accountability" measures as well as the need to "respect limits on the federal spending power" (Conservative Party 2011). The platform thus acknowledged trade-offs, but not how they would be resolved.

By the end of 2011, some of Prime Minister Harper's messages were clear: his government's view of the federal role in health care was based on the pre-eminence of the constitutional distribution of legislative powers, which assigns to provinces broad authority to make laws on health care; and he was keen to shrink the federal state where its involvement was based on the federal spending power. It was for each province to decide what kind of reform was appropriate under its circumstances. By committing to long-term funding, and clarifying its role, the federal government was creating the conditions that would enable provincial governments to do what needed to be done. It was up to the provincial governments to decide. Choosing not to hold meetings with the premiers on health-care reform was apparently the last piece of the federal government's strategy. Prime Minister Harper, in referring to provincial governments, stated (CBC 2012),

> Now what they're wrestling with is how to make that system effective, how to lower wait times, and you know, they're the ones who deliver the service. They're the ones who are responsible. So I think that, you know, we don't just trust them, we understand they have the responsibility, and we want to make sure that we work with them. We're not ... we made it a point, as you know, as a federal government, of not pointing the fingers at the provinces and trying to blame them for problems in the health-care system, but trying to work with them to see how we can make it better. And I think that's been a better method than in the past trying to pretend there is some overarching national standards, and then wave the finger at them for perceived slights. I don't think that's been effective. I think what we're doing is more effective ...

Federal-provincial relations were a major influence on the kind of medicare system that Canadians created for themselves in post–Second World War Canada. Once created, there was an ongoing interaction between medicare and federal-provincial fiscal relations. During P2, the dynamic intensified. The national health-care budget, if only by virtue of its sheer size, could not help but influence federal-provincial fiscal and political relations. And the latter in turn influenced health-care reform. Arguably, however, the feedback arrow from health care to FPT relations was thicker than the arrow from FPT relations to health care. We return to this issue in the last chapter.

The *Canada Health Act*

At end of P2, the *Canada Health Act* and the related Canada Health Transfer remained as ongoing legacies from P1. There are three kinds of criticism levelled at the *CHA* in P2. First is that it is not enforced properly. Critics claim that many infractions of the *CHA* are routinely ignored by the federal government. Examples of this kind of criticism can be found on the websites of the Canadian Health Coalition and the Council of Canadians. On this point, we do not know the facts. There is no public record to analyze, and how much this matters is uncertain. Referring to the case studies done for this project, Gildiner writes,

> The case studies suggest that the terms of the *Canada Health Act*, having been incorporated into provincial legislation, had come to exert legacy and feedback effects primarily at the provincial level. The federal government needed only to maintain the Act, without effort to update it to capture changing conditions on the ground, and even without maintaining its fiscal commitments, to reap the benefits of being seen to support the Act's principles. The provinces, on the other hand, were much more vulnerable to battles with interest groups empowered by the terms of the core bargains—hospitals and physicians—and to punishment by voters, for whom public health insurance was not only a major social benefit but a nation-defining commitment. (2006, 32)

A second criticism is that the absence of transparency in how the federal government interprets the *CHA* has the effect of blocking reforms that are not in fact prohibited by the statute or the principles that lie behind it (Boychuk 2003). Whatever the merits of this argument, it calls on the federal government to play a role that it does not want to play. By clarifying points that may be in doubt, it would be treading on territory it does not wish to enter.

The third criticism is that the *CHA* covers a shrinking share of health expenditures and thus its influence is shrinking. This issue is easier to measure and is considered in the last chapter with other aspects of federal-provincial relations.

Medical Associations

Chapter 8 described the role played by provincial medical associations in P1 with particular attention to master agreements between provincial health ministries and medical associations, and the joint management committees they created to oversee them.

During P2, provincial medical associations continued to shape health-care reforms. Based on a reading of the master agreements alone, it appears that the relationships between the provincial medical associations and provincial health ministries became more intertwined—but not necessarily more amicable. In Ontario, for example, the 2008 agreement between the Ontario Medical Association (OMA) and the Ministry of Health and Long-Term Care (MOHLTC) was longer and broader than the 2000 agreement. It created a more elaborate committee structure to oversee the provisions. In Saskatchewan, the 2011 agreement was much longer than the 2001 agreement (up from 9 pages to 42). The Saskatchewan agreement of 2011 included such new (since P1) measures as parental leave, rural on-call programs, and a specialist retention program, among many others. At least six new joint boards or committees were created. The 2003 agreement between the government of Alberta, the Alberta Medical Association, and the regional health authorities (which were still in place then) is also of interest. In this agreement, "the minister offered an expanded and an enhanced role and relationship to the association regarding how to improve the health care delivery system" (Alberta 2003). The agreement then pointed to the primary care initiative, the physician office system, and electronic health records as ways in which such improvements could be made. Agreement on primary care reform was reached through this mechanism in 2005.

Of the six issues we studied, APP was the one where provincial medical associations were most influential in P2. In this regard, Table 11.1 notes that in Alberta, Ontario, and Quebec there was a momentum shift toward P1 goals during P2.

Physicians also had a greater influence on macro-policy during P2 than they had in P1 through their national body, the Canadian Medical Association (CMA). The CMA is a bottom-up organization that advocates on behalf of Canadian physicians on Canada-wide issues. To become eligible for CMA membership, a physician must be a member of a provincial or territorial association. The provincial and territorial divisions and specialist societies choose both the CMA's 300-member general council and 27-member board of directors. The CMA presidency is rotated among the various provincial/territorial divisions. The general council meets annually and provides policy guidance and direction to the association and the board of directors. The board guides the CMA between annual meetings.

The CMA did not play a direct role in the six issues that underpin this book because these issues were largely or entirely within provincial/territorial jurisdiction.[11] During P1 the CMA focused on issues like the Canada-wide fiscal framework. As the effects of provincial retrenchment took hold (1992–1996), the CMA lobbied Ottawa to increase its transfers to the provinces and territories. It did not succeed, as evidenced by the 1995 federal budget cuts on transfers notionally intended for health care. The CMA persisted and then accelerated its efforts. In 2001 it informed the Romanow Commission and the Kirby Committee that "as a result of the relentless cost-cutting of the 1990s, we are now in the midst of a crisis of sustainability" (CMA 2001, ii).

In 2002 it offered its "Prescription for Sustainability" with policy proposals on many issues, in particular health human resources, primary care and, most of all, access (CMA 2002). Among its proposals was a call for a Patient Wait Times Guarantee. Initially there was some cross-fertilization between the CMA's ideas and the 2001 Mazankowski report, which recommended the Patient Wait Times Guarantee (Premier's Advisory Council 2001, 43). Neither the Government of Alberta nor the Romanow report endorsed it, but the concept gained some credibility when the Senate Committee did so in its October 2002 final report (Standing Senate Committee 2002b, chap. 5, "The Health Care Guarantee"). As mentioned above, in its 2006 election platform the Conservative Party pledged to work with the provinces to develop a Patient Wait Times Guarantee (Conservative Party 2006, 30). In its March 2007 budget, the federal government committed up to an additional $612 million for jurisdictions that implemented guarantees in at least one priority area. The Conservative Party platform was silent on this issue in 2008, but progress on reducing wait times was part of the 2011 program (Conservative Party 2011, 30).

Organizations like the Council of Canadians (2012) and the Canadian Health Coalition (2012b), and their provincial and local counterparts, as well as the Canadian Doctors for Medicare (2012), saw the CMA's policies as a way of advancing privatization. This interpretation gained further support when, in 2007/08 and 2008/09, the CMA elected presidents with proprietary interests in for-profit clinics. The *Canadian Medical Association Journal* and influential medical journals outside of Canada, including the *New England Journal of Medicine* and *The Lancet*, periodically included articles on the differences within the CMA on the privatization issue (for example, Angell 2008; Steinbrook 2006). The CMA submission to the Romanow Commission dealt with this issue in the following terms:

> Health care is delivered mainly by private providers including physicians, pharmacists, private not-for-profit hospitals, private long-term care facilities, private diagnostic and testing facilities, rehabilitation centres....

This significant level of private-sector delivery has served Canada well. Accordingly, the CMA supports a continuing and major role for the private sector in the delivery of health care. *However, we are not proposing a parallel private system.* (CMA 2002, 38; emphasis added)

In 2010, the CMA released a wide-ranging policy statement, *Health Care Transformation in Canada*. The culmination of almost 10 years of homework, the *Transformation* document is the vehicle through which the CMA is currently engaging the public and other interest groups. The document notes that although Canada's health-care system is valued by its citizens,

> it is increasingly recognized that the system is inadequate to meet 21st Century needs and is in urgent need of reform. Canadians wait too long for care. Care providers feel overworked and discouraged. There are insufficient mechanisms to monitor system performance. Technical support needs modernizing. (iv)

A crucial part of the diagnosis involves value for money:

> Canada's care system is under-performing on several key measures, such as timely access, despite the large amounts we spend on health care. Experts agree that Canada's current health care system is not delivering the level of care that other industrialized countries now enjoy.... New governance models should be considered to improve both system effectiveness and accountability. (4)

The CMA's cure involves modernizing the *Canada Health Act* (putting more teeth into the existing five principles); adding new principles (patient-centred care and sustainability); creating a charter of patient-centred care; changing incentives to enhance access and improve quality of care; enhancing patient access along the continuum of care including universal access to prescription drugs and continuing care outside acute care facilities; helping providers help patients by ensuring Canada has an adequate supply of health human resources and more effective adoption of health information technologies; and building accountability/responsibility at all levels with the need for system accountability and system stewardship (2010, 7). In releasing the report, the CMA proclaimed its "readiness to take a leadership position in confronting the hard choices required to make health care work better for Canadians" (2011b, iii).

Between January and June 2011, the CMA held a national public dialogue online (www.healthcaretransformation.ca) and a series of six forums in partnership with *Maclean's*, *L'actualité*, and the cable Public Affairs Channel. The CMA action plan was thrown off course when the federal government announced, in December 2011, its intention to renew the Canada Health Transfer until 2024 without federal-provincial discussion or public consultation.

The CMA and provincial medical associations are not without their critics (for example, Lewis 2010). Critics argue that the physician community, as the most powerful force in the Canadian health-care system, attempts to influence the direction of reform without recognizing that their behaviour plays a large role in the performance of the health-care system. We saw earlier that among the six cases that mattered most to physicians, all were decided within the parameters of what the doctors found acceptable.

The CMA's *Transformation* document calls for massive reform including the opening up of existing federal and provincial law. It seems a stretch to expect such a result. Yet organized medicine has assets that governments lack: the trust of the public, the knowledge of how things work on the ground, and a time horizon that is not determined by four-year election cycles at best. As the steps to date indicate, the CMA is not short of money in the pursuit of its goals. It is unlikely that government, or any other institution, would be able to lead a substantial reform without the backing of the physician community. But no government seems to be thinking about reform on the scale that the CMA has been advocating.

CONCLUSIONS

Two factors—newly elected governments with strong election commitments and fiscal crisis—interacted in P1 to encourage certain types of reform, particularly those focused on cost containment or efficiency. In P2, with the exception of the Ontario Liberal Party, newly formed governments made few campaign commitments to reform health care. The fiscal motive was also lacking. Indeed, the fiscal conditions experienced through most of P2 might have led governments to widen the scope of Canada-wide insurance to include catastrophic drug costs or home care, if not both. The Kirby Committee and Romanow Commission had recommended such action, and governments had money. In fact, the 2003 First Ministers' Accord on Health Care Renewal, in reflecting on the work of these and other bodies, declared that "these studies reflect a great convergence on the value of our publicly funded health system, the need for reform, and on the priorities for reform: particularly primary health care, home care, catastrophic drug coverage…" (First Ministers' Meeting 2003, 1). The emphasis on insuring drug coverage and home care was repeated in the First Ministers' 2004 Accord. But the trend from left to right did not support what fiscal conditions allowed. In fact, the scope of Canada-wide health insurance was not expanded during P2. However, the trend to the political right did not lead to a significant shift toward counter-consensus reform. The new conservative governments were careful not to stir up public opinion, which was still seen as very protective of the core principles of the *Canada Health Act* and the values embedded in it.

During P1, public opinion worked to minimize changes to medicare except those that would enlarge it. In P2, the public was more open to a role for private for-profit clinics and hospitals *within* a publicly funded system rather than a parallel track in competition with the public system. On insurance it still preferred single payer but appeared open to flexibility in exceptional circumstances.

In sum, the absence of strong political commitments, a fiscal situation that did not demand reform, and a Supreme Court decision that did not have much influence beyond Quebec, meant that exogenous factors were a lesser spur to efficiency and effectiveness reforms (those in the governance and financial arrangements cluster) in P2 than they were in P1. At the same time, the shift in public opinion allowed slightly more room for reform in the delivery and program content cluster.

Endogenous factors were largely the same in P2 as in P1. Federal-provincial relations were less confrontational, but this did not seem to have much impact on health reform. The intertwining of provincial medical associations and provincial health ministries continued and seemingly intensified. This relationship signalled incrementalism as the most likely path for health-care reform. Indeed, while the Canadian Medical Association urged transformation of Canada's health-care system, as 2012 drew to a close, it could not find a government partner that was willing and able to dance with it.

NOTES

1. Ontario developed an alternative mechanism for funding hospitals but chose not to introduce it except at the margin during P2.
2. The Quebec legislation also creates some space for purely private-for-profit delivery. The constraints on that option suggest that it may grow slowly, if at all.
3. In P2, there was one change in government in each province except in Newfoundland and Labrador, which had two (election of a new Conservative government in 2003 led by Danny Williams and election of Kathy Dunderdale as Conservative leader in 2010). Although falling within the 2011 frame, Alison Redford's government is excluded. She was elected as leader of the Progressive Conservative Party in Alberta in October 2011, leaving little time to introduce reforms. In P1, Quebec had four changes of government (Parizeau, Bouchard, and Landry PQ premiers from 1994 to 2003 and election of the Liberals in 2003). Newfoundland and Labrador had three governments (election of Liberals in 1989 under Clyde Wells followed by premiers Brian Tobin and Roger Grimes). Ontario also had three governments (election of NDP under Bob Rae in 1990, election of Progressive Conservatives in 1995 under Mike Harris and then under Ernie Eves in April 2002, until defeated in October 2003). Saskatchewan had two changes (election of NDP in 1991

under Roy Romanow and in 2001 under Lorne Calvert). The formation of the Klein government was the sole change in Alberta.

4.   There were fewer changes of party leaders within governing parties in P2 compared to P1.

5.   It would have been ideal to have similar studies done at the end of 2003, but we are not aware of others of similar scope and quality that coincided with the end of P1.

6.   In 1988 and 1998 it asked Canadians, Americans, and Britons which of the following three statements about their health-care system best reflected their views: "On the whole, the health care system: 1) works pretty well and only minor changes are necessary; 2) There are some good things in our health care system but fundamental changes are needed; 3) Our health care system has so much wrong that we need to completely rebuild." In 1988, 56 percent of Canadians identified with the first category. In the US and UK, the comparable figures were 10 and 27 percent. In 1998, the US and UK figures were 17 and 25 percent. In Canada, the spending freeze had seemingly taken its toll and the figure had declined to 20 percent (Mendelsohn 2002, Figure 19). What Canadians wanted was for the problem to be fixed.

7.   When the Regina Qu'Appelle Regional Health Authority entered into a contract to have surgeries contracted out and issued a request for proposals for a contract on imaging, the CUPE local argued that these actions violated the terms of the employer-employee collective agreement, leading to arbitration. At issue, in part, was whether the RHA approach was cost-effective. The arbitration award came down on the employer side for the short run but not for the long term (Ish 2010).

8.   The Alberta Friends of Medicare, for example, actively encouraged members to be in touch with all candidates for the leadership of the Alberta Progressive Conservative Party during its 2011 leadership contest.

9.   The Ontario Health Coalition (2010) urged the McGuinty government to make fundamental structural changes to the Local Health Integration Networks.

10. The argument was not accurate. The federal cuts were announced in 1995 and began to take effect in 1996/97 whereas public concerns about service had begun earlier. The period of provincial retrenchment that began in 1991/92 was more closely linked with complaints about health-care services.

11. Indirectly, however, the CMA played a major role in the wait-times issue by sponsoring and financing the annual Taming of the Queue conferences and creating the Wait Times Alliance (http://www.waittimealliance.ca/index.htm).

CHAPTER 12

PROSPECTS FOR HEALTH-CARE POLICY REFORM

HARVEY LAZAR AND PIERRE-GERLIER FOREST

INTRODUCTION

This book began with a series of questions about the difficulties in reforming health care in Canada. The underlying assumption about the
meagre extent of reform was confirmed in each of the four policy domains
we studied. To shed light on why this was so, we undertook several kinds
of comparisons: by factor (or influence), by issue, by phase, by direction
(consensus or counter-consensus reform), by province, and by technical
complexity. As expected, the paucity of reform was due mainly to the
resistance of those actors in each of the four domains who benefited
most from the status quo. These actors had the political clout to hang on
to the turf they occupied or, where they could not, they generally were
able to steer the direction of the reform process to a destination that was
acceptable to the interests they represented and at a pace that minimized
the disruption to those interests.

The comparative analysis suggested several patterns in the decision
process. One was in the factors associated with the different policy reform
domains. Elites dominated the governance arrangements and financial
arrangements domains. Indeed, on some issues in that grouping, the
public and media were scarcely aware that there were important reform
matters to be decided. When it came to the delivery arrangements and
policy content domains, however, public opinion and civil society groups
purporting to speak for large sectors of the public played a significant role.

There was also a pattern in the factors associated with the different
phases of reform. The media, civil society groups, and the public were
key actors in causing issues in the delivery arrangements and policy
content domains to reach the governmental agenda. They had less influence on policy choice in this grouping and on issues that had substantial
technical content.

The comparative analysis pointed to key variables associated with the relatively few cases of large reforms. These variables included the political commitment of newly formed governments before gaining office (election commitment), quick action on the promise once in office, and fiscal crisis or perceived crisis.

The evidence also suggested that political ideology had a limited influence on the 30 cases we studied.

We extended our 1990–2003 analysis backward to 1945–1989 in chapter 10 and forward to 2004–2011 in chapter 11. In this chapter we consider the future. We do not predict, forecast, or express a preference for what will happen. The focus is on the broad reform trajectories associated with the issues we have examined and the reform possibilities associated with those trajectories.

In this last chapter, the past thus speaks to the future. What do our studies of health-care policy reform in the past suggest about the prospects for health-care policy reform going forward? In asking this question, we recall that policy reform is only one of several ways in which health care in Canada can and does change. New breakthroughs in medical science and medical technology can and do improve diagnosis and treatment without government involvement except, importantly, for paying most of the bills. Developments in information and communications technology create different tools for managing health systems and coordinating case files. These kinds of structural factors are always present, creating possibilities for improvements in health care in Canada.

The evidence in this book suggests that the chances of reform on a very large scale—the proverbial big bang—are slim at best. Some of the conditions that might enable such transformative events to occur are also ones that a majority of Canadians would not vote for if they had a choice. It took the Great Depression and the Second World War to create the political climate in Canada that enabled a new innovative postwar social contract among Canadians. The case study evidence suggests that, in the future, ideologically driven, large-scale reform of this ilk is most unlikely and in any event impossible to predict with a level of certainty that is useful to policy makers. The most that we would venture beyond this generalization is that breakthroughs in medical science or technology (Schipper, Pai, and Swain 2008), or breakthroughs in the management of highly complex systems, may well create health-care policy choices that could overcome political ideologies linked to the status quo. We saw how difficult it was to introduce for-profit delivery in Alberta and Ontario despite the predispositions of the Klein and Harris/Eves governments (chapters 3 and 5). The cases also suggest that political commitment and administrative preparedness were stronger predictors of policy direction than left/right political orientation (chapter 9).

Health policy was one of a long list of big reforms that Ottawa proposed to the provinces and the country at the Dominion-Provincial

Reconstruction Conference in 1945. Ottawa's public health proposals and its offer to help expand delivery capacity of the health sector were well received by affected interests and provinces. In contrast, the health insurance proposals were contentious, especially with provincial governments. Ottawa's call for universal, comprehensive, publicly financed and provincially administered hospital services, medical services, home care ("visiting nurses"), prescription drugs, dental care, and laboratory testing won support only from the governments of Saskatchewan and Manitoba (and Manitoba's position did not last long). Almost all remaining provinces were opposed (including Alberta, Ontario, and Quebec) or appeared to be (using their apparent opposition to try to improve the financial arrangements Ottawa was proposing). There was some resistance by health-care providers and institutions. It took a quarter century to achieve a *portion* of what was proposed in 1945—Canada-wide hospital and medical insurance.

Fast-forwarding, none of the other health-care services that were raised at the 1945 conference continue to have a prominent place on the Canada-wide agenda today (2013).[1] These issues have not necessarily become unimportant. But for any of them to reappear on a Canada-wide agenda, the surrounding narrative would have to reflect contemporary reality. The arguments of principle may not have changed much, but the setting has.

The last substantial Canada-wide government-led effort to reform health-care policy on a large scale came apart when the federal Liberal government lost the 2006 general election. At the provincial level, the Ontario Liberal government under the leadership of Dalton McGuinty (2003–2013) was the sole party among the five provinces that we studied that had a wide and substantial reform agenda in the 2004–2011 period.

Looking beyond government for national leadership, the Canadian Medical Association (CMA) and the Canadian Health Coalition (CHC) have been promoting large reform for more than a decade. Beginning with its 2002 proposals to the Romanow Commission and the Senate Committee chaired by Senator Kirby, the CMA developed a wide-ranging set of proposals that (it contends) represent transformative change (chapter 11, 302-4). The CMA subsequently sponsored cross-country consultations (CMA 2011a). But it has not yet found a government willing to seriously debate its sweeping proposals. As for the CHC, it has long fought to protect Canada-wide health-care benefits and to safeguard the status of unionized health-care workers by resisting calls for more for-profit delivery. At the time of the Romanow and Kirby reports and subsequently, it called for an extension of health-care benefits (universal drug coverage, home care, more provision for needs of seniors, etc.). The CHC had fewer financial resources with which to sell its proposals to the Canadian public than the CMA, but it did have a wide network of affiliates. The CHC and its affiliates have been better at protecting their turf than extending it, however.

Without reform on a grand scale, there is still much room for substantial government-led and government-supported reform, especially at the provincial level. The size and sensitivity of health care mean that provincial governments will always have some health-care issues on their agendas. Some reform proposals will be blocked by established interests, and others will lead to minor adjustments of the status quo. Some reforms will begin small but accumulate over time, while others will fade. A few may be on a scale that resembles what we have called comprehensive reform, but our research suggests that they are likely to be rare.

The rest of this chapter proceeds as follows. First we discuss key points from the 15 cases in the "elite" cluster. It will be recalled that we used this term in characterizing governance and financial arrangements. Reforms in these two domains were dominated by leaders in government, medical associations, and the research community to the exclusion of civil society groups, the media, and public opinion. For this grouping of cases, our main focus is on the lack of transparency in the decision process. The transparency issue in the governance and financial arrangements cluster merits attention by those interested in the future of health care in Canada.

Delivery arrangements and program content are part of the same cluster because they touch people directly, unlike the governance and financial arrangements cluster. However, delivery arrangements and program content are also different enough from one another to merit discussion under separate headings below.

Our analysis for program content is more detailed than it is for the other policy domains. Macro-level data enable us to see which policy paradigms (specifically payment paradigms) have been growing in relative terms and which have been declining. Each paradigm represents a set of values that is distinct from the others and thus conveys a values-influenced direction. We were struck by the role that default positions and tipping points, in conjunction with constitutional considerations, played in this process. We explore these patterns from a historical perspective in annex 3. In this chapter, we consider possible trajectories of the payment paradigms going forward.

Finally, we discuss the relationship between federalism and program reform. The Conservative government has been pursuing a different approach to health-care reform than its predecessors dating all the way back to 1945. What difference has it made? What difference might it make for policy reform in the years to come?

GOVERNANCE AND FINANCIAL ARRANGEMENTS POLICY DOMAINS

Analysis in earlier chapters showed that policy reforms relating to the governance of health care and its financial arrangements were mainly influenced by elites. The elites with influence varied from one policy issue to another.

In the governance domain, we studied regionalization. On this issue, provincial political leaders, with the support of their public servants, exercised a strong influence on policy reform. The differences in provincial approaches to regionalization were based less on broad principle than on conditions within individual provinces at a moment in time. Where there was resistance it was mainly from some hospital elites (not all), and they were more powerful in some provinces (e.g., Ontario) than in others (e.g., Quebec). Provincial medical associations by and large were not visibly involved. But medical associations were known to be firmly opposed to the regionalization of provincial medical care budgets. Rather than face this opposition and slow the regionalization process, provincial governments chose to retain medical care budgets at the provincial level.

We studied two issues in the financial arrangements domain: needs-based funding and alternative payment plans. Political elites exercised broad oversight over needs-based funding. Within this framework the research community played a very large role in working through the substantive aspects of this issue owing to its technical complexity. The level of complexity will likely continue to shape policy reform on this issue going forward.

The alternative payment plans (APP) issue was our window into the wider concern about primary care reform. On this issue, reform was determined by the interactions between political leaders and provincial medical associations. The evidence suggested that it was the medical associations that determined the nature and pace of reform. We enlarge on the influence of provincial medical associations here.

Physicians have significant influence on health-related policy in most countries. But in Canada, they exercise an unusual degree of influence owing to decisions of provincial governments that date back to the 1960s and early 1970s. At that time, provincial governments bought into the fee schedule of insurance companies owned or approved by the provincial medical associations. We have seen how that one decision inexorably led to second and third decisions on such issues as the number of physicians able to bill governments and the intensity of physician usage of the fee schedule. Master agreements between medical associations / unions and health ministries now fill dozens of pages describing large and complex relationships. Writing 15 years ago, Tuohy (1999, 30) observed that Canadian medicare

> rested from its inception in the 1960s on a fundamental accommodation between the medical profession and the state, under which physicians retained their status as independent professionals, trading off a degree of entrepreneurial freedom (particularly over price...) in order to retain substantial collective and individual autonomy in clinical matters.

Our findings are similar to Tuohy's and the earlier work by Lomas, Charles, and Grew (1992).

Exclusivity and insufficient transparency *appear* to be the main governance-related policy reform issues arising from the relationship between the medical profession and the provincial state. We italicize *appear* to draw attention to the fact that, regrettably, we do not know what we do not know. There is some degree of accountability: physician fee schedules are generally available to the public even if not easy for the lay person to understand. Moreover, the close relationship between provincial medical associations and provincial health ministries helps to make health care work. Our concern is the exclusivity and opaqueness of physician-ministry arrangements. For example, how does the public assess broad mandates set out in master agreements between provincial health ministries and provincial medical associations that call on medical associations and ministry staffs to work together to improve health care and accountability? Physician representatives are also a part of more specific mandates like the manner in which primary care is structured, methods of compensation, rural health, Aboriginal health, telehealth, and electronic records. At a minimum, these relationships provide the medical associations with insider status in respect of policy and program changes that affect physician interests. Such insider knowledge is not available to other provider organizations or to the public. Even the physicians' voice acknowledges that something is askew. The CMA Advisory Panel on Resourcing Options used the terms "unaware" and "in the dark" to describe the public's knowledge of evolving payment arrangements for physician compensation and hospital budgeting (CMA 2011a, 9).

Chapter 8 showed that provincial medical associations effectively blocked some consensus reforms that directly affected physician interests and steered others to destinations that were safe ground for physicians. Chapter 9 showed that there was little or no transparency on the three governance and financial issues that we studied. During a period of big reform, these arrangements were a part of the price that was paid to ensure the continuing commitment of physicians to their practices. In particular, provincial governments adopted fee schedules approved by the medical associations to reassure physicians that their remuneration and professional autonomy were not in jeopardy (Tuohy 1999, 55-56, 204-7).

With respect to the future role of physicians in the governance of health care, the CMA's Advisory Panel wrote,

> Reform clearly cannot be effective without their buy-in and co-operation, but we look to them to carry out a more positive role. We believe physicians have insights into how the system could provide greater value for money. At the same time, *they must embark on change within their own ranks* [emphasis added]. Central to this will be examining such issues as their interaction with the system, the organization of their practices, and their status—unique among OECD countries—as independent agents in a publicly funded health care system. (CMA 2011a, 6)

The evidence of this book points in a similar direction. Canadian physicians are accustomed to practicing medicine in a certain way that reflects their history. Calls for reform, such as more group multidisciplinary practices and fewer solo practices, have been around for a long time. The evidence shows that these calls had little influence on physician practice during our study period. Support for reform grew during the update years, although more in some provinces (Ontario and Alberta) than in others (Saskatchewan).

The Canadian Medical Association, through its Advisory Panel, has recognized the need for change in the ranks of physicians. Canadians should pay attention to the way in which the physician community responds to this challenge. They should also insist on enhanced transparency in relations between provincial health ministries and medical associations.

DELIVERY ARRANGEMENTS

For-Profit Delivery

Little reform occurred on this issue during our study period (1990–2003), and the reality did not change much during the update years (2004–2011). The newly elected, mainly conservative provincial governments of the early and mid-2000s were cautious about tackling this issue, possibly wary of an adverse political reaction. Certainly, civil society groups were vigilant in resisting change. Unionized health-care providers were an important part of these civil society groups. They had as much reason to protect their interests in the status quo as did physicians. Where for-profit delivery reforms were introduced, it was typically in locations with shortages in beds or imaging equipment. In some such cases, regional authorities entered into contracts with for-profit clinics or testing facilities to supply some of the delivery capacity that was lacking in the public sector (e.g., Saskatchewan Surgical Care Network initiatives). The for-profit firms were not normally able to charge more than the amount received by not-for-profit hospitals for comparable services. In this sense, the for-profit suppliers were part of the public sector and not its competitors.

Wait Times

Some progress has occurred since the first ministers made wait times a priority in the 2003 and 2004 health accords. At that time they also agreed on five procedures that should receive immediate attention. On those procedures there was further agreement on performance indicators and benchmark time frames. The 2004 accord called on the Canadian Institute for Health Information to "report on progress on wait times across jurisdictions" (First Ministers' Meeting 2004, 3).

But almost a decade later, CIHI (2013, 7) reported,

> More Canadians received priority procedures in 2012 than in any other year, with notable increases in joint replacement and radiation therapy. Yet the proportions receiving care within benchmark time frames have not improved since 2010. Provinces did not attain the target—90% of priority procedures—within the benchmark time frames in any priority area except radiation therapy.

CIHI also found that Canada was still lagging other developed countries on wait times (2013, 1). The physician-led Wait Times Alliance has proposed more ambitious benchmark targets than the ones that health ministries are using.

Program Content

Here we discuss factors that may influence health-care program reform going forward. Our focus is on "who" pays and for "which" services. Since the 1940s, three competing payment paradigms have been present in our health-care systems. As outlined at the beginning of this book (chapter 1, p. 14), the paradigms can be seen as two intersecting axes of policy choice with public payment and private payment at opposite ends of a political left/political right continuum and various mixes of public payment and private payment occupying intermediate points. For cases where public payment is salient, a second axis reflects the question of who decides. Is it each jurisdiction alone, or does the decision-making involve the federal government in partnership with provinces and territories?

The three payment paradigms are private payment, provincial/territorial payment, and Canada-wide public payment. A Canada-wide private payment system was introduced in the 1950s and 1960s through the Canadian Medical Association and its provincial divisions. It became redundant, however, after the federal *Medical Care Act* was passed in 1966.

The Values Embedded in the Paradigms

Canada-wide public payment is the paradigm that has governed hospital and medical services for decades. Expenses are first-dollar covered, and access to services is not income-related. Priority of access is determined by urgency of need and not financial wherewithal. Equal access is in this sense the holy grail of medicare. The revenue for these services comes mainly from provincial consolidated-revenue funds. High-income households contribute more than low-income households to these funds, and so the expenditure side of medicare programs is broadly redistributive.

The extent of redistribution is, however, based on a host of other factors unique to each jurisdiction including its distribution of income before and after taxes and transfers.

Around 20 percent of provincial/territorial (P/T) health-care funding comes from the federal government in the form of the Canada Health Transfer.[2] Since Ottawa collects more revenue per capita from the more affluent provinces than the less affluent, this interjurisdictional realloca-tion adds to the progressivity of the Canada-wide paradigm. Furthermore, for the most part, provinces and territories accept the criterion in the *CHA* that makes medicare benefits "portable" from jurisdiction to jurisdiction.[3] The combination of interjurisdictional reallocation through Ottawa and the portability provisions of the *CHA* has served to strengthen the idea that there are social rights of Canadian citizenship and thus the building of Canada as a nation politically.

Private payment speaks to the importance of values like personal re-sponsibility and personal choice, and the efficiencies inherent in markets. Private payments include out-of-pocket payments by households and payments by insurance companies.[4] Private payments were the source of funds for 30.3 percent of total health-care expenditures in 2010 (CIHI 2012, 11). Out-of-pocket private payments were estimated to constitute a larger share of expenditures under this paradigm (49.1 percent) than insurance payments (39.8 percent). The insurance share grew faster, however (ibid., 17).

Notwithstanding its focus on the word "private," the private payment paradigm involves a role for government in at least two ways. First is through the income tax system. Among other things, the income tax sys-tem includes non-refundable tax credits that allow taxpayers to exclude a portion of their expenses for health-care premiums and uninsured health-care services from their income taxes otherwise payable. It also includes several disability-related provisions. This tax relief is determined mainly at the federal level. Second, provincial governments pay for all or some of the health-care costs of many persons who are unable to pay for care that is not covered by medicare. In 2010, prescription drugs, dental care, and institutional care other than care delivered by hospitals were the three largest uses of private funds (CIHI 2012, 20).

The *provincial/territorial payment* paradigm involves health services, other than hospital and medical services, that provinces and territories pay for. These services do not involve first-dollar coverage and are paid for mainly by a combination of P/T and private payers. Accessibility to these services is often linked to a household income test that includes premiums, deductibles, and copayments. Our case studies of drug coverage showed a range of ways that P/T and private funding can be combined to pay for health-care costs. These health-care services reflect the constitutional role assigned to the provinces and territories rather than the nation-building objectives associated with hospital and medical insurance.

In sum, the Canada-wide payment paradigm can be thought of as redistributive among individuals and across provinces, and as aimed politically at nation building. Private payment aims to encourage self-reliance and political choice. The provincial/territorial payment paradigm emphasizes the constitutional distribution of powers and the autonomy of the individual jurisdictions. It can be more or less redistributive.

Inaction Is Not Neutral

The trend among these three payment paradigms is one way of getting a sense of the trajectory of health-care reform.[5] Based on CIHI data, Table 12.1 displays the trends in health-care expenditure among the three paradigms beginning in 1975. This is a convenient starting point for us because by then the Canada-wide hospital and medical programs were both up and running.

TABLE 12.1
Shares of Total Health Expenditures Allocated to Private Payment, Provincial/Territorial Payment, and Canada-wide Public Payment

Year	Canada-wide Public Payment	Private Payment	P/T Payments*
1975	57.0	23.8	19.3
1980	53.0	24.5	22.5
1990	50.4	25.5	24.0
2000	40.2	29.8	30.0
2005	39.1	29.9	31.0
2010	40.5	29.5	30.0

Note: *The data in this column include expenditures on all "public sector sources other than Canada-wide." Around 93–94 percent of these amounts are provincial/territorial (P/T), and we use these percentages as a proxy for actual P/T expenditure. The remaining 6 to 7 percent includes items such as direct federal, municipal, and social security funds; capital investment; and federal expenditures on research.

Source: CIHI (2011b), *National Health Expenditure Trends, 1975 to 2011*, and calculations provided by CIHI researchers dated 3 July 2013.

In 1975 public expenditures on hospital and medical insurance accounted for an estimated 57 percent of total health expenditures in Canada. These expenditures were governed by provincial health insurance statutes that reflected the criteria set out in the *Canada Health Act*. Public expenditures outside the *CHA* framework accounted for 19.3 percent of total health expenditure payments. Almost all of this was accounted for by P/T expenditures. Private payments accounted for 23.8 percent of the total. In 1990, the comparable percentages were 50.4 Canada-wide public payment, 25.5 private payment, and 24.0 P/T payment. During this 1975–1990 period, the share of Canada-wide payments thus fell by 6.6 percentage points. P/T payments grew faster than private payments.

Between 1991 and 2010, the Canada-wide programs fell further in relative terms to 40.5 percent. P/T expenditures rose as a share of the total expenditures to 30 percent, and private expenditures grew to 29.5 percent. In this period the relative decline in Canada-wide payment programs was shared by roughly equal increases in the P/T payment and private payment paradigms. Expenditure shifts among these three paradigms have been relatively small since 2000. However, since health care constitutes almost 12 percent of gross domestic product (it was 7 percent in 1975 and 9 percent in 1990), even small shifts among the paradigms may involve large absolute numbers (CIHI 2012, 9).

The fact that medicare covers all medically necessary hospital and medical services and none of the costs of other services like prescription drugs and home care has adverse consequences for equity among Canadians. Certainly, no knowledgeable person would design the *CHA* and provincial health insurance as it is today if starting from scratch. But Canadians are reluctant to open a debate that touches the *CHA*. Ironically, this public regard for the *CHA* could result in medicare becoming progressively less relevant to our health-care future.

TRAJECTORIES FOR THE THREE PARADIGMS

In this section, we discuss the broad trajectories of these paradigms in recent decades and what they may mean for the future.

Canada-wide Public Payment

When the idea of countrywide, public health insurance was first mooted seriously in the 1940s, it represented a very big change from the policy status quo. The purpose was set out by the minister of national health and welfare at the 1945 Dominion-Provincial Conference on Reconstruction. Ottawa's proposal was that all Canadians be insured against the costs of sickness and injury through a plan that it would jointly finance with the provinces. In a first stage, the plan would cover general practitioner services, hospital care, and visiting nursing services and, in later stages, medical and nursing services not insured in the first stage, dental care, pharmaceuticals, and laboratory tests. The inducement for obtaining provincial concurrence was money. Ottawa would provide grants to the provinces on condition that each province in turn would establish a health insurance plan that met certain conditions. This sweeping proposal aimed "to remove the disparities in standards of health service in different parts of Canada, to avoid the risks of sudden heavy expenditures, and distribute health costs more widely and equitably, and above all, to obtain the benefits of better health for the great majority of our people" (Dominion-Provincial Conference 1946, 90).

In the quarter century that followed, the proponents of Canada-wide public payment had their ups and downs. The existing literature provides much detail (Maioni 1998; Martin 1985; Taylor 2009; Tuohy 1999). The point we want to emphasize here is that the policy reforms that led to Canada-wide hospital and medical insurance were not inevitable. In annex 3, we summarize the process that led to the two legislative landmarks, the *Hospital Insurance and Diagnostic Services Act* (1957) and the *Medical Care Act* (1966). The annex shows that each of the three paradigms had significant support and that historical "accident" played an important role in the outcomes. With only a few differences on the ground, the tipping points that were reached for hospital and medical insurance might not have been reached when the reform windows opened. The outcomes might have been very different. Other 1945 proposals, such as Canada-wide insurance for prescription drugs, home care, and dental care, have not been implemented since first proposed many years ago.

It may seem archaic to mention dental care in this discussion as it has been off the federal-provincial governmental agenda for a long time. For universal, Canada-wide, publicly funded dental care, there was no open window or tipping point after the 1945 Green Book on Reconstruction. Some reform causes do not get a second chance. Dental care is perhaps the best example of the private payment paradigm.

In contrast, the idea of creating a countrywide prescription drug program and home care programs did not fall off the federal-provincial agenda entirely. Prescription drugs came close to fruition. The reports of the National Forum on Health, the Senate Committee chaired by Kirby, and the Romanow Commission (late 1990s–early 2000s) proposed the idea of national drug insurance. But by that time federal-provincial fiscal relations had become dysfunctional owing to the ongoing fiscal dispute between federal and P/T governments about the adequacy or inadequacy of federal cash transfer payments to the provinces (Lazar et al. 2005, 41-44; Marchildon 2004, 2-6). Prescription drugs were on the agenda of First Ministers' Meetings in 2000, 2003, 2004, and 2006. In 2003 Ottawa created a new Health Reform Fund (finances incremental to the CHT) targeted at helping provinces meet ongoing needs in three priority areas—primary care, home care, and prescription drugs (First Ministers' Meeting 2003). In 2004, the federal/provincial/territorial first ministers directed their ministers of health to "develop, assess and cost options for catastrophic pharmaceutical coverage" and report by 30 June 2006 (First Ministers' Meeting 2004, 7). But most P/T governments stalled on their commitments, preferring to await the outcome of the ongoing power struggle between the Chrétien and Martin forces within the federal Liberal Party and then the results of the general elections of 2004 and 2006. No new coordinated federal-provincial legislative action on drug insurance has been taken since then.

Around 90 percent (Canadian Centre for Policy Alternatives 2002, 37) or more (Fraser Institute 2002) of Canadians carry some measure of prescription drug insurance through private plans, provincial plans, or federal plans (including for Aboriginal peoples, RCMP, and Canadian Forces). In 2012 the Senate Committee on Social Affairs, Science and Technology reported that all but a few of the smallest jurisdictions had "made efforts to establish universal catastrophic-drug-coverage programs for their citizens" (Standing Senate Committee 2012b, 54). A larger concern, however, was variability in coverage. The Senate Committee cited witnesses who had observed "significant and important disparities in the coverage offered" across jurisdictions (ibid., 54-55). The committee continued (55),

> There is still clear evidence that many Canadians are foregoing filling prescriptions due to their costs.... Witnesses explained that a lack of out-of-hospital drug coverage meant that many were choosing to stay in hospital to avoid these costs. They concluded that this lack of uniform universal catastrophic drug coverage across jurisdictions created inequities that resulted in negative health outcomes for Canadians and undermined the principles of the *Canada Health Act*.

Notwithstanding the Senate Committee, the political incentive for the Government of Canada to launch a new Canada-wide drug insurance program through a targeted federal transfer payment to the provinces is questionable. Much of the monies transferred would simply displace provincial coverage and flow through to the bottom line of the P/T consolidated revenue funds.

It is possible to imagine a Canada-wide drug insurance program in the medium or longer term paid for by the federal government directly. Such a policy would be consistent with the government's focus on clarifying roles and responsibilities. The federal government already has extensive responsibilities for regulating pharmaceuticals, including authorizing their entry to the market based on assessments of drug safety, efficacy, and quality as well as regulating manufacturers' prices through the *Patent Act* and appointment of the Patented Medicines Prices Review Board. The Conservative government has shown little overt interest in publicly funded drug insurance since it came to office in 2006. It is noteworthy, however, that the 2004 Conservative election platform stated that the party would "propose to the provinces a federal program for catastrophic drug coverage" (Conservative Party 2004, 27). But the possibility of a Canada-wide drug plan is just that—a possibility down the road. A Canada-wide drug plan is not on the federal government's current agenda.

The Canada-wide payment paradigm, as reflected in its share of total health-care expenditures, followed a downward slope almost from the time of the inception of Established Programs Financing in 1977 until the late 1990s. Since then it has remained relatively flat, covering approximately 40 percent of total health expenditures in Canada. Another way of describing these trends is that following the cuts in federal health-related transfer payments to the provinces and territories beginning in 1996, and the gradual restoration of this funding starting soon thereafter, the big picture has stabilized. In either interpretation, the above discussion on drugs notwithstanding, the prospects for an extension of the Canada-wide paradigm are not strong.

The Canada-wide paradigm relies on the leadership of the government in Ottawa. The political parties historically most associated with Canada-wide medicare are in a different space now. The federal Liberal party is the third party in the House of Commons. The opposition NDP caucus has more MPs from Quebec than from the rest of Canada, and Quebec has a universal plan (not first dollar). As long as the federal NDP has substantial Quebec representation in its caucus, it is most unlikely to open an issue that raises political sensibilities in that province.[6] As for the Conservative Harper government, it has periodically affirmed its ongoing commitment to many of the health-care policies and programs that were in force when it first came to office. In 2012 this was done in the form of a response to the report of the Standing Senate Committee on Social Affairs, Science and Technology on its review of the 2004 first ministers' 10-year health accord (Government of Canada 2012). The government declared its support for "PT health care delivery through fiscal transfers and targeted programs," its provision of "health care for certain populations," its funding of health research, and its role "in protecting and promoting the health of Canadians" (ibid., 1). This response is interesting both for what it does and does not say. What it does say is that the government is committed to these key status quo policies and programs and in some cases their improvement. What is missing is health-care policy reform. By inaction more than action, there is paradigm freeze in Ottawa.

Private Payment Paradigm

Prior to the mid-1940s, payment for health-care services was mainly determined through private arrangements between persons who required care and health-care providers and institutions that provided these services. There was little health-care insurance available privately or through governments. Out-of-pocket payment was thus common. Sometimes providers lowered their fees or accepted payment in kind for patients who had trouble meeting their bills. Governments sometimes subsidized the expenses of persons with little or no means who required treatment.

Sometimes needed care was not provided. When governments did step in it was the provincial or municipal government that did so, as the Constitution assigned the great bulk of the authority to make laws on health care to the provinces (and municipalities are the legal creatures of provinces). In so doing the provinces were acting as funder of last resort rather than as insurer. Put simply, for most Canadians the *default* position on health care meant private payment—they were responsible for paying their own way.

Private payment was not just about what the private sector should or should not do. It was also about what the private sector could do. In fact, private health-care insurance grew rapidly after it became clear that federal and provincial governments would not act quickly on the Green Book proposals (Taylor 2009, 172-73). Commercial and not-for-profit insurers offered hospital, surgical, and medical insurance both to individuals and groups (employers for their employees). In most provinces, the provincial medical association also sponsored its own not-for-profit insurer (Taylor 2009, 171). From the mid-1940s through to the mid-1950s, private insurers had some wind in their sails.

The introduction of Canada-wide publicly financed hospital insurance had a twofold effect. It eased the burden on persons who were paying out-of-pocket for health-care services, and it effectively displaced commercial health insurers from their largest health-care market.[7] When Parliament enacted medical insurance, the effect was similar. The loss of the hospital and medical insurance markets was the nadir of the private payment paradigm and the corresponding apex of the Canada-wide paradigm. In 1975, private payments accounted for 23.8 percent of total health-care expenditures in Canada, and more than half of that share consisted of out-of-pocket expenditures.

Despite these setbacks, the share of private payments did not fall. Private insurers continued to compete for business in the markets that remained open to them, such as prescription drugs, dental services, physiotherapy, and vision care. When provincial governments exercised fiscal restraint in the 1990s, the private payment share of total health expenditures grew to 29.8 percent by 2000. As seen in Table 12.1, its share has not fluctuated much since then.

Supporters of a greater role for the private payment paradigm hold their views for disparate reasons. Some simply believe in the residual state. As Church and Neale discuss in chapter 3, this position has been part of the Alberta political culture for the entire period covered in this book. Elsewhere, however, this ideological stand did not garner much backing. Others point to lessons from history and the gradual replacement of universal social programs with targeted ones such as old age security benefits. For example, Bliss (2010, 1) proposes that "reimbursement for healthcare in Canada now be on the basis of financial need, not universality."

The main intellectual support for an enhanced private role in funding health care is found in the public finance literature. It boils down to an argument that without transferring some share of what is now publicly funded to private provision, public deficit and debt levels will become increasingly difficult to sustain. Health costs will continue to increase faster than the growth in public revenues and accordingly will require higher levels of taxation. Higher taxation will adversely influence economic growth, resulting in a self-inflicted downward spiral in public finances. This vicious cycle will be reinforced by related factors such as the aging of the population and the introduction of new technologies that result in better treatment of illness but at a high price. This chain of reasoning is captured by the term "sustainability" (variously taken to mean economic sustainability, political sustainability, or a combination of the two). This thesis logically leads to the conclusion that increasing the role of private finance in health care is a necessity (Dodge and Dion 2011, among others).

The sustainability thesis has attracted much attention from those who worry about levels of taxation in Canada including finance ministries and much of the business community. Yet Table 12.1 shows no growth in the relative role of private finance in health care since 2000, and more detailed CIHI numbers indicate that the private share in financing health care has been more or less constant since 1997 (CIHI 2012, 12). Plainly, the ideological, historical, and most importantly public finance arguments in support of sustainability have not been able to tip the balance. In a classical "he says she says" debate, supporters of a public finance paradigm, especially the Canada-wide paradigm, counter each of the points made in the sustainability thesis. For example, it is true that health-care expenditures have risen as a share of P/T expenditures but because of tax cuts not growth in medicare costs (Canadian Doctors for Medicare 2011, 1-4). Public sector health-care costs in Canada are not high compared to such costs in other countries (CIHI 2012, 67). The highest rate of increase in health-care expenditures has been in pharmaceuticals, which are not part of the Canada-wide medicare system (CIHI 2011e). It has also been argued that the rising costs of health care will remain affordable because they will be offset by productivity increases in other less labour-intensive sectors (Baumol 2012).The "he says she says" debate suggests that paradigm freeze is an apt description for policy issues in the financing of health care in recent decades.

Recent (2012 and 2013) provincial budgets suggest that provincial governments are determined to slow the growth of health-care spending but not necessarily by relying on for-profit insurers or delivery agents. How sustainable this provincial effort turns out to be remains to be seen. For those who prefer the private payment paradigm, it must be disappointing that after a decade of right-of-centre, mainly conservative governments in Canada, there has been such limited reform in financing. Recalling that the evidence of this book associates large reforms with a change of government that has committed to reform when in opposition, the actors in the sustainability camp ought now be trying to convince opposition parties as well as governments to commit to an enhanced role for private finance. But the Canadian experience of recent decades is that no party, whether right or left leaning, seeks office promising to leave more of the costs of health care to the family and private sector.

The private payment paradigm seems unlikely to make large gains in the absence of crisis or at least the perception of crisis.

Provincial Payment Paradigm

At the end of the Second World War, governmental decisions about health-care governance, finance, and delivery rested mainly with provincial governments. If there was to be publicly funded health insurance, it would require provincial legislation. (The federal government had some important health responsibilities, including the operation of a number of hospitals for war veterans.)

Backers of the provincial payment paradigm held their views for one of three reasons. One was simply that provincial payment was their preferred position. This represented the position of the government of Quebec on many issues including hospital and medical insurance. Others were attached to the idea of Canada-wide public payment for health care but were willing to settle on provincial payment as preferable to continuing with whatever private payment arrangements were in place. The government of Saskatchewan provides examples in the hospital insurance case and again in medical care. The third reason was the opposite. A backer of provincial payment did so to pre-empt the possibility of a new Canada-wide program. The government of Quebec legislated drug reform in 1996 not only for domestic reasons but also to make it harder for the federal government to start a new shared-cost program and occupy this space.

There were grey zones. The "contracting out" arrangements for an established program, jointly funded by federal and provincial governments, provide an example. Under federal law passed in 1965, a provincial government could choose to receive a transfer payment from Ottawa through the transfer of tax room instead of cash.[8]

On the hypothetical political left/political right axis we referred to earlier, there were many intermediate points. The most common were deductibles and copayments on those who qualified for a provincial program. The Ontario and Quebec drug cases are examples. Provincially mandated private coverage of health care is another example with the Quebec drug case again an illustration.

The government of Quebec has arguably been the most consistent of Canada's jurisdictions in its approach to the trade-offs associated with these two axes of policy choice. Over the decades, it has consistently given more weight to the provincial payment/Canada-wide axis than the public payment/private payment axis (Quebec 1998). Protecting Quebec's constitutional status has taken precedence over trade-offs between public payment and private payment for health care.

The government of Alberta has also consistently favoured provincial payment to Canada-wide payment. It has also been most consistent in preferring more private arrangements than other jurisdictions.

The Maritime provinces, too, paid a lot of attention to this same inter-governmental axis but for different reasons. During the early public debates about the creation of hospital and medical insurance, these provinces often resisted federal cost-sharing initiatives. They did so in part, however, as a negotiating tactic to ensure that the federal funding formula that might eventually be adopted would recognize their relatively weak fiscal capacity and thus include some measure of equalization. The stances of other provinces have been less consistent, reflecting changes of government and events of the moment.

Perhaps paradoxically, the change in government attitudes toward the provincial payment paradigm has been largest at the federal level. For almost all of the post–Second World War years, the federal Liberals have attempted to "own" medicare as their issue, the pioneering work of the Saskatchewan Commonwealth Co-operative Federation (CCF) and New Democratic Party (NDP) notwithstanding. While the Liberal govern-ment of St. Laurent was reticent to act on hospital insurance, the Liberal caucus of the time effectively forced his hand (annex 3). Since then, the Liberals have consistently advocated for medicare even if not acting on their advocacy (e.g., 1995 federal budget). They have also maintained that the conservative parties to their political right were enemies of medicare. For their part, the parties to the right (mainly Progressive Conservative and Conservative) have neither run for office on anti-medicare platforms (Mulroney famously referring to it as a "sacred trust"[9]) nor behaved that way while in office. It has been only with the Harper government that a Conservative government has come out strongly and explicitly in favour of a form of classical federalism that would limit if not eliminate the use of the federal spending on a conditional basis. The federal Conservative government's dislike of jointly managed programs suggests that the provincial payment paradigm may have its most effective supporter in Ottawa. At the same time, actions matter more than words; to date the Conservatives have by and large accepted the status quo.

Reform by Default

We found meagre policy reform in our case studies. Yet Table 12.1 shows a substantial shift in the relative positions of the three paradigms. The reports of the provincial commissions and task forces showed what kinds of reforms in public policy were desirable. When the policy response to these calls for reform is inadequate, the status quo does not necessarily prevail. The direction and extent of reform may be determined by other factors. The default position in Canadian health-care insurance falls to individuals, families, and voluntary groupings (e.g., workplace-related arrangements, charitable organizations) not the state. The default position in delivery falls to the goodwill of health-care providers, including physicians and nurses, whether on a voluntary basis (a version of the pre–Second World War models) or otherwise. For those who want to preserve and expand medicare, therefore, strong health-care policy action is needed. For those who wish to see individuals and markets play a bigger role in health care, health-care policy action may be less needed. Policy inaction alone, or more likely in the context of a fiscal crisis or perceived crisis, may move the Canadian health-care model closer to their wishes. In all cases, where there is the political will for governmental action, the Constitution points to provincial governments as the decision makers, not the federal government.

It is about a half century since universally accessible, publicly financed medical care became available to Canadians. Other health services have grown in importance over these decades and as a share of health expenditures. But the political centre and left-centre have not been able to persuade governments to include payment for any of these services, such as prescribed drugs and home care, within the existing Canada-wide framework or any alternative national framework. If new forms of health care emerge that do not already fit firmly under the hospital or medical insurance headings, they too may remain outside the framework. Like other interests, medicare supporters are better able to protect what they have won than to secure new victories. These macro-level observations about the financing domain of health care mirror the meagre reforms found in our case studies.

FEDERALISM AND POLICY REFORM

Federalism helped to shape the manner in which Canada's health-care model was developed, and it continues to do so. The constitutional allocation of legislative powers made provincial governments responsible for the provision of health-care services to Canadians; nonetheless, the federal spending power enabled Ottawa to play a leading role in the creation of Canada-wide hospital and medical care services. How that power is used going forward and what it may mean for health-care reform are the issues we consider here.

During the period of Liberal government from 1993 to 2006, the Liberals cut cash transfers to the provinces and territories as part of their successful effort to improve federal finances. Within Liberal ranks, there was a concern that restoring transfers would inflate the remuneration of health-care providers and not achieve reforms. As just noted, the Liberal government tried to "buy" health-care policy reform from the provinces and territories when it began restoring the transfers in the late 1990s. For their part, the provinces and territories made restoration of the federal fiscal transfer their priority. The result was a heavy reform-associated agenda in the 2000, 2003, and 2004 first ministers' health agreements although the amount of reform achieved fell far short of stated aspirations. Whether Ottawa was genuinely expecting to buy reform or just the appearance of reform we shall never know. It is important to note, however, that the federal government gave a lot space to "how to" questions—how to improve performance in the health-care sector. Arguably, this entailed a more interventionist approach to P/T jurisdiction than had previously been the case. In cutting transfers in 1995 and then restoring them subject to new conditions, the Chrétien and Martin Liberal governments (1993–2006) were using fiscal contribution to the provinces and territories as a way of influencing P/T policy reform. The Progressive Conservative governments of Brian Mulroney (1984–1993) had also tightened their cash contributions to the provinces and territories, but the PCs refrained from attempting to steer the provincial ship of state in matters of health care. Indeed, the PCs made a point of emphasizing their respect for provincial jurisdiction in health care.

The election of the Conservative party in 2006 and its re-election in 2008 and 2011 ushered in a new paradigm in federal-provincial health-care relations—one that does not fit neatly with any of the three paradigms. Like the federal governments that preceded it, the Harper government continues to transfer large sums of money to the provinces under the Canada Health Transfer (CHT). The CHT level is set out in legislation up to 2013/14, after which it rises by 6 percent annually as a result of an automatic escalator. In December 2011, the federal government announced that total CHT cash would keep growing at 6 percent until 2016/17. Thereafter, it would grow in line with a three-year moving average of nominal gross domestic product, with funding guaranteed to increase by at least 3 percent per year (Bailey and Curry 2011). But unlike its Liberal predecessors, the Conservative government has not presumed to use its fiscal commitment to the provinces and territories as a policy reform lever. Quite the opposite, since taking office, the Harper government has committed to continuing transfer payments without imposing new conditions. The Conservative view has been that the presence of two orders of government on a specific program or policy detracts from performance by muting accountability. The Conservative government's approach has served to protect the status quo in health-care policy.

The Conservative federal government's commitment to long-term funding of P/T programs without new conditions was not negotiated by the federal government. It was simply announced and then extended by further announcements. What is different in the Harper approach is the balance that the prime minister has struck between two big commitments.

One is the importance of clarity in roles and responsibilities. The second commitment is the Conservative government's frequently announced support for universal hospital and medical care insurance as set out in the *CHA* (Conservative Party 2006, 30-31; 2011, 30). The *CHA* is not seen as a condition but rather a set of principles that all jurisdictions willingly embrace. Thus, the main difference between the Harper approach and that of his Liberal predecessors is not in the transfer itself. It is in the presence or absence of an accompanying federal/provincial/territorial (FPT) reform agenda. Such an agenda was present and politically linked to the restoration of the CHT in the case of the Liberal governments led by Jean Chrétien and Paul Martin. It has not been present in the case of the Conservative governments led by Harper.

The contrast between buying reform through FPT agreements and encouraging reform by clarifying roles and responsibilities is stark. This contrast is reinforced by the difference in processes associated with the two parties. Under the Liberal government, there were numerous FPT meetings of officials, then ministers, leading to first ministers' meetings. The outcomes were negotiated. Under the Conservatives there were no first ministers' meetings. The prime minister and finance minister simply announced what they had decided. There was nothing to negotiate. Federal dollars were available to provincial governments and nothing was required of the provinces, although they were exhorted to keep on improving performance indicators.

Embedded in the Conservative strategy is the idea that intergovernmentalism is a drag on decision-making and in conflict with clarity of roles and responsibilities. Embedded in the Liberal strategy was a strong role for intergovernmentalism in an increasingly interconnected world.

The starkness of the difference in principle on roles and responsibilities notwithstanding, in practice the differences between Conservative and Liberal government policies on health-care reform have been small. The Conservative government has accepted the medicare legacy. It has not made an effort to undo the past. If clarity had been the federal government's overriding commitment, it could have given notice to the provinces that the Canada Health Transfer would be terminated at some future date. In its stead, the federal government would transfer an appropriate amount of tax room to the provinces. Each province would use the tax room according to its priorities. That approach would leave the provinces and territories unambiguously responsible and accountable for health care. The politics of giving notice, however, would mean a major public confrontation with all of the political left, much of the political centre, and even possibly isolated pockets of the centre-right. It is almost certainly not in the cards in the foreseeable future.

The payment paradigm the Harper Conservatives have been following is a blend of the "Canada-wide" (reflecting the legacy) and "provincial" (leaving future policy reform to provinces). Since federal taxpayers contribute to the provincial programs, there is an element of sharing that stretches beyond provincial boundaries. But it is provincial governments alone that make expenditure decisions.

Whether the Conservative approach will yield more reform than the Liberal approach might have done is an open question. The meagre policy reform that characterized the 1990–2003 period did not improve much in the 2004–2011 period. With the federal government's legal fiscal commitment to the provinces running to 2016/17, and its political commitment for a much longer period, the Conservative approach may have time to be well tested.

Final Words

The extensive empirical analysis underpinning this book shows that there has been relatively little fundamental change in Canadian health-care policy over the past four decades. This intransigence—the result of the interaction of ideas, interests, and institutions—has resulted in a paradigm freeze. Without some sort of insurmountable disruptive force, either a major shift in medical science or technology or a catastrophic economic or political crisis, fundamental health policy reform in Canada is unlikely. As Pogo once reminded us, "We have met the enemy and he is us."[10]

NOTES

1.   The Conservative party platform in 2004 stated that the government would "propose to the provinces a federal program for catastrophic drug coverage" (Conservative Party 2004, 27).
2.   It is also arguable that a portion of Equalization is for health. There is no formal string between federal CHT payments to provinces and territories and how the funds are used. These transfers are sometimes described as "notionally" allocated to P/T health expenditures.
3.   Residents moving from one province or territory to another are covered for insured health services by the "home" jurisdiction during any waiting period imposed by the new province or territory. After the waiting period, which must not exceed three months, the new province or territory of residence assumes responsibility for health-care coverage.
4.   Private payments also include non-consumption expenditures such as hospital non-patient revenue, capital expenditures for privately owned facilities, and health research (CIHI 2012, 11).
5.   For a more technical approach to the trajectory, see Dodge and Dion 2011.
6.   Nonetheless, the government of Quebec might accept a new federal initiative on drugs provided that the new transfer had no conditions that Quebec could not readily meet and that the province could opt out with full financial compensation. In other words, the arrangement would essentially be an unconditional grant from Ottawa to the Quebec government.

7. The private market had been eliminated earlier in Saskatchewan and British Columbia.
8. There has been a debate about whether or not to continue to count the tax points transferred to the provinces at the time of EPF. The 20 percent share does not count the tax points.
9. Canada, House of Commons Debates, *Hansard,* 9 December 1983, 44.
10. Walt Kelly, author of a long-running American cartoon strip, http://en.wikipedia.org/wiki/Pogo_%28comic_strip%29.

Annex 1

Analyzing the Nature and Extent of Health-Care Policy Reforms, 1990–2003

Harvey Lazar

Methodology

This volume has assessed the nature and extent of reforms against the benchmarks established by the grey literature produced from the mid-1980s to 2003. As outlined in chapter 8, if all the elements proposed in the grey literature are met for a particular issue, we describe that reform as comprehensive. Other degrees of reform are described as significant, moderate, limited, or none. The purpose of this annex is to define these varying degrees of reform for each issue in relation to specific elements in the grey literature.

Determining the grey literature consensus was not always easy. In some cases there was a clear majority of reports in favour of a reform direction, but in other cases views were divided. When a strong plurality of reports (but less than a majority) supported a certain reform, we accepted the plurality view as our benchmark. For example, where two or three reports supported a reform direction and, say, one rejected that direction (and others were silent), the plurality position became the benchmark. We also decided that all provinces would be subject to the same benchmark. Thus, if the grey literature in a particular province was out-of-step with the grey literature consensus, for our analytical purposes that particular province was still subject to the same standard as other provinces.

It is implicit in this approach that all reforms assessed as limited or higher were *directionally consistent* with the grey literature. Decisions by provincial governments that were opposite in direction to the consensus of the grey literature are described as *counter-consensus reforms*. It bears repeating that we are not expressing a normative preference for reforms that were directionally consistent with the grey literature standard. We are observing and classifying events and non-events, not judging their desirability.

Grey literature refers to reports that are typically prepared by commissions, task forces, and advisory committees appointed by provincial and federal governments. Additional grey literature exists in the form of reports or studies produced by think tanks and stakeholder groups in the health-care field. Given the sheer magnitude of the grey literature, we decided to focus on the broader studies—those that covered at least two of the six issues analyzed in this project. Reports that focused on only one issue (e.g., regionalization, alternative payments plans, for-profit delivery) were also taken into account but on a much less systematic basis.

The main national studies we used, in chronological order, were the following:

- National Forum on Health (1997), *Canada Health Action: Building on the Legacy*
- Institute for Research on Public Policy (IRPP) Task Force on Health Policy (2000), *Recommendations to First Ministers*
- Standing Senate Committee on Social Affairs, Science and Technology (2002), *The Health of Canadians – The Federal Role.* Volume 6, *Recommendations for Reform* (Kirby report)
- Commission on the Future of Health Care in Canada (2002), *Building on Values: The Future of Health Care in Canada* (Romanow report)

We also took into account systemwide reports that were national in scope but not "official," for example, publications emanating from the Canadian Medical Association, the federal-provincial-territorial (FPT) committees, and related sources. These reports were used mainly to corroborate or clarify the grey literature in situations where that literature was thin.

The most significant national report for our purposes was the one by the National Forum on Health, because of its timing. Its final report—an independent, federally sponsored systemwide analysis—was published in 1997. The two other major reports of this era, the Kirby and Romanow reports, were published in 2002—too late to have much direct impact on governments during the period we assessed. Nonetheless, the processes followed by the Senate Committee and Romanow Commission, the evidence they amassed, and the reports they issued prior to their final reports doubtless had some influence. The flow of influence between these national reports and provincially sponsored grey literature was not, however, one way. The national reports were to some extent a response to and a distillation of the provincial reports.

The provincial reports were published in two "waves." We discussed the context and content of these reports in detail in chapter 8. Here we present a list of the reports used in our study.

First Wave

- British Columbia. Royal Commission on Health Care and Costs (1991), *Closer to Home*, chaired by Justice Peter D. Seaton
- Alberta. Premier's Commission on Future Health Care for Albertans (1989), *The Rainbow Report: Our Vision for Health*, chaired by Lou Hyndman
- Saskatchewan. Saskatchewan Commission on Directions in Health Care (1990), *Future Directions for Health Care in Saskatchewan*, chaired by R.G. Murray
- Ontario. Ontario Task Force on the Use and Provision of Medical Services (1990), *Final Report of the Task Force on the Use and Provision of Medical Services*, chaired by Graham Scott
- Quebec. Commission d'enquête sur les services de santé et les services sociaux (1988), *Rapport de la Commission d'enquête sur les services de santé et les services sociaux*, chaired by Jean Rochon
- Nova Scotia. Royal Commission on Health Care (1989), *The Report of the Nova Scotia Royal Commission on Health Care: Towards a New Strategy*, chaired by J. Camille Gallant

Second Wave

- Alberta. Premier's Advisory Council on Health (2001), *A Framework for Reform: Report of the Premier's Advisory Council on Health*, chaired by Don Mazankowski
- Saskatchewan. Commission on Medicare (2001), *Caring for Medicare: Sustaining a Quality System*, chaired by Kenneth Fyke
- Ontario. Ontario Health Services Restructuring Commission (2000), *Looking Back, Looking Forward: A Legacy Report*, chaired by Duncan Sinclair.
- Quebec. Commission d'étude sur les services de santé et les services sociaux (2000), *Report and Recommendations: Emerging Solutions*, chaired by Michel Clair
- Newfoundland and Labrador. Government of Newfoundland and Labrador (2002), *Healthier Together: A Strategic Health Plan for Newfoundland and Labrador*

Note that all of the reports were by bodies at arm's-length from the sponsoring government except the 2002 report by the Government of Newfoundland and Labrador. While these were the main provincially initiated reports used in our study, we also cite other provincial reports in the text.

Some of the standards that we have used for analytical purposes emerged in the first wave and thus, in some sense, governments had a decade or longer to decide whether or not to act on them. Other standards emerged during the second wave, and thus left less time for action. This distinction is taken into account in chapters 8 and 9 where we analyze the extent and nature of reform and the factors that explain reform, and compare performance among jurisdictions.

STANDARDS FOR THE SIX REFORM ISSUES

1. Regionalization

We begin with the issue of devolution to the subprovincial level. This entailed a range of proposals to shift some provincial health-care functions and services to the regional or local level, along with the corresponding authority to manage and operate those services. The proposals called for regional or local authorities to be at least in part regionally or locally elected. Regionalization was not proposed by the National Forum on Health, but in the late 1980s and early 1990s all of the above first-wave provincial reports focused on this issue except Ontario's. (Note that the second-wave Ontario report did recommend devolution.) While the specifics of these reports differed, the commonalities were strong.

Quebec had adopted a regional structure in the 1970s. Twelve regional councils (plus one each for First Nations and Inuit) were established at that time for health and social services. Their roles were mainly advisory with limited coordinating, including resource allocation, responsibilities. The focus of the 1988 Rochon report was to improve on what already existed, not to start from scratch. The report recommended a clarification of roles and responsibilities between the Ministry of Health and Social Services, and regional councils and institutions. It also called for regional councils to be replaced by elected regional boards with three-year mandates. These boards were to be composed in a manner that more closely represented the population being served. The boards were to be invested with the authority to plan, organize, implement, and evaluate health care and social services in the regions based on overarching provincial policy.

Alberta's Rainbow Commission (1989) advocated that the province be divided into nine autonomous administrative areas, accountable through regional health authorities. The scope of the activities to be transferred was broad and included both institutions and physicians. Functions transferred would include planning, resource allocation, coordination, and even the power to raise revenues beyond the amount the province would transfer. Physician remuneration would be negotiated at the regional level. These health authorities would be composed of locally elected trustees. Each authority would be required to report annually to the Department of Health on activities, resource utilization, programs and services, fiscal arrangements, and health status with in its jurisdiction.

The 1989 Nova Scotia Royal Commission report recommended that the province establish a regional health authority (RHA) in each region, based on boundaries to be defined by a Health Council, and appoint the boards of these regional authorities through a public nomination process. The Ministry of Health should transfer financial resources to the regional health authorities for the management of all health-care services.

Reorganization of governance was the central theme of Saskatchewan's Murray report (1990). It saw regionalization as the lynchpin for modernizing and rationalizing the health-care system. This was to be accomplished, first, by making the system accountable through the creation of regional health divisions managed by elected councils. The councils would be responsible for the allocation of resources including the funding of hospitals and, interestingly, payment of health-care professionals. Of note, the report explicitly stated that the financing of health care should remain a responsibility of the provincial government. It did not propose the transfer of revenue-raising authority to the regional level, as did the *Rainbow Report*.[1]

The BC commission (1991) argued that devolution would improve the efficiency and effective use of health-care resources. It therefore proposed development of a regional health services system by transferring control for area-specific health services planning and resource allocation. Under the proposed system, the Ministry of Health would develop systemwide goals, objectives, and standards and would establish budget envelopes in consultation with regions for the allocation of resources. Regional budget envelopes would include funds for all health programs in the region. Funds would come from the Medical Services Plan allocated for the region, as well as capital and other operational monies. Regional budget processes were to be public, allowing consumer and provider input into decision-making.

The 1990 Scott report in Ontario did not offer proposals on regionalization, possibly because his task force was not mandated to investigate the issue. But other grey literature reports from Ontario argued in favour. The 1991 Premier's Council on Health Strategy recommended that responsibility for planning and service delivery including coordination, integration, and resource allocation be devolved from the provincial to the local level. The intent was to create greater opportunities for people living in communities to influence the choices that affected them.

Also worth taking into account is the 1994 *Framework for Evaluating Devolution* by the Task Force on Devolution appointed by the Premier's Council on Health, Well-Being and Social Justice in Ontario. It conceptualized devolution on the basis of three dimensions: scope (the "substantive

---

[1] The original Saskatchewan districts, however, were able to run deficits and borrow money to finance them.

areas of responsibility" being transferred); function (the nature of the activities being transferred such as planning, coordinating, integrating, allocating resources, and delivering services); and authority (the degree to which the local or regional organization can take decisions independently of the provincial government).

Although there was no systemwide report commissioned by the Government of Newfoundland and Labrador during the first half of the assessment period, regionalization as a theme was attracting much attention in such diverse areas as economic development, education, and municipal government as well as hospital board integration. In the case of the hospitals, a former CEO of a hospital in St. John's, Lucie Dobbin, was hired by the health minister to chair a commission to review how hospital boards could be integrated. In March 1993, the *Report on the Reduction of Hospital Boards* was released. It included recommendations on how to reduce and integrate hospital boards. An advantage of regionalizing, according to the Dobbin report, is that it "allows for one body to determine the needs of the area, assess the present level of service, eliminate duplication or inappropriate services, and apply the health dollars available in the most appropriate place" (Dobbin 1993, 15).

Although with the benefit of hindsight the idea of devolving authority for physician remuneration to the regional level may have been a "stretch," a majority of the first-wave reports proposed the transfer of medical budgets as well as institutional budgets. This is reflected in our definitions below.

Four provinces—Alberta, Saskatchewan, Ontario, and Newfoundland and Labrador—did not have substantial autonomous regional structures for health-care planning, integration, and coordination, for or resource allocation at the beginning of the 1990s. All four made their decisions on the nature and extent of their reforms before the second-wave provincial and national reports were published. Thus, it is the first-wave provincial reports that established the benchmark for assessing the extent of reform in the regionalization case study.

Quebec's health-care system was to some degree regionalized in the 1970s with the creation of the regional health and social service councils. They had administrative responsibilities; on policy matters, their role was mainly advisory. Quebec's system of regionalization was subject to ongoing change throughout the period we covered. In 1991, the regional level was enhanced through the creation of regional boards with some executive authority and the termination of the advisory councils. But the main focus of our study involved the 2003 decision of the government to replace the regional boards with "agencies." The agency function was narrower than that held by the boards with authority shifting both upward back to the province and downward to the local networks.

Bearing in mind all of the above, the definition of *comprehensive* for the regionalization case study includes the following elements:

1. Devolution of authority and responsibility for all or a large majority of health-care planning to a subprovincial level with that level (either regional or local) also responsible for management, coordination, and integration of services including for institutional and physician services
2. Resource allocation decisions of all or a large majority of health-care spending within the regions to be done by the regional health authority (RHA) including for institutions and physician services
3. Some method for making the RHA responsive to local needs, likely though not necessarily through election of board members

(Note that this definition is silent on the role of the regional level in respect of drugs as this issue received insufficient attention in the grey literature to establish a consensus.)

Significant. Includes policy reform elements that are broadly consistent in principle with the comprehensive reform but does not include all elements. For example, a significant rating would apply to a province that transfers the same kind of authority and functions as in the comprehensive case but limits the scope of the transfer by excluding physician remuneration. In other words, one important element of the reform proposals is not implemented, but other key elements are acted on.

Moderate. At least two or parts of two of the second and third elements in the comprehensive definition are lacking.

Limited. The role assigned to the authority at the subprovincial level is a planning role only and does not include managing, coordinating, and integrating services. Thus, key parts of the first element and the entire second element are absent. In this situation, the presence or absence of the third element is likely irrelevant.

Counter-consensus. Changes in the regional/local system are in the opposite direction of the consensus definitions. In the Quebec case the reform is labelled counter-consensus because, as a result of 2003 decisions, much of the authority that had been located at the regional level in 1991 was transferred either to the provincial level or to the local level. The result was that the authority at the combined regional and local levels in 2003–2004 was less than it had been in the aftermath of the 1991 decision.

2. Needs-Based Funding

We again look mainly to the first wave of provincial reports to establish our standard for needs-based funding.

In British Columbia, the Royal Commission proposed regional budget envelopes that would include funds for the bulk of health programs in the region, funds from the Medical Services Plan allocated for the region, capital, and other operational monies. These funds were to be transferred from the province to RHAs on a weighted capitation formula that would incorporate local service needs and a broad range of population health-risk indicators. (As with the regionalization case, the report did not recommend transferring out-of-hospital drug budgets.)

The terms of reference of the Ontario report chaired by Graham Scott meant that it did not tackle this issue. The Murray report also gave it little attention, but the Health Services Funding Advisory Committee (1996) appointed by the Government of Alberta argued forcefully in favour of a population-based, needs-adjusted model with provision for ensuring that a regional authority treating a patient from outside its boundaries would be compensated by the patient's home region.

The Alberta *Rainbow Report* recommended that RHAs be allocated global budgets according to needs and priorities. This global funding "could be per-capita based, adjusted for demography, epidemiology, and other socio-economic factors" (Premier's Commission on Future Health Care for Albertans 1989b, 129). Hospitals would be funded by RHAs based on outputs and eventually outcomes, not inputs. Hospitals "would be paid an average cost per case adjusted for severity" (ibid., 125).

Under Quebec's Rochon report, the Ministry would be responsible for the development of an allocation formula for regional envelopes through global budgets on a per-capita basis. The envelopes would reflect the demographics of the region. Regional budgets would cover programs that were the responsibility of the regional board. As well, the budgets would include capital and equipment costs, and funds for the remuneration of health professionals who worked with the programs covered. Regional boards would be responsible for their own deficits and, by the same token, would be allowed to retain any surpluses.

The 1989 Nova Scotia Royal Commission on Health Care proposed that regional health authorities be funded on a capitation formula that would take into account population, demographics, and regional health status.

In short, the British Columbia, Alberta, and Nova Scotia first-wave provincial reports built needs-based funding into their recommendations, and the 1995 Saskatchewan Advisory Committee moved decisively in that direction as well. The Quebec report was less precise on incorporating needs, but it did argue for taking demographics into account.

Based on the above, the definition of *comprehensive* reform that had emerged by the mid-1990s included the following elements:

1. Per capita funding formula for regional authorities based on the distribution of population health needs among the regions, including age and disease distribution

2. The funding formula to apply to all or most of the provincial health budget for institutions and programs (but not out-of-hospital drugs, physician remuneration, highly specialized care, and teaching hospitals)

(Note that this definition does not include medical budgets in the formula even though physician remuneration was included in the "comprehensive" definition for regionalization. Even though the two cases are linked, there was much more explicit support in the grey literature for the inclusion of medical budgets in the regionalization case than in the needs-based funding case. It is understood that this is not entirely logical, but it does reflect the grey literature.)

Significant. Reform includes the first element, but the needs-based funding formula applies to a smaller portion of the provincial health budget.

Moderate. The traditional, historically based system of funding institutions is maintained but with some substantive adjustments to reflect differences in need among regions.

Limited. The traditional, historically based system of funding institutions is maintained with marginal adjustments to reflect differences in need among regions.

Counter-consensus. Reforms entail shifts in a direction that is the opposite of what the grey literature proposed.

3. Alternative Payment Plans

The various national reports suggested that alternative payment plans (alternatives to the widely used fee-for-service) for primary care physicians were desirable, although these reports avoided precise recommendations. Thus, the National Forum on Health advocated strongly for a revamped primary care system but did not make recommendations on physician remuneration. The final report of the Senate (Kirby) Committee argued for reform of primary health-care systems. It recommended federal financial support for provincial reform initiatives to create multidisciplinary teams that would require, among other things, alternative methods of payment to fee-for-service (Standing Senate Committee 2002b, section 4.4). The Romanow Commission similarly suggested that the federal Primary Health Care Transfer should be allocated to provinces and territories to address "implementing new approaches for paying physicians" (Commission on the Future of Health Care 2002, 125).

Turning to the first wave of provincial reports, Quebec's 1988 Rochon report suggested that greater collaboration between physicians and other front-line resources in the community could be achieved by associating physicians with particular programs or population groups. Physician remuneration would be factored into program budgets with physicians paid on a lump-sum basis for their participation in specific programs. Physicians working in institutions would receive some form of fixed remuneration (salary) for the whole of their medical and administrative functions. They could top up their salaries to a predetermined ceiling through fee-for-service payments.

The 1989 Alberta *Rainbow Report* suggested that "methods other than fee-for-service should be investigated and implemented where there is evidence that such a payment system would result in more equitable compensation for providers ... better service to consumers ... and at a cost which is acceptable and affordable to Health Authorities" (Premier's Commission on Future Health Care for Albertans 1989b, 130).

The 1989 Nova Scotia commission recommended the introduction of a mixed system of remuneration for physicians, including fee-for-service, salary, and capitation methods of payment.

The 1990 Murray report was concerned about the existing remuneration system and its tendency to promote "over-medication, excessive recall of patients, inadequate communication and consultation" (Saskatchewan Commission on Directions in Health Care 1990, 107). Although vague on details, the commission concluded that a major restructuring of the payment system was needed to encourage different medical practice models including group practice, and that options to the fee-for-service model should be developed.

The 1990 Ontario Task Force report made no recommendations on the forms of physician compensation, but it did argue that comprehensive reform of medical services could be undertaken only with a reasonable consensus among the principal stakeholders. This view proved to be prophetic.

The 1991 BC Seaton report argued that fee-for-service was an impediment to the kind of reform it saw as desirable, but its recommendations in this regard were not precise apparently due to lack of physician buy-in. Nonetheless, it called on the Ministry of Health to commit to developing alternative health-service-delivery organizations and overseeing the development, coordination, and integration of policies, procedures, and legislation necessary to support them. It also suggested an annual global cap on gross payments to physicians that would respond to population change and price level but not to increased utilization. This would thus create a substantial fiscal incentive for primary care physicians to consider alternatives to fee-for-service.

In summary, at the outset of the decade most provincial reports were suggesting that fee-for-service compensation be replaced by an alternative, although not always well-defined, system (Alberta, Nova Scotia, Saskatchewan, and Quebec). The BC report hinted at such an approach, and Ontario's Scott report considered change desirable but this needed to be worked out with affected interests. There was thus a consensus in favour of reforms at the outset of the decade but ambiguity regarding the details.

By the second wave of reports, there was an even larger measure of consensus. Quebec's 2000 Clair Commission proposed that family physicians within the Family Medicine Groups be placed on a mixed or blended payment system that would include capitation, lump-sum payments for participation in specific programs, and fee-for-service.

In Ontario, the 2000 Sinclair report promoted the idea of primary care reform, advocating funding for primary health-care teams based on three complementary approaches: (a) the majority of funding would be in the form of capitation, age-adjusted and illness-adjusted, supplemented by (b) fee-for-service funding, particularly for preventive/screening/public health services like vaccinations and Pap smears, and (c) sessional fees for service in the local emergency room, on-call in a nursing home, and so on. About one-fourth of the remuneration was to be held back and paid out at the end of the year in the form of a bonus based on satisfaction surveys of people registered with the team, together with other measures like adherence to clinical guidelines. The report favoured comprehensive provincial implementation of the primary health-care reform strategy and recommended that "a structure [be] put in place to support implementation activities" (Ontario Health Services Restructuring Commission 2000, 145).

The 2001 Mazankowski report recommended that the Alberta government take the lead in negotiating new payment arrangements with physicians, that blended approaches to paying primary care physicians should be developed and implemented, and that these should include approaches that combined fee-for-service and rostering.

In Saskatchewan's 2001 Fyke report, primary care reform was top of the agenda. The report argued for the creation of interdisciplinary teams of professionals in health services centres to improve accessibility to primary health services. Drawing on its extensive public consultations, the report noted that "participants in the public and health care provider dialogue suggested that the fee-for-service system for physicians is a barrier that prevents innovative approaches to health services" (Commission on Medicare 2001, 14). The report's vision for primary care practice made clear that it was anticipating a much reduced role for fee-for-service. Nonetheless, the report did not make precise recommendations on physician compensation, suggesting that there were political sensitivities.

No second-wave provincial report recommended abolishing fee-for-service, although the Ontario report came close. Instead, the different reports sought to encourage a larger role for alternative payment plans. The national reports were similar in tone and direction.

Based on the general consensus in these reports, *comprehensive* reform is defined as having three elements:

1. A strong provincial plan and political commitment to eliminate fee-for-service alone as a principal form of remuneration for primary care physicians and to replace it with an alternative payment system, buttressed by an agreement between the provincial government and the physicians' bargaining agent (in most provinces the provincial medical association) that the funds to support the alternative payment system could come from the fee-for-service pool
2. Plan attributes that made it fiscally attractive for physicians to switch from fee-for-service to alternative systems of remuneration relatively quickly
3. A strong administrative commitment to push this alternative (which might potentially be found in special units of the health ministry, or in regional boards to the extent that they were given responsibility for allocating the remuneration of family doctors)

Significant. Reform is based on the same three elements, but without strong political pressure on primary care physicians to make the switch to alternative funding. The fiscal incentive (element 2) would still, however, have to be substantive and the administrative push (element 3) "strong."

Moderate. Reform is based on the same three elements, but the political commitment in element 1 would be long term and have no suggestion of political pressure on physicians. The fiscal incentive in and of itself would not be strong enough to encourage a quick decision by physicians to make the switch, and the administrative commitment would be correspondingly less powerful.

Limited. Includes the last two elements but with the fiscal incentive marginal and the administrative commitment very light.

4. For-Profit Delivery

The case of for-profit delivery of hospital/rehabilitation institutions and related diagnostic services may be interpreted by some as unique in the context of this volume. This is because it envisages a reduced role for the public and not-for-profit sectors in the delivery of hospital/rehabilitation institutions and related diagnostic services whereas the other reform issues we studied were aimed at strengthening the efficiency or equity of such services and other benefits (specifically prescription drugs).

   Given the general support that medicare enjoyed during the years we assessed, it is perhaps not surprising that most government-appointed or government-related commissions, task forces, and committees did not focus on the private for-profit sector as the appropriate vehicle for reform of these institutions and related diagnostic services. Neither the National Forum on Health nor the Romanow Commission, for example, made proposals to strengthen the role of the for-profit delivery system. Indeed, the Romanow report made clear it considered this a bad idea (Commission on the Future of Health Care 2002, 6-9). Similarly, most provincial reports did not make recommendations in this area.

The 2002 Senate Committee report suggested that the patient and the funder/insurer would be served equally well regardless of who owned a health-care institution provided two conditions were met: (a) all institutions in a province were paid the same amount for performing any given medical procedure or service; and (b) all institutions, no matter what their form of ownership, were subject to the same rigorous, independent quality control and evaluation system. The Senate Committee emphasized that it was not pushing for the creation of private, for-profit facilities but that such facilities should not be prohibited, just as they were not prohibited under the *Canada Health Act*. It also stated it fully expected that the overwhelming majority of institutional providers would continue to be privately owned, not-for-profit institutions. The aim of the Senate Committee was to strengthen the single-payer medicare system.

The idea of affording the for-profit sector a greater role was largely ignored in the first-wave provincial reports. By the time of the second wave, the issue of for-profit delivery had acquired a higher profile in the public discourse. Nonetheless, the Saskatchewan (Fyke), Ontario (Sinclair), and Newfoundland and Labrador reports either ignored it or touched on it lightly as an item that needed further analysis. The principal exception to this was the Mazankowski report, which argued that the health system does not provide the right incentives for people to stay healthy and/or economize in their use of health services. The absence of choice or competition meant that the system fails to encourage the most effective or efficient services. The Premier's Advisory Council thus recommended that the Alberta government's multiple roles as insurer, provider, and evaluator of health services should be broken up. The role of government should be strategic planning and direction as the primary but not exclusive source of funding for health authorities. The Mazankowski report recommended that private for-profit sector delivery options be expanded and noted that Alberta had legislation for regulating private sector organizations (whether for-profit or not-for-profit), with standards set by the College of Physicians and Surgeons. At the same time, the RHAs should have the authority to enter into contracts with a range of suppliers, including private for-profit suppliers of insured hospital and related diagnostic services.

While the Mazankowski report was the main second-wave document that emphasized this option, the 2001 Clair report in Quebec was also

open to an enhanced role for the private for-profit sector, setting out
a position that was similar to that subsequently adopted by the Kirby
Committee. Clair recommended that the Government of Quebec establish
a "framework of partnership with the private sector and third sector"
(Commission d'étude sur les services de santé et les services sociaux
2000, 167), noting that the private sector might play a useful role in areas
where there are large capital needs and where rapid technological or
demographic change might require quick adjustments. But this was only
one of 36 recommendations in the Clair report, and it received much less
elaboration than many other recommendations. The role of the private
for-profit sector was certainly not a central theme of the report.

In short, the Mazankowski report argued for an enlarged role for the
for-profit sector, while the Clair and Kirby reports were open to this possibility without pushing it. The remaining national literature and the other
provincial reports were opposed or barely interested. Thus, during the
second half of the period we covered the opposition to this proposal was
weaker but, on balance, the grey literature consensus remained against
this kind of reform direction.

Given that in the grey literature that we searched only the Alberta and
the Senate Committee reports gave significant attention to the issue of
for-profit delivery, we also looked for what other supporters of this idea
had in mind. We examined reports published by the Fraser Institute (such
as Part 2 of the 1996 Fraser Institute volume entitled *Healthy Incentives:
Canadian Health Reform in an International Context* edited by Ramsay,
Walker, and McArthur) and David Gratzer's (1999) *Code Blue* as representative of this literature. In a nutshell, like the Mazankowski report,
they emphasized three elements that are relevant for our purposes here:
a political commitment to a larger role for the for-profit sector; legislative and/or regulatory changes that would create incentives or at least
remove disincentives for investments in the for-profit sector (supply-side
initiatives); and actions that would place more purchasing power in the
hands of patients which, in turn, could be expected to lead to demands
for more patient choice including for for-profit services and institutions.
This demand-side initiative would support the supply-side changes.

Since the consensus of the grey literature was not in favour of these
kinds of reforms, the recommendations that favour for-profit delivery are,
in our analytical perspective, the elements of *counter-consensus reforms*. In
this limited grey literature perspective, we define *comprehensive counter-
consensus* reform to include the following elements:

1.   A legal framework within which all or the great majority of for-profit
     hospital/rehabilitation institutions and related diagnostic services
     would be able to operate on no worse than a level playing field with
     not-for-profit and public facilities

2.   A strong political commitment to a substantial and growing market for the services of for-profit hospital/rehabilitation institutions and related diagnostic services (e.g., periodic tenders for services that would enable for-profits to bid against not-for-profit facilities)
3.   More purchasing power placed in the hands of patients/consumers, possibly through Medical Savings Accounts

Significant counter-consensus. The legal framework and political commitment is similar to the "comprehensive" definition but applied to a narrower range of hospitals/institutions and services. The third element of the comprehensive definition may or may not be present.

Moderate counter-consensus. The legal framework allows diagnostic services and/or remedial services in narrow niches to be provided by for-profit facilities, with a political commitment to create opportunities that will enable for-profit providers to compete.

Limited counter-consensus. The elements are similar to the "moderate" definition, but the legal framework and political commitment are focused on one or two services only.

It follows that *consensus* reform entails steps to protect or reinforce the not-for-profit system against for-profit delivery. In that vein, *comprehensive* reform includes the following:

1.   A new or reformed legal framework that clearly precludes for-profit delivery across all or virtually all services (hospitals, institutions, imaging, lab)
2.   A decisive political stand against for-profit delivery
3.   Rolling back any for-profit delivery that has been part of the existing system (e.g., lab testing)

Significant. Reform includes element 1 in the comprehensive definition across a wide range of services, but not as wide as in comprehensive. Thus, reform might apply to certain types of hospitals and services (e.g., major teaching hospitals but not small community hospitals; imaging services but not lab tests). It also includes element 2, but the tone of the political stance is not quite as decisive.

Moderate. Reform includes element 1 in the comprehensive definition, but it applies only to hospitals and imaging. The political commitment is again softer than in the significant definition.

Limited. Includes a political stance, even a relatively low-key one, against widening the scope of for-profit delivery.

Note that in the last few years, a distinction has emerged between for-profit delivery in which the provider operates on terms that are identical or close to identical to those of not-for-profit providers (no extra-billings by facilities or physicians, and compensation by government at the same rate as not-for-profits) and for-profit delivery without such restrictions. Since this distinction did not apply during most of the period covered, it is not reflected in our definitions.

5. Wait-Time Management

This issue focused on the introduction of formalized processes to manage surgical wait lists. In this case, the national reports played the dominant role in defining the range of reform proposals, although one provincial report also tackled this issue in a major way and a second gave it some attention.

Starting with the national reports, in 1997 the Striking a Balance Working Group of the National Forum on Health discussed the public's concern that waiting times were growing. It observed, however, that "most waiting lists for elective surgery are unstructured, many are padded, few are standardized, and even fewer are evaluated" (National Forum on Health 1997c, 38). It thus recommended "that provincial/territorial agencies together with a national agency ... give priority to developing a set of indicators and benchmarks to be used by all jurisdictions for assessment of the state of access to appropriate health services ... and make this information public at regular intervals" (ibid., 40). In 1998, the federal government released a paper on waiting times and wait-list management (McDonald et al. 1998).

While the first-wave provincial reports were silent on the issue of wait times, presumably because it had not yet emerged as a major issue when they were published, the second-wave reports gave it some attention. In particular, the 2001 Mazankowski report proposed that "all Albertans have guaranteed access to selected health services within 90 days of a diagnosis and recommendation by their physician" (Premier's Advisory Council on Health for Alberta 2001, 43). A regional health authority that could not provide such service would be obliged to purchase it from another jurisdiction. It is also worth noting that in 1996 Premier Klein proposed a Health Charter that would guarantee Albertans access to key health services such as heart surgery and hip and knee replacements within defined periods of time.

The 2001 Fyke report argued that performance measures should drive the health-care system and it specifically pointed to data on wait-list management as a key element of the system. It observed the need for standardized wait lists to keep track of the proportion of people served within a "reasonable" period of time. It did not make specific recommendations, however. Ontario's report argued that developing a health information management system was the "top" priority for building a better health system, but it did not give special attention to wait times. Other provincial reports also passed over this issue.

By the time the interim report of the Standing Senate Committee on Social Affairs, Science and Technology (Kirby Committee) was made public in September 2002, the issue of wait times and their management had acquired greater prominence in public discussion. The committee set out its position that "reasonable access" to insured health services meant "timely" access. It observed, as had the National Forum, that there was a lack of reliable information about the facts. It also discussed options such as a "care guarantee" and "patient's bill of rights" as potential ways of creating pressures that would require provinces to manage wait times effectively (Standing Senate Committee 2002a, 43-47). In its final report (Standing Senate Committee 2002b), the committee opted for the Health Care Guarantee recommending that, for each type of major procedure or treatment, a maximum needs-based waiting time be established and made public. When this maximum time was reached, the insurer (government) would pay for the patient to seek the procedure or treatment immediately in another jurisdiction, including, if necessary, another country. Importantly, the Kirby report argued that this care guarantee should be implemented immediately, even in advance of waiting-list management systems, apparently assuming that the associated cost would create an incentive to implement the system quickly.

In November 2002, although calling for a new Canadian Health Covenant endorsed by governments to reflect the values Canadian share, the Romanow Commission concluded that these particular options (guarantees and charters) were not appropriate and instead called on provincial and territorial governments to take "immediate action to manage wait lists more effectively by implementing centralized approaches, setting standardized criteria [for assessing patients], and providing clear information to patients on how long they can be expected to wait" (Commission on the Future of Health Care 2002, 251). For the commission, the definition of *centralized* varied according to the nature of the intervention (e.g., life-saving surgery as opposed to elective quality-of-life surgery). In some situations it was to be at the regional level within the province, in others provincewide, and in cases of rare surgeries interprovincial.

In summary, wait times emerged as an issue in the second half of the 1990s and had become a major concern by the early years of the new millennium. All of the national grey literature treated it seriously as did two of the provincial reports. Solutions varied. Some focused exclusively on getting the building blocks right. This meant establishing appropriate benchmarks based on standardized and objective criteria for treatment and then implementing the information systems to determine if the benchmarks were being met. This approach essentially required surgeons to follow agreed procedures in determining the priority to be attached to a patient. The assumption was that the publication of reliable data on the extent to which benchmarks were met would put pressure on provinces and territories to improve performance. Others followed a more legalistic and arguably more interventionist and radical course by proposing guarantees to patients when benchmarks were exceeded.

Based on the above, *comprehensive* reform is defined as follows:

1. Scientifically based wait-time standards (i.e., benchmarks for the amount of time a patient might reasonably be expected to wait for treatment based on scientific evidence) for a substantial majority of key surgical services
2. A tracking system for wait times for key surgeries that is centralized and mandatory in the sense that surgeons are expected to follow agreed procedures in ranking patient need and thus urgency
3. Information that is easily available to patients on standards for timely treatment and on length of wait for those treatments
4. Some form of legal guarantee of timely treatment, such as a health care guarantee (possibly in the expectation that this guarantee will create incentives for provincial and territorial governments to complete elements 1, 2, and 3 swiftly)

Significant. Includes the first three elements in the comprehensive definition, and the tracking system covers a reasonably broad range of surgeries.

Moderate. Includes (1) scientifically based wait-time standards for some key surgical services; (2) a tracking system for wait times for those key surgeries (this element is voluntary and therefore unlikely to involve centralization); and element 3 above but for only the surgeries covered.

Limited. A tracking system is implemented across a narrow range of surgeries on a voluntary basis.

Although wait times emerged as an issue in the grey literature in the second half of the period we have analyzed, it is important to recognize that in a small but not unimportant way, reform on the ground preceded the grey literature on this issue. Therefore, even though the grey literature sets our standard, it would probably be an exaggeration to say that the provinces and territories had only a few years to consider whether to act on the grey literature proposals. These ideas were "in the wind" before then. On the other hand, it was only in 2004 (after our assessment period) that the federal government began earmarking some of its cash transfers to the provinces for wait-times management.

6. Drug Coverage

Similar to wait-times, for the prescription drugs issue we had to look mainly to the national grey literature to establish our benchmark, and the literature began to focus on drugs only in the second half of the period studied. The first wave of provincial reports made no recommendations for altering the scope of provincial drug coverage, and only a few reports in the second wave touched on this issue and generally without recommendations. (For example, the Fyke report cautioned against expanding drug coverage in the short term for fear of unaffordable costs, while the Clair report proposed programs to review the use of drugs by seniors including their therapeutic effect.) The lack of attention to drug coverage in provincial reports during the early part of the assessment period was due in part to the very onerous fiscal conditions that prevailed at that time, bearing in mind the high cost of insurance. During the latter part of the assessment period, a major fiscal dispute occurred between federal and provincial governments as a result of the Canada Health and Social Transfer–related cuts in federal cash transfers to provinces. This militated against provinces suggesting that they would undertake major extensions of drug coverage if only because it would undermine their negotiating position that Ottawa's arbitrary cash transfer reductions had unfairly deprived them of revenues to which they were entitled. Given this context, provinces were not likely to appoint commissions, task forces, or advisory bodies with terms of reference that invited them to make recommendations on the scope of drug insurance coverage.

But the national reports did not labour under such constraints. Thus, the National Forum on Health called on "federal, provincial, and territorial governments, health service providers, private payers (employers and unions) and consumers to chart a course leading to full public funding for medically necessary drugs" (1997a, section 1.2.2). The 2000 IRPP report similarly called on the federal government and the provinces and territories to include prescription drugs as "insured services" under the *Canada Health Act*. These were, in effect, calls in one form or other for *universal* coverage for prescription drugs.

But even as these reports emerged there was a concern for affordability, and the two major reports that followed were more cautious in their advice. The Senate Committee proposed that the federal government introduce a program to protect Canadians against catastrophic prescription drug expenses. For all eligible plans, the federal government would agree to pay 90 percent of all prescription drug expenses over $5,000 for those individuals for whom the combined total of their out-of-pocket expenses and the contribution that a province/territory incurred on their behalf exceeded $5,000 in a single year; and 90 percent of prescription drug expenses in excess of $5,000 for members of private, supplementary prescription drug insurance plans for whom the combined total of their out-of-pocket expenses and the contribution that the private insurance plan incurred on their behalf exceeded $5,000 in a single year. The remaining 10 percent would be paid by either a provincial/territorial plan or a private supplementary plan. In this context, what is important is that the Senate Committee saw the federal government as the key funder.

The Romanow Commission argued for a new federal Catastrophic Drug Transfer program. The transfer would cover a portion of the rapidly growing costs of provincial and territorial drug plans. In short, there were two broad views in the national reports. One (National Forum and IRPP) called simply for full public funding of prescription drugs, although with some vagueness about time lines. The second (Kirby and Romanow) proposed a Canada-wide program of protection against catastrophic drug expenses with the federal government either as the main payer or a large payer.

Romanow also called for a major expansion of the public system to cover medication costs of those who were not in hospital but who required prescribed drugs on an ongoing basis to manage chronic conditions ("medication management"). As for the Kirby report, it too proposed an important add-on to the Canada-wide insurance system, recommending a post-acute home care benefit for patients that would cover "all home care services received between the first date of service provision following hospital discharge, if that date occurs within 30 days of discharge, and up to three months following hospital discharge" (Standing Senate Committee 2002b, section 8.4.1). This benefit was to include prescription drugs during this period.

For the five issues considered above, the nature and extent of reform was defined in relation to two or more elements. This issue is different in that "the extent of reform" is defined by only one element, namely, the proximity to universal coverage under public stewardship due to policy change. As just seen, the grey literature contained proposals ranging from universal coverage for prescribed drugs (all provincial/territorial residents), to catastrophic coverage for the same population, to drug benefits for the chronically ill, to benefits for those requiring follow-up treatment including drugs after release from an acute-care hospital. The definitions are thus as follows:

Comprehensive. Reform that provides for inclusion of all or a substantial majority of prescription drugs on a universal basis within the provincial systems of publicly insured health services. (This element does not preclude modest deductibles and copayments). With public stewardship, the drug coverage could be provided from either the public or private (including for-profit) sectors.

Because catastrophic drug transfer reform along the lines proposed by both Kirby and Romanow entails really big change, we define it as *on the border between comprehensive and significant.*

Significant. Reforms along the lines of the Romanow proposals for those with chronic conditions and the Senate ideas for the post-acute period at home.

Moderate. Reforms improve in a noticeable way either the breadth or depth of coverage for a distinct demographic group.

Limited. Small changes in either depth or breadth of coverage.

Counter-consensus. Reductions in coverage. The extent of the reduction determines whether it is limited or comprehensive or somewhere in between.

APPLYING THE METHODOLOGY TO THE 30 CASE STUDIES

Having defined the nature and extent of reform based on the grey literature consensus, the remaining task is to apply these definitions to the case studies. This is done in Table A1.1.

The column on the left that is headed "Elements" refers to the elements that constitute the definitions for each of the six policy issues in the above text. For example, the numbers 1, 2, and 3 immediately below the Elements heading correspond to the three elements that help to define the extent of reform for regionalization. The time frame shown in the left column indicates when the grey literature proposals were published during the 1990–2003 period. For example, "early" indicates that the grey literature was released from the late 1980s to the mid-1990s. The capital letters under the five provincial columns refer to the extent to which each element was found to be present. These *ratings* are defined in the note to the table. Case *assessments* are qualitative roll-ups of each case based on the element ratings.

TABLE A1.1
Nature and Extent of Reform: Applying the Definitions to the Cases

Case (Time)	Elements	Newfoundland and Labrador	Quebec	Ontario	Saskatchewan	Alberta
				Assessment		
Regionalization (Early)	1	B	D	D	B†	B†
	2	B	D	D	B†	B†
	3	D	D	D	C	C
		Moderate	Counter-consensus limited	None	Significant	Significant
Needs-based Funding (Early)	1	D	C‡	D	B	B
	2	D	D**	D	B	B
		None	Limited	None	Significant	Significant
Alternate Payment Plans (Early)	1	D	D	C	D	D
	2	D	C	B	C	C
	3	D	C	B	C	C
		None	Limited	Moderate	Limited	Moderate
For-Profit Delivery (Middle)	1	D	D	-C	B	-C
	2	C	D	-B	A	-B
	3	D	D	D	D	D
		None	None	Counter-consensus moderate	Significant	Counter-consensus moderate
Wait Times (Middle to Late)	1	D	D	C	A	C
	2	D	C††	B	A	C‡‡
	3	D	D	C	A	C
	4	D	D	D	D	D
		None	Limited	Moderate	Significant/ comprehensive	Limited
Drug Coverage	1	D	A	B	-C	C
		None	Comprehensive	Moderate	Counter-consensus limited	Limited

Notes:
A = element found strongly in case
B = element found moderately
C = element found lightly
D = element not present
A minus sign indicates that the element is directionally opposite to the consensus of the grey literature.
† Physicians are excluded
‡ Theoretical consideration of population needs but largely ignored in practice
** Physical health is excluded
†† Voluntary, decentralized
‡‡ Voluntary

Annex 2

Independent Variables Referred to in 30 Case Studies That Best Help to Explain Nature and Extent of Reforms

Harvey Lazar and Julia Diamond

The purpose of this annex is to outline some of the steps that were taken to identify the independent variables (also referred to as "factors" and "influences") that best help explain the decisions made in each of the 30 cases. The results are shown in Tables A2.1 and A2.2.

In Table A2.1, the independent variables are identified under four headings according to the role they played relative to the grey literature consensus benchmark:

- facilitated reform in the direction of the grey literature (pro-reform)
- hindered reform recommended by the grey literature (anti-reform)
- facilitated reform in a different direction from that recommended by the grey literature (counter-consensus reform)
- worked as both pro- and anti-reform at the same time ("middle territory")

Variables were identified as occupying middle territory when the actors involved were seen to be attempting to mediate between the comprehensive reform proposals in the grey literature and outright opposition to such proposals. A good and common example is that in some provinces the medical associations neither rejected fully nor endorsed completely the grey literature proposal to do away quickly with fee-for-service compensation methods. Instead the associations negotiated with government to define a workable compromise that would allow medical practitioners who preferred an alternative compensation method to fee-for-service (such as capitation) to be paid on that basis while permitting other physicians (in all provinces a majority) to continue with fee-for-service. What was particularly significant was that the associations agreed that a part of the fee-for-service pool of money could be diverted into the alternative payment stream.

The list of independent variables reflects the authors' analyses of the 30 cases. As described in chapter 2, the authors used a common methodology. To reinforce this commonality in research method, the 30 cases were read and analyzed by the project's principal investigator and then discussed with the case authors. In turn, the case study authors vetted Tables A2.3 to A2.7 to ensure they reflected the substantive content of their case studies. Through this process, eight broad categories of independent variables were formed and organized based on whether they were endogenous or exogenous to the decision process.[1]

As noted in chapter 8, in the roll-ups we "unpacked" the "3I's" (ideas, interests, and institutions) and "E" (exogenous) categories and did some modest rearranging. This was only done after the case studies were complete (so the individual case studies do not reflect the rearrangement). The reasons for the unpacking are noted here. First, in the ideas category we decided to examine the impact of *knowledge* separately from *values*. There is much interest in evidence-based decision-making, and we wanted to form a view of how relevant evidence was in government decision-making. Second, we decided to include *major reports* and *interjurisdictional learning* as part of this separate knowledge category as channels for communicating evidence to decision makers. During the period we studied, these reports were often shaped by leaders and researchers who were inside the health-care system, or close to it. Third, the role of civil society, including advocacy groups that represent segments of civil society, was separated from other interests and categorized with public opinion. We found that the views of advocacy groups were much closer to public opinion than to the positions of other interests, such as organizations representing the medical profession, hospital boards, and pharmaceutical products. These provider organizations are grouped under the heading *insider interests*.

Another point worth noting is that most "large" reforms (those assessed as "comprehensive" or "significant") were undertaken by newly formed, first-time governments that had committed to reform prior to taking office and that acted swiftly on their commitments once in office. These governments are treated as external to the health sector and as "exogenous" influences on the decision processes during the first half

---

[1] Technological change was excluded as it did not surface often enough to be included as a category on its own, nor did it fit logically within any other category. However, it is important in a few cases and is included as a ninth category in chapter 9.

of their first mandate (under the heading *change in government/leader* in the tables). To the extent that they come to office with reform ideas and act on them, we decided to think of them as "outsiders." Over time, of course, they became insiders. Since many reforms were launched early in the first term of new governments, relatively few observations were assigned to "elected government officials."

Finally, physician groups generally worked to moderate or oppose reforms that they perceived to be in conflict with their core bargain with the provincial state. This bargain involved "public payment/private delivery" and professional self-regulation. In trying to understand how to deal with this influence from a methodological perspective, we considered three choices: categorize this influence as *insider interest*, as *institutional* rules of the game, or as both interest and institution since the influence of medical associations reflects both. We chose the first option, although this was a "close call" because the core bargain itself is the product in part of interest group activity. Without those interests working vigilantly to secure the bargain, the bargains would not have occurred or would have been less advantageous to physicians. It is important for the reader to bear in mind this methodological choice and that it results in some understatement of institutional influence. A similar choice was made in respect of the core bargain between the provincial state and hospital boards and management to the extent that such bargains existed.

Note that any reader who is not comfortable with any of the above methodological choices can "re-pack" the variables by referring to the five provincial tables below (Table A2.3 to Table A2.7). They provide enough detail for this to be done.

This method has enabled us to do comparative analysis in three ways. First, it helped clarify why some reforms fared better than others within a single province. Second, it helped clarify why, in aggregate, some provinces achieved more reform than others, as discussed in chapter 8. Third, it facilitated the cross-provincial and cross-issue comparisons in chapter 9.

Notwithstanding all of the above, we would not argue that the numbers in the tables are "objective" to the point that they cannot be challenged. It is indeed a judgment call about how to describe some of the variables (for example, some may understand physician opposition to alternative payment plans as an "interest" at work, whereas others may classify it as an "institution").

So, with these kinds of qualifications, Table A2.1 provides the five-province roll-up based on the 30 case studies.

TABLE A2.1
Independent Variables Observed as Influences on Policy Outcomes in 30 Case Studies: Five Province Roll-up

Category	Variable	Pro-Reform	Middle Territory	Anti-Reform	Counter-Consensus Reform	Total
Exogenous						
Change in Government/ Leader	Election of first term governing party/political leader (premier) with electoral commitment to reform	8 (6)	3	3	2 (1)	*16 (7)*
	Political champion with strategic policy reform decision in first half of mandate	10 (5)		5	3 (1)	*18 (6)*
Fiscal Crisis/ Near Crisis		9 (6)	2 (2)	10 (4)	3 (1)	*24 (13)*
Public Opinion and Civil Society	Public opinion	7 (2)	1 (1)		1	*9 (3)*
	Citizen groups	10 (3)		1		*11 (3)*
	Policy entrepreneurs	3 (2)		5	1 (1)	*9 (3)*
Media		11 (3)	1		3 (1)	*15 (4)*
Technological Change		2 (2)	1		2	*5 (2)*
Exogenous and Endogenous						
Values	Egalitarianism/national sharing	23 (11)				*23 (11)*
	Markets, personal choice, personal responsibility, corporate accountability	4	1	1	6 (5)	*12 (5)*
Knowledge	Major reports[a]	13 (4)	3 (2)			*16 (6)*
	Research/information	7 (3)	4		1	*12 (3)*
	Interjurisdictional learning	10 (3)	1			*11 (3)*
	Adequacy of information			2		*2*

TABLE A2.1
(Continued)

Category	Variable	Pro-Reform	Middle Territory	Anti-Reform	Counter-Consensus Reform	Total
Exogenous and Endogenous (continued)						
Institutional Arrangements	Policy networks	10 (6)	2			*12 (6)*
	Legislative provisions	4		2	2	*8*
	Government structures/administrative factors	9		2		*11*
	Federal-provincial relations/federal government	11 (3)	4			*15 (3)*
	Policy legacies	2	2 (1)	3 (1)		*7 (2)*
Endogenous						
Insider Interests	Physician interests[b]	3	6 (4)	8 (6)	1	*18 (10)*
	Hospital interests	4 (1)	1	7 (3)	1	*13 (4)*
	Pharmaceutical interests	7	3 (1)			*10 (1)*
	Other private interests	1 (1)				*1 (1)*
	Elected government official	4 (2)	5 (2)	1 (1)	2 (2)	*12 (7)*
	Public service	14 (4)	5	6		*25 (4)*
	Insider champion	3				*3*
Other		4		1		*5*
Total		*193 (67)*	*45 (13)*	*57 (15)*	*28 (12)*	*323 (107)*

Note: Figures outside parentheses refer to the number of times that a variable was observed as a factor, whether major or not, in accounting for a reform. Figures in parentheses indicate the number of times that the variable was observed as a *major* factor in accounting for a reform.

[a] The major reports are listed in annex 1.
[b] The political activities of physician groups in protecting and/or advancing their core bargains with provincial governments (public payment/private delivery) are reflected here and not under the institutions heading.

Table A2.1 includes 27 different independent variables. For purposes of understanding the overall extent of reform and similarities and differences among provinces, 27 variables are simply too many. Table A2.2 is derived from Table A2.1. It rolls up variables into broader groupings that take account of the interests, institutions, ideas, and exogenous factors discussed earlier. It also excludes all independent variables that were cited less than 10 times unless they are part of a broader grouping. If a variable or grouping of variables was not cited at least 10 times or in one-third of the 30 cases, no matter how important that variable may be in a particular case, it is difficult to argue that it had an overarching impact on the nature and extent of reform or on the interprovincial comparisons. None of the variables that were dropped included a high proportion cited as major. In total, only 10 of the 323 variables included in Table A2.1 were excluded from Table A2.2

Table A2.2 lists eight categories of independent variables. The table distinguishes between categories made up of factors that are exclusively or mainly exogenous to the health-care system decision process, categories that contain exogenous and endogenous influences in roughly equal proportions, and a category that is exclusively or mainly endogenous.

The first two categories in the table, "change in government/leader" and "fiscal crisis/near crisis," are exclusively *exogenous*. These factors and conditions were essential in opening reform windows in certain cases, especially in the governance and financial arrangements domains. Without their presence, it is likely that there would have been little or no reform. "Public opinion and civil society" were very important in the cases involving delivery or program content and worked closely with the "media." Public opinion and civil society were influenced by and had a reciprocal relationship with "values." Values also influenced other categories—for example, the political stance of a new government in moving from opposition to the governing benches. Some values associated with health care have been around for at least three decades and, as such, can be viewed as endogenous values. Other values, outside of health care, periodically posed a challenge to the status quo and thus can be perceived as exogenous. As for "knowledge," in some cases it was an essential part of the background that led political actors to adopt the stances that they did. In other cases, knowledge had to be created in order for reform to proceed. "Institutional arrangements" in many cases were the formal manifestation of the success of ideas and/or interests.

The remaining *endogenous* category, "insider interests," came into play once the windows were opened. Insider interests sought to protect the existing institutional or other arrangements from which they benefited. When this proved politically impossible, the interests sometimes attempted to move to the head of the parade and lead reform to a destination that was acceptable to their members.

In addition to the link between political values and both public opinion/civil society and opposition parties, in some cases there was a symbiotic relationship among values, insider interests, and institutional arrangements.

TABLE A2.2
Categories of Independent Variables That Influenced Policy Reform Decisions in 30 Case Studies: Five Province Roll-up

Category	Pro-Reform	Middle Territory	Anti-Reform	Counter-Consensus Reform	Total
Exogenous					
Change in government/ leader	18 (11)	3	8	5 (2)	34 (13)
Fiscal crisis/near crisis	9 (6)	2 (2)	10 (4)	3 (1)	24 (13)
Public opinion and civil society	20 (7)	1 (1)	6	2 (1)	29 (9)
Media	11 (3)	1		3 (1)	15 (4)
Exogenous and Endogenous					
Values	27 (11)	1	1	6 (5)	35 (16)
Knowledge	30 (10)	8 (2)	2	1	41 (12)
Institutional arrangements	36 (9)	8 (1)	7 (1)	2	53 (11)
Endogenous					
Insider interests	36 (8)	20 (7)	22 (10)	4 (2)	82 (27)
Total	*187 (65)*	*44 (13)*	*56 (15)*	*26 (12)*	*313 (105)*

Note: Figures outside parentheses refer to the number of times that a variable was observed as a factor, whether major or not, in accounting for a reform. Figures in parentheses indicate the number of times that a variable was observed as a *major* factor in accounting for a reform. A modified version of this table appears in chapter 8 (Table 8.2).

TABLE A2.3
Independent Variables Observed as Influences on Policy Outcomes in Alberta Case Studies

Category	Variable	Pro-Reform	Middle Territory	Anti-Reform	Counter-Consensus Reform	Total
Exogenous						
Change in Government/ Leader	Election of first term governing party/political leader (premier) with electoral commitment to reform	**1, 2**				2 (2)
	Political champion with strategic policy reform decision in first half of mandate	**1, 2**			4	3 (2)
Fiscal Crisis/ Near Crisis		**1, 2, 3,** 5			4	5 (3)
Public Opinion and Civil Society	Public opinion	**5**				1 (1)
	Citizen groups	**4,** 6				2 (1)
	Policy entrepreneurs			4, 5	**6**	3 (1)
Media		3, **5**	4			3 (1)
Technological Change					4	1
Exogenous and Endogenous						
Values	Egalitarianism/national sharing	1, **2,** 3, **4,** 5				5 (2)
	Markets, personal choice, personal responsibility, corporate accountability	1, 2, 3	5		**4, 5, 6**	7 (3)
Knowledge	Major reports	1, 5				2
	Research/information	3, **5**	5		4	4 (1)
	Interjurisdictional learning	**2,** 3, 5				3 (1)
	Adequacy of information					

TABLE A2.3
(Continued)

Category	Variable	Pro-Reform	Middle Territory	Anti-Reform	Counter-Consensus Reform	Total
Exogenous and Endogenous (continued)						
Institutional Arrangements	Policy networks	**2, 3**	5			3 (2)
	Legislative provisions	4				1
	Government structures/administrative factors	1, 2				2
	Federal-provincial relations/federal government	**4, 5, 6**	3, 6			5 (2)
	Policy legacies		3	3		2
Endogenous						
Insider Interests	Physician interests	4	**3, 5**	**1**		4 (3)
	Hospital interests			1		1
	Pharmaceutical interests					
	Other private interests					
	Elected government officials		3, 5		**4**	3 (1)
	Public service	1, **2**, 3, 5	6			5 (1)
	Insider champion					
Other						
Total		41 (19)	12 (2)	5 (1)	9 (5)	67 (27)

Notes:

The values that appear in the table refer to the six issues/case studies as follows:

1 = regionalization

2 = needs-based funding

3 = alternative payment plans

4 = for-profit delivery

5 = wait-times management

6 = drug coverage

Bolded values indicate that a variable was a *major* factor in explaining a case outcome. Unbolded values indicate that a variable was an observable (but not a major) factor in explaining the case outcome. In the "Total" column/row, the first figure indicates the total number of times the variable was observed as a factor (major or non-major). The second figure in parentheses indicates the number of times the variable was observed as a major factor.

TABLE A2.4

Independent Variables Observed as Influences on Policy Outcomes in Saskatchewan Case Studies

Category	Variable	Pro-Reform	Middle Territory	Anti-Reform	Counter-Consensus Reform	Total
Exogenous						
Change in Government/Leader	Election of first term governing party/political leader (premier) with electoral commitment to reform	**1, 2, 3**				3 (3)
	Political champion with strategic policy reform decision in first half of mandate	**1, 2**, 3, 4, 5				5 (2)
Fiscal Crisis/Near Crisis		**1, 2, 3**			6	4 (4)
Public Opinion and Civil Society	Public opinion	**5**	**3**			2 (2)
	Citizen groups	4				1
	Policy entrepreneurs	**5**		4		2 (1)
Media		**5**				1 (1)
Technological Change						
Exogenous and Endogenous						
Values	Egalitarianism/national sharing	**1, 2**, 3, **4, 5**				5 (4)
	Markets, personal choice, personal responsibility, corporate accountability					
Knowledge	Major reports	1, 3, 5				3
	Research/information	2, **5**				2 (1)
	Interjurisdictional learning	**2**, 3, **5**				3 (2)
	Adequacy of information					

TABLE A2.4
(Continued)

Category	Variable	Pro-Reform	Middle Territory	Anti-Reform	Counter-Consensus Reform	Total
Exogenous and Endogenous (continued)						
Institutional Arrangements	Policy networks	1, **2, 5**				3 (2)
	Legislative provisions	4				1
	Government structures/ administrative factors	2, 3				2
	Federal-provincial relations/federal government	4, 5				2
	Policy legacies	4	3	3		1
Endogenous						
Insider Interests	Physician interests			**3**		1 (1)
	Hospital interests			**1**		1 (1)
	Pharmaceutical interests	4	3			2
	Other private interests					
	Elected government officials	**4,** 5				2 (1)
	Public service	1, **2, 3,** 4, **5**	3			6 (3)
	Insider champion	1, 2, 5				3
Other						
Total		48 (24)	3 (1)	3 (2)	1 (1)	55 (28)

Notes:

The values that appear in the table refer to the six issues/case studies as follows:

1 = regionalization
2 = needs-based funding
3 = alternative payment plans
4 = for-profit delivery
5 = wait-times management
6 = drug coverage

Bolded values indicate that the variable was a *major* factor in explaining the case outcome. Unbolded values indicate that the variable was an observable (but not a major) factor in explaining the case outcome. In the "Total" column/row, the first figure indicates the total number of times the variable was observed as a factor (major or non-major). The second figure in parentheses indicates the number of times the variable was observed as a major factor.

TABLE A2.5
Independent Variables Observed as Influences on Policy Outcomes in Ontario Case Studies

Category	Variable	Pro-Reform	Middle Territory	Anti-Reform	Counter-Consensus Reform	Total
Exogenous						
Change in Government/ Leader	Election of first term governing party/political leader (premier) with electoral commitment to reform	6	3	1, 2	4	5
	Political champion with strategic policy reform decision in first half of mandate			1	4	2
Fiscal Crisis/ Near Crisis		3		**1, 2, 6**		4 (2)
Public Opinion and Civil Society	Public opinion	4, 5				2
	Citizen groups	**4,** 5, **6**				3 (2)
	Policy entrepreneurs	**5**				1 (1)
Media		4, **5,** 6			4	4 (1)
Technological Change		**6**			4	2 (1)
Exogenous and Endogenous						
Values	Egalitarianism/national sharing	3, **4, 5, 6**				4 (3)
	Markets, personal choice, personal responsibility, corporate accountability			2	**4**	2 (1)
Knowledge	Major reports	1, **3**				2 (1)
	Research/information	**3**	2, 5			3 (1)
	Interjurisdictional learning					
	Adequacy of information					

TABLE A2.5
(Continued)

Category	Variable	Pro-Reform	Middle Territory	Anti-Reform	Counter-Consensus Reform	Total
Exogenous and Endogenous (continued)						
Institutional Arrangements	Policy networks	**3, 5**	6			3 (2)
	Legislative provisions	3, 4		3	4	4
	Government structures/administrative factors	1, 2, 3				3
	Federal-provincial relations/federal government	3, 6	4			3
	Policy legacies	5	**3**			2 (1)
Endogenous						
Insider Interests	Physician interests	4	**3, 5**	1		4 (1)
	Hospital interests	4		1, 2		3
	Pharmaceutical interests	4				1
	Other private interests					
	Elected government officials	5	**6**		4	3 (2)
	Public service	6		1, 2		3
	Insider champion					
Other		3,[a] 4, 5				3
Total		37 (12)	9 (3)	13 (2)	7 (2)	66 (19)

Notes:

The values that appear in the table refer to the six issues/case studies as follows:

1 = regionalization
2 = needs-based funding
3 = alternative payment plans
4 = for-profit delivery
5 = wait-times management
6 = drug coverage

Bolded values indicate that the variable was a *major* factor in explaining the case outcome. Unbolded values indicate that the variable was an observable (but not major) factor in explaining the case outcome. In the "Total" column/row, the first figure indicates the total number of times the variable was observed as a factor (major or non-major). The second figure in parentheses indicates the number of times the variable was observed as a major factor.

[a] Willingness of Ontario Medical Association to split physician fee-for-service pool to fund alternative payments.

TABLE A2.6
Independent Variables Observed as Influences on Policy Outcomes in Quebec Case Studies

Category	Variable	Pro-Reform	Middle Territory	Anti-Reform	Counter-Consensus Reform	Total
Exogenous						
Change in Government/ Leader	Election of first term governing party/political leader (premier) with electoral commitment to reform	2, **6**	3, 4	2	**1**	6 (2)
	Political champion with strategic policy reform decision in first half of mandate	4, **6**		5	**1**	4 (2)
Fiscal Crisis/ Near Crisis			**2, 6**	2, 3, 5	4	6 (2)
Public Opinion and Civil Society	Public opinion	5, 6			4	3
	Citizen groups	1, 4, 6		3[a]		4
	Policy entrepreneurs			4, 5		2
Media		4, 5, 6			4, **6**	5 (1)
Technological Change		**6**	5			2 (1)
Exogenous and Endogenous						
Values	Egalitarianism/national sharing	1, **2**, 3, 4, 5, **6**				6 (2)
	Markets, personal choice, personal responsibility, corporate accountability	1			**1,** 4	3 (1)
Knowledge	Major reports	*1, 2*, 3, **6**	1, **4,** 5			7 (5)
	Research/information	3, 5	1			3
	Interjurisdictional learning	2, 3, 4	1			4
	Adequacy of information			2, 5		2

TABLE A2.6
(Continued)

Category	Variable	Pro-Reform	Middle Territory	Anti-Reform	Counter-Consensus Reform	Total
Exogenous and Endogenous (continued)						
Institutional Arrangements	Policy networks	1, 3				2
	Legislative provisions				4	1
	Government structures/administrative factors	1, 2				2
	Federal-provincial relations/federal government	**6**	4			2 (1)
	Policy legacies					
Endogenous						
Insider Interests	Physician interests		**3**, 5	**5**	1	4 (2)
	Hospital interests	6	2	**5**	1	4 (1)
	Pharmaceutical interests	1, 4	2, **6**			4 (1)
	Other private interests	**6**				1 (1)
	Elected government officials		1, **6**			2 (1)
	Public service	2, 3, 5	1, 6			5
	Insider champion					
Other				2[b]		1
Total		*41 (10)*	*20 (7)*	*13 (2)*	*11 (4)*	*85 (23)*

Notes:
The values that appear in the table refer to the six issues/case studies as follows:
1 = regionalization
2 = needs-based funding
3 = alternative payment plans
4 = for-profit delivery
5 = wait-times management
6 = drug coverage
Bolded values indicate that the variable was a *major* factor in explaining the case outcome. Unbolded values indicate that the variable was an observable (but not major) factor in explaining the case outcome. In the "Total" column/row, the first figure indicates the total number of times the variable was observed as a factor (major or non-major). The second figure in parentheses indicates the number of times the variable was observed as a major factor.
[a] Coalition Solidarité Solide.
[b] Impact on Montreal budget.

TABLE A2.7
Independent Variables Observed as Influences on Policy Outcomes in Newfoundland and Labrador Case Studies

Category	Variable	Pro-Reform	Middle Territory	Anti-Reform	Counter-Consensus Reform	Total
Exogenous						
Change in Government/ Leader	Election of first term governing party/political leader (premier) with electoral commitment to reform					
	Political champion with strategic policy reform decision in first half of mandate	1		2, 3, 5		4
Fiscal Crisis/ Near Crisis		1		2, **3**, 5, **6**		5 (2)
Public Opinion and Civil Society	Public opinion	4				1
	Citizen groups	6				1
	Policy entrepreneurs	3				1
Media		5, 6				2
Technological Change						
Exogenous and Endogenous						
Values	Egalitarianism/national sharing	1, 2, 4				3
	Markets, personal choice, personal responsibility, corporate accountability					
Knowledge	Major reports	1, 6				2
	Research/information					
	Interjurisdictional learning	1				1
	Adequacy of information					

TABLE A2.7
(Continued)

Category	Variable	Pro-Reform	Middle Territory	Anti-Reform	Counter-Consensus Reform	Total
Exogenous and Endogenous (continued)						
Institutional Arrangements	Policy networks	1				*1*
	Legislative provisions			6		*1*
	Government structures/ administrative factors			2, 6		*2*
	Federal-provincial relations/federal government	3, 4, 6				*3*
	Policy legacies			**2**, 5		*2 (1)*
Endogenous						
Insider Interests	Physician interests	4		**1, 2,** 3, **5**		*5 (3)*
	Hospital interests	1, **2**		2, **5**		*4 (2)*
	Pharmaceutical interests	1, 3, 4				*3*
	Other private interests					
	Elected government officials	**1**		**2**		*2 (2)*
	Public service	1	3	2, 3, 4, 6		*6*
	Insider champion					
Other		4				*1*
Total		26 (2)	1	23 (8))		50 (10)

Notes:
The values that appear in the table refer to the six issues/case studies as follows:
1 = regionalization
2 = needs-based funding
3 = alternative payment plans
4 = for-profit delivery
5 = wait-times management
6 = drug coverage
Bolded values indicate that the variable was a *major* factor in explaining the case outcome. Unbolded values indicate that the variable was an observable (but not major) factor in explaining the case outcome. In the "Total" column/row, the first figure indicates the total number of times the variable was observed as a factor (major or non-major). The second figure in parentheses indicates the number of times the variable was observed as a major factor.

ANNEX 3

SOME OBSERVATIONS ON THE HISTORICAL DEVELOPMENT OF MEDICARE

HARVEY LAZAR

The purpose of this annex is to comment on the factors that led to the *Hospital Insurance and Diagnostic Services Act* (1957) and *Medical Care Act* (1966). By shedding light on the processes that led to those two policy reforms, we will provide additional context for the reform outlook going forward.

As explained in chapter 1, health insurance was a priority for Canadians after the Second World War. The dominion government outlined its proposal in the 1945 Green Book on Reconstruction (Dominion-Provincial Conference 1946). Supporters of the Green Book included much of the political centre (including much of the federal Liberal Party), the social democratic and socialist left (the CCF), the union movement, and the Canadian Federation of Agriculture. They were aided by the mood of the era which saw government in matters relating to the economy and social justice as the *solution* and not the *problem*. Despite the breadth of its backing, the Canada-wide public payment paradigm lost round one. Ottawa's Green Book proposals were stymied by the forceful opposition of the governments of Ontario, Quebec, and Alberta and the doubts of the Maritimes. Only Saskatchewan and Manitoba supported Ottawa. The federal Liberals and others who had sought national and universal health insurance thus failed on first attempt.

As time passed, new sources of resistance to Canada-wide publicly financed heath care showed up, some more predictable than others. Predictably, the medical associations and health insurance companies were a big piece of the opposition. Less predictably, the prime minister was opposed. Louis St. Laurent led the Liberal Party to victory in the 1949 and 1953 elections, winning a substantial majority of seats both times. St. Laurent favoured private insurance. So too did most of the cabinet (Lamarsh 1969, 338-40; Martin 1985, 226). But a substantial majority of the federal Liberal caucus favoured the 1945 proposals (Maioni 1998, 102-3; Martin 1985, 226). Not wanting an open rift in the party, St. Laurent stalled. During the two general election campaigns, he made the federal government's 1945 policy stance conditional on receiving a large measure of provincial support (the precise "rule" seeming to change over time). Since a majority of provinces, including the two largest, were still opposed to the 1945 Ottawa initiative at the beginning of the 1950s, St. Laurent was able to keep his Liberal caucus at bay for some time (Maioni 1998, 94, 103; Martin 1985, 220-47).

By the early 1950s, British Columbia, Alberta, Saskatchewan, and Newfoundland and Labrador were in favour of a countrywide, federal-provincial cost-sharing regime for hospital services. All four were already paying for hospital insurance to one degree or other and would be fiscally advantaged if Ottawa paid for a share of hospital costs. There was also likely to be some interest from one or more of the Maritime provinces if their costs could be adequately subsidized. Only Quebec was unlikely to agree under any foreseeable circumstances, which left Ontario as key to opening the hospital insurance door.

The Progressive Conservative government of Ontario had led the opposition to the 1945 Green Book proposals. Although its leader, Premier George Drew, had stepped down in 1949, his successor, Premier Leslie Frost, continued Ontario's opposition. The federal Liberals, when under pressure in the House of Commons, blamed the government of Ontario for the inaction. These attacks were echoed in the Ontario legislature by the opposition Liberals and CCF. In late 1954, with an Ontario provincial general election approaching, Frost changed his tune. He soon became the lead spokesman for those provinces and territories that supported a national hospital insurance program, and he pushed St. Laurent hard for a federal-provincial national approach to hospital insurance (Martin 1985, 229-45; Taylor 2009, chap. 3). Once Frost declared for national health insurance, the jig was up. St. Laurent was caught in the crossfire: opposition to his position from a substantial majority of his own caucus who favoured Canada-wide hospital insurance and feared loss of their ridings, opposition parties in the House of Commons, and now the premier of Ontario. St. Laurent yielded. The federal Hospital Insurance and Diagnostic Services Act was passed in 1957 with wide support from MPs in all parties.

It had taken more than a decade following the 1945 Green Book proposals to achieve Canada-wide hospital insurance. Insiders who supported private insurance were well ensconced in positions of authority in both the federal and provincial orders of government. Had Frost not shifted his stance when he did, Canada's hospital insurance outcome might well have been much different. In fact, the Ontario window opened only briefly. A few years after the Hospital Insurance and Diagnostic Services Act was passed, the government of Ontario fought tenaciously against the Medical Care Act (Canada-wide medical care) and two decades later it vigourously opposed the *Canada Health Act.* The Ontario Progressive Conservatives were the governing party throughout this period (until 1985). Historical accident, as well as the competition of interests and institutions, played a role in what was enacted in 1957.

The dynamics of the Canada-wide medical care insurance reform had some similarities to hospital insurance and some differences. One similarity was that the NDP government of Saskatchewan pioneered medical insurance in 1962 as its predecessor, the CCF, had done on hospital insurance in 1947. In both cases Saskatchewan acted alone although encouraging the idea that there should be a countrywide program. At the beginning of the 1960s, the four largest provinces were firmly opposed to federal medical care legislation. Three of them—the governments of Alberta, British Columbia, and Ontario—were in the private payment camp. They saw a residual role for government (helping persons who lacked the financial means to pay their own way), but only for provincial government. Working with the health and life insurance industry, the Canadian Medical Association and its provincial divisions, these provincial governments had enacted and put into effect private "medicare" legislation, or were about to do so, when Ottawa tabled its bill in the House of Commons (Taylor 2009, 338-41). As for Quebec, the Liberal Party government was not opposed to the idea of public payment. But it rejected entirely the idea of the federal government having any role in what Quebecers would decide for themselves. The Liberal government of Quebec was first and foremost a defender of provincial autonomy. These were the early years of the Quiet Revolution in Quebec.

Other provincial governments were less strident in their positions. But Saskatchewan alone favoured the idea of universal, publicly financed, Canada-wide medical insurance.

Events were also unfolding at the federal level. The Diefenbaker Progressive Conservative government, elected in 1957, appointed a royal commission in 1961 to

> inquire into and report upon the existing facilities and the future need for health services for the people of Canada and the resources to provide such services, and to recommend such measures, consistent with the constitutional division of legislative powers in Canada, as the Commissioners believe will ensure that the best possible health care is available to all Canadians. (Health Canada 2004)

Chaired by Justice Emmett Hall, the two reports issued in 1964 recommended a national health policy and a comprehensive health-care program for three main areas: health services; health personnel, facilities, and research; and financing and priorities (Royal Commission 1964, 17-18). The result was a stunning endorsement of the Canada-wide paradigm. The Progressive Conservatives were no longer in power when the Hall report was released. They were in the process of tearing themselves apart on matters unrelated to health care. Their internal divisions left them a small actor in what followed.

The federal Liberal Party led by Lester Pearson had promised a national medical insurance plan in the general elections of 1962 (it lost), 1963 (in which it won a minority government), and 1965 (once again won a minority). As a minority government it might have had second thoughts about fulfilling its promise, especially since there was much opposition within the Liberal government itself (Maioni 1998, 126-28), but the left of the cabinet prevailed. Legislation was introduced and passed with the support from the federal NDP members of Parliament. Resistance from the more conservative side of the cabinet did not disappear, however. Indeed, finance minister Mitchell Sharp was able delay implementation for a year (Kent 1988, 369; Taylor 2009, 368-69).

Unlike the *Hospital Insurance and Diagnostic Services Act*, for which St. Laurent had required a measure of provincial consensus before introducing legislation, Pearson did not (Kent 1988, 364-69). Federal cost sharing would be available to any province that met the broad conditions of the legislation—universality, provincial administration, comprehensiveness (meaning primary care physicians and medical specialists), and portability among provinces (Kent 1988, 367). Public opinion turned in Ottawa's favour despite the opposing public relations campaign waged by the Canadian Medical Association (Taylor 2009, 334). Ottawa gambled that no provincial government would take the political risk of refusing the federal offer once it was law. It turned out that the federal government was right. Provincial political leaders were unable to walk away from the fiscal incentive that Ottawa had put in front of them.

Publicly financed medical insurance was apparently an idea whose time had come or so it may seem looking backward. Although almost all MPs voted for the legislation as it worked its way through the House of Commons (only two MPs voted against on final reading), the reality was more complex. The four largest provinces had initially been strongly opposed, and they had their own ideas of what medicare should look like. If the federal Liberal government had waited until it won a majority before acting, which it did win in the 1968 general election, events might well have run a different course. Provincial medical schemes would have had more time to sink roots. The economy softened in the late 1960s and early 1970s and then worsened. Affordability would have probably loomed larger as a constraint. Indeed, provincial governments had barely begun to implement the medical insurance program with the allure of federal matching grants when the federal government began ratcheting back on its cost sharing. The window of opportunity had not been wasted. Canada-wide medical care was the product of political forces at a moment in time.

References

Abelson, J., M. Mendelsohn, J.N. Lavis, S.G. Morgan, P.-G. Forest, and M. Swinton. 2004. "Canadians Confront Health-Care Reform." *Health Affairs* 23 (3): 186-93.

Action démocratique du Québec. 2007. *Une vision. Un plan. Une parole. Un plan A pour le Québec.* Action démocratique du Québec.

Adams, D. 2001a. "Canadian Federalism and the Development of National Health Goals and Objectives." In *Federalism, Democracy and Health Policy in Canada*, edited by D. Adams. Montreal and Kingston: McGill-Queen's University Press for Institute of Intergovernmental Relations.

—. 2001b. "Conclusions: Proposals for Advancing Federalism, Democracy and Governance of the Canadian Health Care System." In *Federalism, Democracy and Health Policy in Canada*, edited by D. Adams. Montreal and Kingston: McGill-Queen's University Press for Institute of Intergovernmental Relations.

—. 2001c. "The White and the Black Horse Race: Saskatchewan Health Reform in the 1990s." In *Saskatchewan Politics: Into the Twenty-First Century*, edited by H. Leeson, 267-93. Regina, SK: Canadian Plains Research Centre.

Agnew, G.H. 1974. *Canadian Hospitals, 1920 to 1970: A Dramatic Half Century.* Toronto: University of Toronto Press.

Alberta. 1962. *Submission to the Royal Commission on Health Services.*

—. 2003. Master Agreement Regarding the Trilateral Relationship and Budget Management Process for Strategic Physician Agreements. http://www.health.alberta.ca/documents/trilateral-agreement-2004.pdf.

Alberta Health. 1989. *Report of the Advisory Committee on the Utilization of Medical Services* (Watanabe Committee).

—. 1991a. *Partners in Health: The Government of Alberta's Official Response to the Premier's Commission on Future Health Care for Albertans.* Edmonton: Alberta Health.

—. 1991b. "Discussion Paper: Ambulatory Care Services in Alberta." 14 February.

—. 1991c. *Accountability in Alberta Health.* Edmonton: Alberta Health.

—. 1992. *Health Vision: Turning Ideas into Reality* [newsletter]. Vol. 1, Issue 2 (June).

—. 1993. *Palliative Care: A Policy Framework.* Edmonton: Alberta Health.

—. 1994. *A Three Year Business Plan.* 24 February.

—. n.d. Letter of Understanding between the Minister of Health of the Government of Alberta and the President of the Alberta Medical Association.

Alberta Health and Wellness. 1995–2004. *Public Surveys about Health and the Health System in Alberta.* A series of individual yearly reports.

—. 1999a. *Summary of Consultations with Public, November 1998 to March 1999.* Edmonton.

—. 1999b. *Healthy Aging: New Directions for Care. Part II: Listening and Learning.* Final report of the Policy Advisory Committee on Long-Term Care, Edmonton.

Alberta Health Planning Secretariat. 1993. *Starting Points: Recommendations for Creating a More Accountable and Affordable Health System.* Edmonton: Government of Alberta.

Alberta Human Resources and Employment. 2002. *Annual Report 2001/02.* Edmonton.

Alford, R.R. 1975. *Health Care Politics: Ideological and Interest Group Barriers to Reform.* Chicago: University of Chicago Press.

AMA (Alberta Medical Association). 1993. *The President's Newsletter.*

—. 1996. *You Told Us Where It Hurts: A Summary of Comments Received during the Alberta Medical Association's 1995 Public Awareness Campaign.* Edmonton: Alberta Medical Association.

—. n.d. *Alternative Remuneration for Primary Care: Fee for Comprehensive Care.*

Angell, M. 2004. "Excess in the Pharmaceutical Industry." *CMAJ* 171 (12), 7 December.

—. 2008. "Privatizing Health Care Is Not the Answer: Lessons from the United States." *CMAJ* 179 (21 October): 916-19. http://www.cmaj.ca/search?fulltext=Angell&submit=yes&x=9&y=9.

Archer, D.G. 1991. *Annual Report of the Provincial Auditor of Ontario for the Year Ended March 31, 1991.* Toronto: Queen's Printer.

Archibald, T., and A. Jeffs. 2004. "Physician Fee Decisions, the Medicare Basket and Budgeting: A Three-Province Survey." Paper presented at Canadian Health Services Research Foundation-funded project, Toronto, 30 November. Toronto.

Armstrong, W. 2000. *Canada's Canary in the Mineshaft: The Consumer Experience with Cataract Surgery and Private Clinics in Alberta.* Edmonton: Consumers' Association of Canada (Alberta).

Aucoin, P. 1990. "Administrative Reform in Public Management: Paradigms, Principles, Paradoxes and Pendulums." *Governance* 3 (2): 115-37.

—. 2002. "Beyond the 'New' in Public Management: Catching the Wave." In *The Handbook of Canadian Public Administration,* edited by C. Dunn, 37-52. Toronto: Oxford University Press.

Bachrach, P., and M.S. Baratz. 1970. *Power and Poverty: Theory and Practice.* New York: Oxford University Press.

Bailey, I., and B. Curry. 2011. "In Surprise Move, Flaherty Lays Out Health-Spending Plans til 2024." *Globe and Mail,* 19 December. http://www.theglobeandmail.com/news/politics/in-surprise-move-flaherty-lays-out-health-spending-plans-til-2024/article4247851/.

Banting, K., and R. Boadway. 2003. "Defining the Sharing Community: The Federal Role in Health Care." In *Money, Politics and Health Care: Reconstructing the Federal-Provincial Partnership,* edited by H. Lazar and F. St-Hilaire. Montreal and Kingston: McGill-Queen's University Press.

Banting, K., and S. Corbett. 2002. "Health Policy and Federalism: An Introduction." In *Health Policy and Federalism: A Comparative Perspective on Multi-Level Governance,* edited by K. Banting and S. Corbett. Montreal and Kingston:McGill-Queen's University Press.

Barer, M., J. Lomas, and C. Sanmartin. 1996. "Re-minding our Ps and Qs: Medical Cost Controls in Canada." *Health Affairs* 15 (2): 216-34.

Barer, M., and G. Stoddart. 1991. "Toward Integrated Medical Resource Policies for Canada: Background Document." Centre for Health Services and Policy Research, University of British Columbia, Vancouver.

—. 1999. "Improving Access to Needed Medical Services in Rural and Remote Canadian Communities: Recruitment and Retention Revisited." Discussion paper prepared for the Federal/Provincial/Territorial Advisory Committee on Health Human Resources, Ottawa.

Barnes, M. 2006. *Ontario Primary Health Care Transition Fund Initiative*. Ottawa: Primary Health Care Transition Fund.

Barr, J.J. 1974. *The Dynasty: Rise and Fall of the Social Credit in Alberta*. Toronto: McClelland and Stewart.

Barrie, D. 2004. "Ralph Klein." In *Alberta Premiers of the Twentieth Century*, edited by B.J. Rennie, 255-79. Regina, SK: Canadian Plains Research Centre, University of Regina.

Baumol, W., with D. de Ferrati, M. Malch, A. Pablos-Mendez, H. Tabish, and L. Gomory Wu. 2012. *The Cost Disease: Why Computers Get Cheaper and Health Care Doesn't*. New Haven, CT: Yale University Press.

Bégin, J.-F. 1998. "Oui à un rôle accru du privé dans la santé." *La Presse*, 29 septembre, A1.

Bégin, M. 2002. "Revisiting the *Canada Health Act* (1984): What Are the Impediments to Change?" Institute for Research on Public Policy. http://www.irpp.org/events/archive/020218e.pdf.

Bell, E. 1992. "Reconsidering Democracy in Alberta." In *Government and Politics in Alberta,* edited by A. Tupper and R. Gibbons, 85-108. Edmonton: University of Alberta Press.

Bergeron, P., and F. Gagnon. 2003. "La prise en charge étatique de la santé au Québec: émergence et transformations." In *Le système de santé du Québec : organisations, acteurs et enjeux*, 2nd ed., edited by V. Lemieux, P. Bergeron, C. Bégin, and G. Bélanger (7-33). Sainte-Foy, QC: Les Presses de l'Université Laval.

Bernier, J., and M. Dallaire. 2000. *Le prix de la réforme du système de santé pour les femmes: La situation au Québec*. Montreal: Centre d'excellence pour la santé des femmes/Consortium Université de Montréal.

Bhatia, V. 2002. "Literature Review." McMaster University Centre for Health Economics and Policy Analysis, Hamilton.

Birch, S., and S. Chambers. 1993. "To Each According to Need: A Community-Based Approach to Allocating Health Care Resources." *CMAJ* 149 (5): 607-12.

Bird, R.M. 1979. *Financing Canadian Government: A Quantitative Overview*. Toronto: Canadian Tax Foundation.

Blake, R. 1994. *Canadians at Last: Canada Integrates Newfoundland as a Province*. Toronto: University of Toronto Press.

Bliss, M. 2010. "Critical Condition: A Historian's Prognosis on Canada's Aging Healthcare System." Toronto: C.D. Howe Institute. http://www.cdhowe.org/critical-condition-a-historians-prognosis-on-canadas-aging-healthcare-system/4446.

Boase, J.P. 1994. *Shifting Sands: Government-Group Relationships in Health Care*. Montreal: McGill-Queen's University Press.

Botting, I. 2000. *Health Care Restructuring and Privatization from Women's Perspective in Newfoundland and Labrador*. St. John's: Memorial University of Newfoundland Coasts under Stress Project.

Boychuk, G.W. 2003. "The Changing Political and Economic Environment of Health Care." In *The Fiscal Sustainability of Health Care in Canada*. The Romanow Papers, Vol. 1. Edited by G.P. Marchildon, T. McIntosh, and P.-G. Forest. Toronto: University of Toronto Press.

Boyle ,T. 2002. "Tories Taking Offers for MRI Clinics." *Toronto Star*, 16 November, A06.

Bozeman, B., and S. Panday. 2004. "Public Management Decision Making: Effects of Decision Content." *Public Administration Review* 64 (5): 553-65.

Bradford, N. 1999. *Commissioning Ideas*. Toronto: Oxford University Press.

—. 2003. "Public-Private Partnership? Shifting Paradigms of Economic Governance in Ontario." *Canadian Journal of Political Science* 36 (5): 1005-33.

British Columbia. Royal Commission on Health Care and Costs. 1991. *Closer to Home*. Chaired by Justice P.D. Seaton. Victoria.

Brownsey, K. 2005. "The Post-Institutionalized Cabinet: The Administrative Style of Alberta." In *Executive Styles in Canada: Cabinet Structures and Leadership Practices in Canadian Government*, edited by L. Bernier, K. Brownsey, and M. Howlett, 208-24. Toronto: University of Toronto Press.

Burns, R.M. 1980. *The Acceptable Mean: The Tax Rental Agreements, 1941–1962.* Toronto: Canadian Tax Foundation.

Cairns, A.C. 1988. *Constitution, Government, and Society in Canada.* Toronto: McClelland and Stewart.

Canada. 1945. "White Paper on Employment and Income."

Canadian Centre for Policy Alternatives. 2002. "Canadian Health Care Reform: Trade Treaties and Foreign Policy." http://www.policyalternatives.ca/sites/default/files/uploads/publications/National_Office_Pubs/putting_health_first.pdf.

Canadian Doctors for Medicare. 2011. "Neat, Plausible, and Wrong: The Myth of Health Care Unsustainability." http://www.canadiandoctorsformedicare.ca/.

—. 2012. "Taking Action on Health Equity in Canada." http://www.canadiandoctorsformedicare.ca/images/stories/TakingActionHealthEquity.pdf.

Canadian Health Coalition. 2001. "Extendicare Is Not a Model for Medicare." Submission to the Standing Senate Committee on Social Affairs, Science and Technology. http://healthcoalition.ca/wp-content/uploads/2010/09/Extendicare-Brief-2001.pdf.

—. 2012a. "About the Canadian Health Coalition." http://healthcoalition.ca/main/about-us/contact-us.

—. 2012b. "Leading Economist Shatters Myth That Health Care Is Unsustainable." http://medicare.ca/.

—. 2012c. "Medicare Sustainability: Facts and Myths." http://medicare.ca/medicare-sustainability-facts-myths.

Canadian Intergovernmental Conference Secretariat. 2000. "First Ministers' Meeting Communiqué on Health." News release, 11 September. http://www.scics.gc.ca/english/conferences.asp?a=viewdocument&id=1144.

Canadian Labour and Business Centre and the Canadian Policy Research Networks. 2005. *Canada's Physician Workforce: Occupational Human Resources Data Assessment and Trends Analysis.* Report to Task Force II. Ottawa: Physician HHR Planning for Canada.

Canadian Policy Research Networks. 2004. *The Taming of the Queue: Wait Time Measurement, Monitoring and Management.* Colloquium report. http://www.cprn.org/documents/28648_en.pdf.

Canadian Public Health Association. 2012. *This Is Public Health: A Canadian History.* http://www.cpha.ca/en/programs/history/book.aspx.

Carter, G.E. 1971. *Canadian Conditional Grants since World WAR II.* Toronto: Canadian Tax Foundation.

CBC. 2012. Transcript of conversation with Prime Minister Harper. 16 January. http://www.cbc.ca/news/politics/story/2012/01/17/pol-mansbridge-interview-harper-transcript.html.

Church, J., and P. Barker. 1998. "Regionalization of Health Services in Canada: A Critical Perspective." *International Journal of Health Services* 28 (3): 467-86.

Church, J., and T. Noseworthy. 1999. "Fiscal Austerity through Decentralization." In *Health Reform: Public Success, Private Failure,* edited by D. Drache and T. Sullivan, 186-203. New York: Routledge.

Church, J., and N. Smith. 2006. "Health Reform and Privatization in Alberta." *Canadian Public Administration* 49 (4): 486-505.

—. 2007. "The Introduction of APPs in Alberta." Project case study.

—. 2008. "Health Care Reform in Alberta: The Introduction of Regional Health Authorities." *Canadian Public Administration* 51 (2): 217-38.

—. 2009. "Health Reform and Wait Times Policy in Alberta under the Klein Government." *Canadian Political Science Review* 3 (4): 63-84. http://ojs.unbc.ca/index.php/cpsr/article/view/194.

CIHI (Canadian Institute for Health Information). 1998. *Waiting for Health Care in Canada: What We Know and What We Don't Know.* Ottawa: CIHI.

—. 2005. "Canada's Healthcare Providers: 2005 Chartbook." Accessed January 2012. https://secure.cihi.ca/estore/productFamily.htm?pf=PFC568&lang=en&media=0.

—. 2008. *Physicians in Canada: The Status of Alternative Payment Programs, 2005–2006.*

—. 2011a. "Canada's Health Care Providers 2009 Provincial Profiles: A Look at 24 Health Occupations." Accessed January 2012. http://secure.cihi.ca/cihiweb/products/ProvProf2009EN.pdf.

—. 2011b. "National Health Expenditure Trends, 1975 to 2011." Accessed March 2012. http://secure.cihi.ca/cihiweb/products/nhex_trends_report_2011_en.pdf.

—. 2011c. "National Physician Database, 2009–2010 Data Release." Accessed January 2012. https://secure.cihi.ca/estore/productFamily.htm?locale=en&pf=PFC1678.

—. 2011d. "Physician Supply Increasing Twice as Quickly as Canadian Population." News release, 15 December. Accessed March 2012. http://www.cihi.ca/CIHI-ext-portal/internet/en/Document/spending+and+health+workforce/workforce/physicians/RELEASE_15DEC11.

—. 2011e. "Health Care Cost Drivers: The Facts." https://secure.cihi.ca/free_products/health_care_cost_drivers_the_facts_en.pdf.

—. 2012. "National Health Expenditure Trends: 1975 to 2012."

—. 2013. "Wait Times for Priority Procedures in Canada, 2013." https://secure.cihi.ca/free_products/wait_times_2013_en.pdf.

CMA (Canadian Medical Association). 2001. "Getting the Diagnosis Right: Toward a Sustainable Future for Canadian Health Care Policy." Part 1 of a two-part brief to the Royal Commission on the Future of Health Care in Canada, 31 October.

—. 2002. "A Prescription for Sustainability." 6 June. Ottawa.

—. 2010. *Health Care Transformation in Canada.* http://www.cma.ca/multimedia/ CMA/Content_Images/Inside_cma/Advocacy/HCT/HCT-2010report_ en.pdf.

—. 2011a. *Report of the Advisory Panel on Resourcing Options for Sustainable Health Care in Canada.* http://www.cma.ca/multimedia/CMA/Content_Images/ Inside_cma/Annual_Meeting/2011/AdvisoryPanelReport_en.pdf.

—. 2011b. *Voices into Action: Report on the National Dialogue on Health Care Transformation.* http://www.cma.ca/multimedia/CMA/Content_Images/ Inside_cma/Advocacy/HCT/HCT_townhalls_en.pdf.

Coleman, W.D., and G. Skogstad. 1990. *Policy Communities and Public Policy in Canada: A Structural Approach.* Mississauga, ON: Copp Clark Pitman.

Collège des médecins de famille du Canada. 2000. Soins de première ligne et médecine familiale au Canada : une ordonnance de renouvellement. Accessed 29 janvier 2008. http://www.cfpc.ca/uploadedFiles/Resources/Resource_ Items/Health_Professionals/SOINS%20DE%20PREMIERE%20LIGNE% 20ET%20MED%20FAM%202000.pdf.

Comité de gestion des listes d'attente en cardiologie tertiaire et F. Grenier. 1993. *Gestion des listes d'attente en cardiologie tertiaire. Rapport du comité - version finale.* Quebec: Ministère de la Santé et des Services sociaux.

Comité de révision de la circulaire «Malades sur pied». 1994. *De l'assistance à l'assurance.* Quebec: Ministère de la Santé et des Services sociaux.

Comité d'experts sur l'assurance médicaments. 1996. *L'assurance médicaments : des voies de solution.* Quebec: Comité d'experts sur l'assurance medicaments.

Comité sur la réévaluation du mode de budgétisation des centres hospitaliers de soins généraux et spécialisés. 2002. *La budgétisation et la performance financière des centres hospitaliers.* Quebec: Ministère de la Santé et des Services sociaux.

Comité sur la réévaluation du mode de budgétisation des CLSC et des CHSLD. 2002. *L'allocation des ressources et la budgétisation des services de CLSC et de CHSLD.* Quebec: Ministère de la Santé et des Services sociaux.

Commission d'enquête sur la santé et le bien-être social. 1967. *Rapport / Commission d'enquête sur la santé et le bien-être social.* Éditeur officiel du Québec.

Commission d'enquête sur les services de santé et les services sociaux. 1988. *Rapport de la Commission d'enquête sur les services de santé et les services sociaux.* Chaired by J. Rochon. Publications du Québec.

Commission d'étude sur les services de santé et les services sociaux. 2000. *Report and Recommendations: Emerging Solutions.* Chaired by M. Clair. Quebec City: Gouvernement du Québec.

Commission on the Future of Health Care in Canada. 2002. *Building on Values: The Future of Health Care in Canada – Final Report.* R. Romanow, Commissioner. Ottawa: Health Canada.

Commission on Medicare. 2001. *Caring for Medicare: Sustaining a Quality System.* Chaired by K.J. Fyke. Regina: Government of Saskatchewan.

Conference of Provincial/Territorial Ministers of Health. 1997. *A Renewed Vision for Canada's Health Care System.* January.

Conservative Party of Canada. 2004. "Demanding Better." Election platform. http://www.cbc.ca/canadavotes2004/pdfplatforms/platform_e.pdf.
—. 2006. "Stand Up for Canada." Election platform. http://www.cbc.ca/canada votes2006/leadersparties/pdf/conservative_platform20060113.pdf.
—. 2008. "The True North Home and Free." Election platform. http://www.scribd.com/doc/6433355/Conservative-Party-of-Canada-2008-Election-Platform-English.
—. 2011. "Here for Canada." Election platform. http://www.scribd.com/doc/52594069/Conservative-Party-of-Canada-2011-Election-Platform.
Contandriopoulos, D., and A. Brousselle. 2010. "Reliable in Their Failure: An Analysis of Healthcare Reform Policies in Public Systems." *Health Policy* 95 (2-3): 144-52.
Contandriopoulos, D., R. Hudon, F. Martin, and D. Thompson. 2007. "Tensions entre rationalité technique et intérêts politiques : l'exemple de la mise en œuvre de la Loi sur les agences de développement de réseaux locaux de services de santé et de services sociaux au Québec." *Administration publique du Canada* 50 (2): 219-43.
Council of Canadians. 2011. "The Council of Canadians: 25 Years of Action." http://www.canadians.org/about/history/index.html.
—. 2012. "Wait Time Success Stories in the Public System." http://canadians.org/healthcare/documents/wait_time_successes.pdf.
Council of the Federation. 2004. "Premiers' Action Plan for Better Health Care: Resolving Issues in the Spirit of True Federalism." Press communiqué, 30 July. Niagara on the Lake. Accessed 9 August 2011. http://www.councilofthe federation.ca/pdfs/HealthEng.pdf.
David, M. 2001. "Il faut sauver le soldat Trudel." *Le Devoir*, 30 octobre, A3.
Davies, R.F. 1999. "Waiting Lists for Health Care: A Necessary Evil?" *CMAJ* 160 (10): 1469-70.
Demers, V., M. Melo, C. Jackevicius, J. Cox, D. Kalavrouziotis, S. Rinfret, K.H. Humphries, H. Johansen, J.V. Tu, and L. Pilote. 2008. "Comparison of Provincial Prescription Drug Plans and the Impact on Patients' Annual Drug Expenditures." *CMAJ* 178 (4): 405-9.
Denis, J.-L. 1997. "Trois modèles et trois terrains pour penser la décentralisation." In *La santé demain: vers un système de soins sans murs*, edited by J.-P. Claveranne, C. Lardy, G. De Pouvourville, A.-P. Contandriopoulos, and B. Experton, 49-66. Paris: Economica.
Department of Finance Canada. 2013. "What Is the Canada Health Transfer (CHT)?" http://www.fin.gc.ca/fedprov/cht-eng.asp.
Derworiz, C. 2010. "Health Board Tries New Funding Model." *Calgary Herald*, 18 February. http://www2.canada.com/calgaryherald/news/story.html?id=4f326f1a-c8f5-4610-abbd-0858ced9613c.
Dickerson, M.O., and G.L. Flanagan. 1995. "The Unique Fiscal Situation of Alberta: Can Alberta's Deficit Reduction Model Be Exported?" Paper presented at the annual meeting of the Canadian Political Science Association, Montreal, May.
Dion, S. 2005. "Fiscal Balance in Canada." In *Canadian Fiscal Arrangements: What Works, What Might Work Better*, edited by H. Lazar. Published for the Institute of Intergovernmental Relations and the School of Policy Studies. Kingston, ON: McGill-Queen's University Press.
Dobbin, L.C. 1993. *Report on the Reduction of Hospital Boards.* St. John's, NL: Carrick Consulting Services.

Dodge, D., and R. Dion. 2011. "Chronic Healthcare Spending Disease: A Macro Diagnosis and Prognosis." C.D. Howe Institute, Toronto, 6 April. http://www.cdhowe.org/chronic-healthcare-spending-disease-a-macro-diagnosis-and-prognosis/9268.

Doern, B.D. 1998. *Changing Regulatory Institutions in Britain and North America.* Toronto: University of Toronto Press.

Dominion Bureau of Statistics. "Life Expectancy by Sex, at Selected Ages, Canada, Census Years, 1871 to 1971." Series B65-74. http://www.statcan.gc.ca/pub/11-516-x/sectionb/4147437-eng.htm.

—. "Number of Physicians, Dentists and Nurses, Population per Physician, Dentist and Nurse, Number of Graduates of Medical and Dental Schools, Canada, 1871 to 1975." Series B82-92. http://www.statcan.gc.ca/pub/11-516-x/sectionb/4147437-eng.htm.

—. "Rated Bed Capacity in Reporting Hospitals, Canada, 1932 to 1975." Series B141-188. http://www.statcan.gc.ca/pub/11-516-x/sectionb/4147437-eng.htm.

Dominion-Provincial Conference 1945. 1946. *Dominion and Provincial Submissions and Plenary Conference Discussions* (Green Book on Reconstruction). Ottawa: Edmond Cloutier, King's Printer.

Douglas, R. 1993. *Unfinished Business.* Auckland, NZ: Random House.

Dufour, V. 2000. "Radio-oncologie: Le CHUM obtient la moitié de 61 millions pour réduire les listes d'attente." *Le Devoir*, 3 juin, A2.

Duplantie, J.-P. 2001. "À petits pas ... De la Commission Rochon à la Commission Clair." *Ruptures, revue transdisciplinaire en santé* 8 (1): 88-97.

Dutil, R. 2002. "La médecine familiale ou prendre le temps de bien faire." *Le Soleil*, 11 janvier, A15.

Dyck, R. 1996. *Provincial Politics in Canada: Towards the Turn of the Century.* Toronto: McClelland and Stewart.

Economic Council of Canada. 1988. *Back to Basics.* Ottawa: Minister of Supply and Services.

Ekos Research Associates. 1994. "Rethinking Government." Ottawa.

Elkins, D., and R. Simeon. 1980. "Regional Political Cultures." In *Small Worlds*, edited by D. Elkins and R. Simeon. Toronto: Methuen Press.

Epp, J. 1985. Letter from Minister of Health Jake Epp to Provincial and Territorial Ministers of Health, 18 June. Annexed to the annual reports on the administration of the *Canada Health Act.*

Evans, J.R. 1987. *Toward a Shared Direction for Health in Ontario.* Report of the Ontario Health Review Panel. Toronto: Ontario Ministry of Health.

Evans, R.G. 2000. "Canada." *Journal of Health Politics, Policy and Law* 25 (5): 889-97.

Eyles, J., and S. Birch. 1993. "A Population Needs-Based Approach to Health-Care Resource Allocation and Planning in Ontario: A Link between Policy Goals and Practice?" *Canadian Journal of Public Health* 84 (2): 112-17.

Eyles, J., S. Birch, S. Chambers, J. Hurley, and B. Hutchison. 1991. "A Needs-Based Methodology for Allocating Health Care Resources in Ontario, Canada: Development and an Application." *Social Science and Medicine* 33(4): 489-500.

Farrell, C., and J. Morris. 2003. "The Neo-bureaucratic State: Professionals, Managers and Professional Managers in Schools, General Practices and Social Work." *Organization* 10 (1): 129-56.

Federal/Provincial/Territorial Advisory Committee on Health Services. 1995. "The Victoria Report on Physician Remuneration: A Model for the Reorganization of

Primary Care and the Introduction of Population-Based Funding: A Discussion Document." Victoria, BC.

Federal/Provincial/Territorial Advisory Committee on Population Health. 1994. *Strategies for Population Health: Investing in the Health of Canadians*. Report prepared for the meeting of the Ministers of Health, 14–15 September, Halifax. http://www.phac-aspc.gc.ca/ph-sp/pdf/strateg-eng.pdf.

Fédération des médecins omnipraticiens du Québec. 2001. "Les groupes de médecine de famille: il ne faut pas jeter le bébé avec l'eau du bain!" *Nouvelles de la FMOQ* 21 (2): 1-4.

Finance Canada. 1996. "The Atlantic Groundfish Strategy." http://www.gov.nl.ca/publicat/tags/text/content.htm.

First Ministers' Meeting. 2003. "First Ministers' Accord on Health Care Renewal." 5 February. http://www.scics.gc.ca/CMFiles/800039004_e1GTC-352011-6102.pdf.

—. 2004. "A 10-Year Plan to Strengthen Health Care." 2004. First Ministers' Meeting on the Future of Health Care, 16 September. http://www.scics.gc.ca/CMFiles/800042005_e1JXB-342011-6611.pdf.

Flood, C.M., and T. Sullivan. 2005. "Supreme Disagreement: The Highest Court Affirms an Empty Right." *CMAJ* 173 (2). http://www.cmaj.ca/content/173/2/142.full.

Forest, P.-G. 2007. "Santé: en finir avec la chaise vide." In *Reconquérir le Canada: un nouveau projet pour la nation québécoise*, edited by A. Pratte (261-85). Éditions voix parallèles.

—. Forthcoming. "Be Careful What You Wish for… Policy Development and the Federal Role in Canadian Health Care." In *Bending the Cost Curve*, edited by G. Marchildon and L. di Matteo. Toronto: University of Toronto Press.

Fraser Institute. 2002. "Drug Expense Coverage in the Canadian Population: Protection from Severe Drug Expenses." http://www.frasergroup.com/downloads/severe_drug_e.pd.

Freddi, G., and J.W. Bjorkman, eds. 1989. *Controlling Medical Professionals: The Comparative Politics of Health Governance*. Sage Modern Politics Series. Thousand Oaks, CA: Sage Publications.

Gafni, A., S. Birch, and B. O'Brien. 1994. "Paying the Piper and Calling the Tune: Principles and Prospects for Reforming Physician Payment in Canada." Centre for Health Economics and Policy Analysis (CHEPA) Working Paper Series, No. 1994-16. http://ideas.repec.org/p/hpa/wpaper/199416.html.

Gagné, J.-P. 1999. La médecine privée gagne du terrain." *Les Affaires*, 11 septembre, 6.

"Getting a Handle on Hospital Costs." 1991. *Toronto Star*, 28 November, A22.

Gildiner, A. 2001. "What's Past Is Prologue: A Historical-Institutionalist Analysis of Public-Private Change in Ontario's Rehabilitation Health Sector, 1985–1999." PhD diss., University of Toronto.

—. 2006. "Did the Centre Hold? A Comparative Analysis of Health Care Policy-Making and Privatization in Five Provinces." Working Paper 2013. Institute of Intergovernmental Relations, Queen's University. http://www.queensu.ca/iigr/WorkingPapers.html.

Gillet, J., B. Hutchison, and S. Birch. 2001. "Capitation and Primary Care in Canada: Financial Incentives and the Evolution of Health Service Organizations." *International Journal of Health Services* 31 (3): 583-603.

Gilmour, J.M. 2003. "Regulation of Free-Standing Health Facilities: An Entrée for Privatization and For-Profit Delivery in Health Care." Special issue, *Health Law Journal*: 131-52.

Glynn, P., M. Taylor, and A. Hudson. 2002. *Surgical Wait List Management: A Strategy for Saskatchewan*. A report to Saskatchewan Health.

Government of Canada. 1998. "Status Update on Reinvestment Plans under the National Child Benefit – March 12, 1998." Accessed 16 August 2005. http://www.nationalchildbenefit.ca/ncb/status2_e.shtml.

—. 2005. "National Child Benefit. Description of Reinvestments." Accessed 16 August 2005. http://www.nationalchildbenefit.ca/ncb/progdesc.shtml.

—. 2012. "Taking Action to Improve the Health of Canadians." The Government of Canada response to the report of the Standing Senate Committee on Social Affairs, Science and Technology, *Time for Transformative Change: A Review of the 2004 Health Accord*. 12 September.

Government of Newfoundland and Labrador. 1966. *Royal Commission on Health*. Chaired by Lord Brain. St. John's, NL: Queen's Printer.

—. 1984. *Report of the Royal Commission on Hospital and Nursing Home Costs*. St. John's, NL: Queen's Printer.

—. *The Atlantic Groundfish Strategy*. St. John's, NL: Department of Finance, Economics and Statistics Branch. http://www.gov.nl.ca/publicat/tags/text/content.htm.

—. 2002a. *Health Scope: Reporting to Newfoundlanders and Labradorians on Comparable Health and Health Systems Indicators*. St. John's, NL: Department of Health and Community Services.

—. 2002b. *Healthier Together: A Strategic Health Plan for Newfoundland and Labrador*. St. John's, NL: Department of Health and Community Services.

—. 2003. *Royal Commission on Renewing and Strengthening Our Place in Canada*. St. John's, NL: Queen's Printer.

Government of Newfoundland and Labrador Health Study Group. 1973. *Health Care Delivery: An Overview*. St. John's, NL: Queen's Printer.

Government of Ontario. 2002. *Ontario Budget 2002: Ontario's Prosperity – A Growing Economy*. Toronto: Government of Ontario.

Gow, I. 2004. *A Canadian Model of Public Administration*. Canadian School of Public Service.

Gratton, D. 1996. "1,1 million de Québécois n'ont pas d'assurance-médicaments." *Le Droit*, 29 août, 4.

Gratzer, D. 1999. *Code Blue: Reviving Canada's Health Care System*. Toronto: ECW Press.

Grootendorst, P. 2002. "Beneficiary Cost Sharing under Canadian Provincial Prescription Drug Benefit Programmes: History and Assessment." *Canadian Journal of Clinical Pharmacology* 9 (2): 79-99.

Groupe de travail. 1999. *La complémentarité du secteur privé dans la poursuite des objectifs fondamentaux du système public de santé au Québec* (Arpin Report). Quebec: Gouvernement du Québec/Ministère de la Santé et des Services sociaux.

Groupe de travail sur la chirurgie générale et orthopédique au Québec. 1993. *Rapport préliminaire*. Quebec: Ministère de la Santé et des Services sociaux.

Groupe de travail sur l'allocation des ressources financières. 1993. *Cadre de référence sur l'allocation des ressources dans le contexte de la gestion par programmes et de la décentralisation des activités: rapport*. Quebec: Ministère de la Santé et des Services sociaux.

Groupe de travail sur le financement du système de santé. 2008. *En avoir pour notre argent : des services accessibles aux patients, un financement durable, un système productif, une responsabilité partagée.* Quebec: Groupe de travail sur le financement du système de santé.

Guest, D. 1997. *The Emergence of Social Security in Canada.* 3rd ed. Vancouver: University of British Columbia Press.

Hanrahan, H., B. Mackenzie, C. Orridge, J. Saunders, K. Worthington, and R.B. Deber. 1992. "Heritage, Votes, Money and Medicine: Rural Health Care in Alberta." In *Case Studies in Canadian Health Policy and Management,* edited by R.B. Deber, 143-54. Ottawa: Canadian Hospital Association Press.

Hastings, J.E.F. 1972. "The Community Health Centre in Canada: Report of the Community Health Centre Project to the Conference of Health Ministers." Special issue, *CMAJ* 107: 361-80.

Health Canada. 2003. *Canada Health Act – Annual Report.* Annual report on the administration and operation of the *Canada Health Act* for the fiscal year that ended 31 March 2003.

—. 2004. "Royal Commission on Health Services, 1961 to 1964." http://www.hc-sc.gc.ca/hcs-sss/com/fed/hall-eng.php.

—. 2009. *Canada Health Act – Annual Report.* Annual report on the administration and operation of the *Canada Health Act* for the fiscal year that ended 31 March 2009. http://www.hc-sc.gc.ca/hcs-sss/alt_formats/pdf/pubs/cha-ics/2010-cha-ics-ar-ra-eng.pdf.

Health Council of Canada. 2010. *How Do Canadians Rate the Health Care System: Results from the 2010 Commonwealth Fund International Health Policy Survey.* Toronto: Health Council of Canada.

—. 2012. *Progress Report 2012: Health Care Renewal in Canada.* Toronto: Health Council of Canada. http://www.healthcouncilcanada.ca/rpt_det.php?id=377.

Health Services Funding Advisory Committee. 1996. *Funding Regional Health Services in Alberta.* Edmonton: Government of Alberta.

Hillier, J., and P. Neary. 1980. *Newfoundland in the 19th and 20th Centuries.* Toronto: University of Toronto Press.

Hornick, J.P., R.J. Thomlison, and L. Nesbitt. 1988. "Alberta." In *Privatization and Social Services in Canada,* edited by J.S. Ismael and Y. Vaillancourt, 41-74. Edmonton: University of Alberta Press.

Howell, T.S. 2010. "Private Health-Care Hospital on Life Support." *Fast Forward Weekly,* 20 May. http://www.ffwdweekly.com/article/news-views/news/private-health-care-hospital-on-life-support-5717/.

Howlett, M., and M. Ramesh. 2003. *Studying Public Policy: Policy Cycles and Policy Subsystems.* 2nd ed. Oxford: Oxford University Press.

Howlett, M., M. Ramesh, and A. Perl. 2009. *Studying Public Policy: Policy Cycles and Policy Subsystems.* 3rd ed. Oxford: Oxford University Press.

Houston, S.C. 2002. *Steps on the Road to Medicare: Why Saskatchewan Led the Way.* Montreal and Kingston: McGill-Queen's University Press.

Hutchison, B.G., J. Abelson, and J.N. Lavis. 2001. "Primary Care Reform in Canada: So Much Innovation, So Little Change." *Health Affairs* 20 (3): 116-31.

Hutchison, B., J.-F. Levesque, E. Strumpf, and N. Coyle. 2011. "Primary Health Care in Canada: Systems in Motion." *Milbank Quarterly* 89 (2): 256-88.

Immergut, E.M. 1992. "The Rules of the Game: The Logic of Health Policy-Making in France, Switzerland, and Sweden." In *Structuring Politics: Historical*

Institutionalism in Comparative Analysis, edited by S. Steinmo, K. Thelen, and F. Lonstreth, 57-89. Cambridge: Cambridge University Press.

Ipsos Reid. 2010. *2010 National Report Card: Final Report*. Submitted to the Canadian Medical Association. August. http://www.cma.ca/multimedia/CMA/Content_Images/Inside_cma/Media_Release/2010/report_card/2010-National-Report-Card_en.pdf.

—. 2011. *2011 National Report Card: Final Report*. Submitted to the Canadian Medical Association. August. http://www.cma.ca/multimedia/CMA/Content_Images/Inside_cma/Media_Release/2011/reportcard/2011National-Report-Card_en.pdf.

IRPP Task Force on Health Policy. 2000. *Recommendations to First Ministers*. Montreal: Institute for Research on Public Policy.

Ish, D. 2010. In the Matter of an Expedited Arbitration between: Regina Qu'appelle Health Region Employer and Canadian Union of Public Employees, Local 3967. Arbitration decision. http://cupe.ca/updir/100929_Arbitration_decision.pdf.

Kaminski, V.L., W.J. Sibbald, and E.M. Davis. 1989. *Investigation of Cardiac Surgery at St. Michael's Hospital, Toronto, Ontario: Final Report*. Toronto: Government of Ontario.

Kapur, V., and K. Basu. 2005. "Drug Coverage in Canada: Who Is at Risk?" *Health Policy* 71 (2): 181-93.

Kent, T. 1988. *A Public Purpose: An Experience of Liberal Opposition and Canadian Government*. Kingston and Montreal: McGill-Queen's University Press.

Keon, W.J. 1991. *Provincial Working Group on Cardiovascular Services: Final Report*. Toronto: Government of Ontario.

Kilshaw, M. 1995. *The Victoria Report on Physician Remuneration: A Model for the Reorganization of Primary Care and the Introduction of Population-Based Funding*. Report to the Federal, Provincial and Territorial Advisory Committee on Health Services. Victoria: Queen's Printer for British Columbia.

Kingdon, J.W. 1995. *Agendas, Alternatives, and Public Policies*. New York: Harper Collins.

—. 2003. *Agendas, Alternatives, and Public Policies*. 2nd ed. New York: Addison-Wesley Educational Publishers.

—. 2006. "The Reality of Public Policy Making." In *The Ethical Dimension of Health Policy*, edited by M. Danis, C.M. Clancy, and L.R. Churchill, 97-116. Oxford: Oxford University Press.

—. 2010. *Agendas, Alternatives, and Public Policies*. Update edition, with an Epilogue on Health Care. New York: Longman.

Kralj, B., and J. Kantarevic. 2012. "Primary Care in Ontario: Reforms, Investments and Achievements." *Ontario Medical Review* (February): 18-24.

Labonte, R., M. Polanyi, N. Muhajarine, T. McIntosh, and A. Williams. 2005. "Beyond the Divides: Towards Critical Population Health Research." *Critical Public Health* 15 (1): 5-17.

Laframboise, H.L. 1986. "Outflanking Dominant Elites." *Policy Options* (July): 36-41.

Lalonde, M. 1974. *A New Perspective on the Health of Canadians* (The Lalonde Report). Ottawa: Minister of Supply and Services Canada. http://www.phac-aspc.gc.ca/ph-sp/pdf/perspect-eng.pdf.

Lavis, J.N. 2002. *Political Elites and Their Influence on Health-Care Reform in Canada*. Commission on the Future of Health Care in Canada, Discussion Paper No. 26, October.

—. 2004. "Political Elites and Their Influence on Health-Care Reform in Canada." In *The Governance of Health Care in Canada*, edited by T. McIntosh, P.-G. Forest, and G. Marchildon, 257-79. Toronto: University of Toronto Press.

Lavis, J.N., S.E. Ross, J.E. Hurley, J.M. Hohenadel, G.L. Stoddart, C.A. Woodward, and J. Abelson. 2002. "Examining the Role of Health Services Research in Public Policymaking." *Milbank Quarterly* 80 (1): 125-54.

Lavis, J.N., J.A. Røttingen, X. Bosch-Capblanch, R. Atun, F. El-Jardali, L. Gilson, S. Lewin, S. Oliver, P. Ongolo-Zogo, and A. Haines. 2012. "Guidance for Evidence-Informed Policies about Health Systems: 2. Linking Guidance Development to Policy Development." *PLoS Medicine* 9 (3): e1001186. doi:10.1371/journal. pmed.1001186.

Lazar, H., F. St-Hilaire, and J.-F. Tremblay. 2004a. "Federal Health Care Funding: Toward a New Fiscal Pact." In *Money, Politics and Health Care: Reconstructing the Federal-Provincial Partnership*, edited by H. Lazar and F. St-Hilaire. Montreal and Kingston: McGill-Queen's University Press for the Institute for Research on Public Policy and the Institute of Intergovernmental Relations.

—. 2004b. "Vertical Fiscal Imbalance: Myth or Reality." In *Money, Politics and Health Care: Reconstructing the Federal-Provincial Partnership*, edited by H. Lazar and F. St-Hilaire. Montreal and Kingston: McGill-Queen's University Press for the Institute for Research on Public Policy and the Institute of Intergovernmental Relations.

Lee, R.L. 2003. "Family Health Networks in Ontario." *CMAJ* 168 (2): 152.

Léger Marketing/Journal de Québec. 2007. *Les Québécois et l'accès aux soins de santé*. Léger Marketing, Québec.

Lessard, D. 1995. "À la maison après l'opération: Québec vise la «chirurgie d'un jour» pour réduire les frais d'hospitalisation." *La Presse*, 25 mars, A28.

—. 2001. "Le ministre au site internet." *La Presse*, 16 juin, B5.

—. 2005. "Les Québécois favorables au privé: 69% des moins de 35 ans l'approuvent." *La Presse*, 30 juin, A4.

Lessard, D., and J.-F. Bégin. 2000. "De l'espoir pour les cardiaques: Marois débloque 25 million pour réduire les listes d'attente en cardiologie." *La Presse*, 20 mai, A1.

Lewis, S. 2010. "CMA Emerges Dazed from Cave, Writes Report." In *Essays*, Longwoods.com. http://www.longwoods.com/content/21904.

Lewis, S., C. Donaldson, C. Mitton, and G. Currie. 2001. "The Future of Health Care in Canada." *BMJ (British Medical Journal)* 323 (7318): 926-29.

Liberal Party of Canada. 2004. "Moving Canada Forward: The Paul Martin Plan for Getting Things Done." Election platform.

Lisac. M. 1995. *The Klein Revolution*. Edmonton: NeWest Press.

Living in Canada. 2012. "Canadian Salary Survey." http://www.livingin-canada. com/wages-for-health-jobs-canada.html.

Lomas, J., and M.L. Barer. 1986. "And Who Shall Represent the Public Interest? The Legacy of Canadian Health Manpower Policy." In *Medicare at Maturity: Achievements, Lessons and Challenges*, edited by R.G. Evans and G.L. Stoddart, 221-86. Calgary, AB: University of Calgary.

Lomas, J., C. Charles, and J. Grew. 1992. "The Price of Peace: The Structure of and Process of Physician Fee Negotiation in Canada." Paper 92-17, Centre for Health Economics and Policy Analysis, McMaster University, Hamilton.

Lomas, J., J. Wood, and G. Veenstra. 1997. "Devolving Authority for Health Care in Canada's Provinces: 1. An Introduction to the Issues." *CMAJ* 156 (3): 371-77.

Lukes, S. 2005. *Power: A Radical View*. 2nd ed. Toronto: Macmillan.

Macpherson, C.B. 1962. *Democracy in Alberta: Social Credit and the Party System*. 2nd ed. Toronto: University of Toronto Press.

Madore, O. 2005. *The* Canada Health Act: *Overview and Options*. Ottawa: Library of Parliament. http://www.parl.gc.ca/Content/LOP/ResearchPublications/944-e.htm.

Madore, O., and M. Tiedemann. 2005. *Private Health Care Funding and Delivery under the* Canada Health Act. Library of Parliament: Parliamentary Information and Research Service.

Maioni, A. 1998. *Parting at the Crossroads: The Emergence of Health Insurance in the United States and Canada*. Princeton: Princeton University Press.

Mansell, R. 1997. "Fiscal Restructuring in Alberta: An Overview." In *A Government Re-invented: A Study of Alberta's Deficit Elimination Programme*, edited by C.J. Bruce, R.D. Kneebone, and K.J. McKenzie. Toronto: Oxford University Press.

Marchildon, G.P. 2004. "Three Choices for the Future of Medicare." Caledon Institute of Social Policy, Ottawa.

Marchildon, G.P., and K. O'Fee. 2007. *Health Care in Saskatchewan: An Analytic Profile*. Regina, SK: Canadian Plains Research Centre Press.

Martin, D. 2003. *King Ralph: The Political Life and Success of Ralph Klein*. Toronto: Key Porter Books.

Martin, P. 1985. *A Very Public Life*. Vol. 2: *So Many Worlds*. Toronto: Deneau.

Martin, E., M.-P. Pomey, and P.-G. Forest. 2010. "One Step Forward, One Step Back: Quebec's 2003–04 Health and Social Services Regionalization Policy." *Canadian Public Administration* 53 (4): 453-74.

Maxwell, J., K. Jackson, B. Legowski, S. Rosell, and D. Yankelovich, with P.-G. Forest and L. Lozowchuk. 2002. *Report on Citizens' Dialogue on the Future of Health Care in Canada*. Prepared for the Commission on the Future of Health Care in Canada. http://www.collectionscanada.gc.ca/webarchives/20071220010304/http://www.hc-sc.gc.ca/english/pdf/romanow/pdfs/dialogue_e.pdf.

Maxwell, J., S. Rosell, and P.-G. Forest. 2003. "Giving Citizens a Voice in Healthcare Policy in Canada." *British Medical Journal* 326: 1031-33.

McArthur, D. 2007. "Policy Analysis in Provincial Governments in Canada." In *Policy Analysis in Canada: The State of the Art*, edited by L. Dobuzinski, M. Howlett, and D. Laycock, 238-65. Toronto: University of Toronto Press.

McDonald, P., S. Shortt, C. Sanmartin, M. Barer, S. Lewis, and S. Sheps. 1998. *Waiting Lists and Waiting Times for Healthcare in Canada: More Management!! More Money??* Ottawa: Health Canada.

McGregor, M.J., and L.A. Ronald. 2011. "Residential Long-Term Care for Canadian Seniors: Nonprofit, For-Profit or Does It Matter?" Institute for Research on Public Policy, Montreal. January.

McIntosh, T., and M. Ducie. 2009. "Private Health Facilities in Saskatchewan: Marginalization through Legalization." *Canadian Political Science Review* 3 (4): 47-62.

McIntosh, T., M. Ducie, M. Burka-Charles, J. Church, J. Lavis, M.-P. Pomey, N. Smith, and S. Tomblin. 2010. "Population Health and Health System Reform: Needs-Based Funding for Health Services in Five Provinces." *Canadian Political Science Review* 4 (1): 42-61.

McIntosh, T., M. Ducie, and C. England. 2007. "Managing Wait Times in Saskatchewan." Project website. http://www.queensu.ca/iigr/apps/secure/main.php?dirPass=4_-_Case_Studies.

McIntosh, T., B. Jeffery, and N. Muhajarinel. 2010. "Moving Forward on Critical Population Health Research." In *Redistributing Health: New Directions in Population Health Research in Canada*, edited by T. McIntosh, B. Jeffery, and N. Muhajarine, xi-xxv. Regina, SK: Canadian Plains Research Centre Press.

McKillop, I., G.H. Pink, and L.M. Johnson. 2001. *The Financial Management of Acute Care in Canada: A Review of Funding, Performance, Monitoring and Reporting Practices*. Ottawa: Canadian Institute for Health Information.

Mechanic, D. 1991. "Sources of Countervailing Power in Medicine." *Journal of Health Politics, Policy and Law* 16 (3): 485-97.

Mendelsohn, M. 2002. *Canadians' Thoughts on Their Health Care System: Preserving the Canadian Model through Innovation*. Commission on the Future of Health Care in Canada. http://www.queensu.ca/cora/_files/MendelsohnEnglish.pdf.

Ministère de la Santé et des Services sociaux. 1989. *Pour améliorer la santé et le bien-être au Québec: orientations*. Quebec: Gouvernement du Québec/Ministère de la Santé et des Services sociaux.

—. 1990. *Une réforme axée sur le citoyen*. Quebec: Gouvernement du Québec.

—. 1992. *La politique de la santé et du bien-être*. Quebec: Ministère de la Santé et des Services sociaux.

—. 1995a. *Mise en place d'un régime universel de base d'assurance médicaments au Québec: Analyse de la faisabilité*. Quebec: Ministère de la Santé et des Services sociaux.

—. 1995b. *Plan d'action sur l'accessibilité des services en chirurgie*. Quebec: Ministère de la Santé et des Services sociaux.

—. 1999. *Relever ensemble le défi des urgences: Plan d'action issu du Forum sur la situation dans les urgences*. Quebec: Ministère de la Santé et des Services sociaux.

—. 2004. *L'intégration des services de santé et des services sociaux: Le projet organisationnel et clinique et les balises associées à la mise en oeuvre des réseaux locaux de services de santé et de services sociaux*. Ministère de la Santé et des Services sociaux, Québec.

—. 2006. *Garantir l'accès: un défi d'équité, d'efficience et de qualité*. Quebec: Ministère de la Santé et des Services sociaux.

—. 2008. "Accès aux services médicaux spécialisés." Accessed 29 January 2008. http://wpp01.msss.gouv.qc.ca/appl/g74web/default.asp.

—. 2009. "Répertoire des établissements." Accessed 1 October 2009. http://wpp01.msss.gouv.qc.ca/appl/M02/index.asp.

MOHLTC (Ministry of Health and Long-Term Care). 2004. "Health Results Team – Local Integration Networks." Bulletin No. 2, 20 October. Toronto, Ontario.

—. 2005. *Health Results Team: First Annual Report 2004–05*. Toronto: Government of Ontario. http://www.health.gov.on.ca/en/common/ministry/publications/reports/health_results_team/hrt_annual_05.pdf.

—. 2007. *Health Results Team: Third Annual Report 2006–07. A Focus on Results and Sustainability*. Toronto: Government of Ontario. http://www.health.gov.on.ca/en/common/ministry/publications/reports/hrt_annual_06/hrt_2006_ar_20070907.pdf.

Moisan, M. 2002. "Sondage CROP-Le Soleil-La Presse: Les riches devraient payer pour la santé." *Le Soleil*, 5 octobre, A3.

Monaghan, B., C. Morgan, B. Shragge, L. Higginson, M. Vimr, and J. Trypuc. 2001. "Through the Looking Glass: The Cardiac Care Network of Ontario 10 Years Later." *Hospital Quarterly* 4 (3): 30-38.

Moralis, M. 1996. "Cardiac Care Network Takes Heart." Accessed 16 January 2004 from the Ontario Hospital Association website. No longer available.

Nanos Research. 2012. "Jobs/Economy Pulls Away from Healthcare." CTV News/Globe and Mail/Nanos Poll. http://www.nanosresearch.com/library/polls/2012-01-IssueE.pdf.

National Forum on Health. 1997a. *Canada Health Action: Building on the Legacy.* Vol. 1. Final report of the National Forum on Health. Ottawa: Health Canada.

—. 1997b. "Directions for a Pharmaceutical Policy in Canada." In *Canada Health Action: Building on the Legacy.* Vol. 2, *Synthesis Reports and Issues Papers.* http://www.hc-sc.gc.ca/hcs-sss/pubs/renewal-renouv/1997-nfoh-fnss-v2/index-eng.php.

—. 1997c. "Striking a Balance Working Group Synthesis Report." In *Canada Health Action: Building on the Legacy.* Vol. 2, *Synthesis Reports and Issues Papers.* http://www.hc-sc.gc.ca/hcs-sss/pubs/renewal-renouv/1997-nfoh-fnss-v2/index-eng.php.

Naylor, C.D. 1986. *Private Practice, Public Payment.* Montreal: McGill-Queen's University Press.

—. 1991. "A Different View of Queues in Ontario." *Health Affairs* 10 (3): 110-28.

—. 1999. "Health Care in Canada: Incrementalism under Fiscal Duress." *Health Affairs* 18 (3): 9-26.

Naylor, C.D., C.M. Levinton, S. Wheeler, and L. Hunter. 1993. "Queueing for Surgical Coronary Surgery During Severe Supply-Demand Mismatch in a Canadian Referral Centre: A Case Study of Implicit Rationing." *Social Science & Medicine* 37 (1): 61-67.

NDP (New Democratic Party). 1991. "Renewing the Saskatchewan Community: A New Democratic Vision for the 90's." Regina.

Newfoundland and Labrador Health Board Council. 1972. *A Concept of Regionalization of Health Care Services in the Province of Newfoundland.* St. John's: Newfoundland and Labrador Health Board Council.

Newfoundland and Labrador Health Boards Association. 2001. *Funding Model for the Health System of Newfoundland and Labrador.* St. John's.

Newfoundland and Labrador Hospital and Nursing Home Association. 1993. *Guidelines for Hospital Boards to Improve Recruitment and Retention of Physicians in Rural Newfoundland and Labrador.* St. John's.

"Newfoundland Rural PCR Talks Stalled." 2001. *The Rural News,* 13 (16), 1 July.

Normand, G. 1996. "Réduction de 669 millions à la Santé et aux Services Sociaux." *La Presse,* 28 mars, B4.

Nova Scotia. Royal Commission on Health Care. 1989. *The Report of the Nova Scotia Royal Commission on Health Care: Towards a New Strategy.* Chaired by J.C. Gallant. Halifax: Government Printer.

OECD (Organization for Economic Co-operation and Development). 2011. "Country Profile, Canada." Accessed January 2012. http://www.oecd-ilibrary.org/content/table/20752288-table-can.

O'Fee, K. 2002a. "Grey Literature 1980s–2003: Synthesis Paper." Project research report. http://www.queensu.ca/iigr/apps/secure/main.php?dirPass=2.2_-_Grey_LiteratureOn-line.

—. 2002b. "Grey Literature 1980s–2003: Report Summaries." Project research report. http://www.queensu.ca/iigr/apps/secure/main.php?dirPass=2.2_-_Grey_Literature.

Ontario. Premier's Council on Health Strategy. 1991. *Local Decision-Making for Health and Social Services.* Final report of the Integration and Coordination Committee. Toronto: Queen's Printer.

Ontario. Premier's Council on Health, Well-Being and Social Justice. 1994a. *A Framework for Evaluating Devolution.* Report prepared by ARA Consulting Group for the Task Force on Devoloution. Toronto: Queen's Printer.
—. 1994b. *Devolution of Health and Social Services in Ontario: Refocusing the Debate.* Toronto: Queen's Printer.
Ontario Association of Radiologists. 2002. *CT/MRI Needs Assessment Report: Expansion Plan for CT/MRI Services in Ontario Hospitals.* Accessed November 2002. http://www.oar.info/html/CTMRINEEDSASSESSMENTRPT2.pdf.
Ontario Family Health Network. 2005. *Your Family Health Network, Your Doctor, and More...* Toronto: Ministry of Health and Long-Term Care.
Ontario Health Coalition. 2010. Open Letter to Premier McGuinty. 11 August. http://www.web.net/ohc/mcguintyletter11august2010.pdf.
Ontario Health Services Restructuring Commission. 1999. *Primary Health Care Strategy: Advice and Recommendations to the Honourable Elizabeth Witmer, Minister of Health.* Toronto: Government of Ontario.
—. 2000. *Looking Back, Looking Forward: A Legacy Report.* Chaired by D. Sinclair. Toronto: Government of Ontario.
Ontario Liberal Party. 2003. *Government That Works for You: The Ontario Liberal Plan for a More Democratic Ontario.* http://www.leonarddomino.com/news/platform-ontarioliberal2003.pdf.
Ontario Medical Association (OMA) and Ministry of Health and Long-Term Care (MOHLTC). 2000. OMA-MOHLTC 2000–2004 Agreement. http://www.srpc.ca/PDF/OMA-MOHLTC.pdf.
Ontario Progressive Conservative Party. 1995. "The Common Sense Revolution."
Ontario Task Force on the Use and Provision of Medical Services. 1990. *Final Report of the Task Force on the Use and Provision of Medical Services.* Chaired by G. Scott. Toronto: Ministry of Health.
O'Reilly, P. 2001. "The Federal/Provincial/Territorial Health Conference in Canada." In *Federalism, Democracy and Health Policy in Canada,* edited by D. Adams. Montreal and Kingston: Institute of Intergovernmental Relations.
Osborne, D., and T. Gaebler. 1992. *Reinventing Government.* Boston: Addison-Wesley.
Pal, L.A. 1992. "The Political Executive and Political Leadership in Alberta." In *Government and Politics in Alberta,* edited by A. Tupper and R. Gibbons. Edmonton: University of Alberta Press.
Papp, L. 1994. "Protestors Demand Help to Pay for AIDS Drugs." *Toronto Star,* 8 March, A11.
Paré, I. 2001. "Les médecins fuiront la 'galère' de Trudel: Le projet des groupes de médecine de famille démarre mal." *Le Devoir,* 13 juin, A1.
Parliamentary Task Force on Federal-Provincial Fiscal Arrangements. 1981. *Fiscal Federalism in Canada.* Ottawa: Supply and Services Canada.
Parti libéral du Québec. 2002. *Partenaires pour la santé: Donner les soins et des services sociaux en tout temps et partout au Québec.* Québec.
—. 2003. *Un gouvernement au service des Québécois. Ensemble réinventons le Québec. Plan d'action du prochain gouvernement libéral.* Québec.
—. 2007. *S'unir pour réussir le Québec de demain. Plan d'action 2007–2012.* Deuxième mandat du gouvernement du Parti libéral du Québec – Plateforme électorale, Québec.
—. 2008. "Le parti – les valeurs libérales." Accessed 29 January 2008. http://www.pq.org/?menu=2&menu2=b1&q=node/1270.

Parti Québécois. 1993. *Des idées pour mon pays.* Québec.

—. 2008. "Le parti – la vision." Accessed 29 January 2008. http://www.pq.org/?menu= 2&menu2=b1&q=node/1270.

Patented Medicine Prices Review Board. 2012. Home page. http://www.pmprb- cepmb.gc.ca/english/View.asp?x=1433.

Philippon, D.J., and S.A. Wasylyshyn. 1996. "Health Care Reform in Alberta." *Canadian Public Administration* 39 (73): 70-84.

Pierson, P. 1993. "When Effect Becomes Cause: Policy Feedback and Political Change." *World Politics* 45: 595-628.

—. 1995. "Fragmented Welfare States: Federal Institutions and the Development of Social Policy." *Governance* 8 (4): 449-78.

—. 2000. "Increasing Returns, Path Dependence, and the Study of Politics." *American Political Science Review* 94 (2): 251-67.

Pink, G.H., and P. Leatt. 2003. "The Use of 'Arms-Length' Organizations for Health System Change in Ontario, Canada: Some Observations by Insiders." *Health Policy* 63 (1): 1-15.

Pomey, M.-P., P.-G. Forest, H. Palley, and E. Martin. 2007. "Public/Private Part- nerships for Prescription Drug Coverage: Policy Formulation and Outcomes in Quebec's Universal Drug Insurance Program, with Comparisons to the Medicare Prescription Drug Program in the United States." *Milbank Quarterly* 85 (3): 469-98.

Pomey, M.-P., E. Martin, and P.-G. Forest. 2005. "Making Decisions about Prescrip- tions Drugs in Quebec: Implementing the Public Prescription Drug Insurance Regime in 1996–1997." Project website. http://www.queensu.ca/iigr/apps/ secure/main.php?dirPass=4_-_Case_Studies.

Premier's Advisory Council on Health for Alberta. 2001. *A Framework for Reform: Report of the Premier's Advisory Council on Health.* Chaired by D. Mazankowski. http://www.assembly.ab.ca/lao/library/egovdocs/alpm/2001/132279.pdf.

Premier's Commission on Future Health Care for Albertans. 1989a. *The Rainbow Report: Our Vision for Health.* Vol. 1. Chaired by L. Hyndman. Edmonton: Gov- ernment of Alberta.

—. 1989b. *The Rainbow Report: Our Vision for Health.* Vol. 2. Edmonton: Govern- ment of Alberta.

Premiers' Council on Canadian Health Awareness. 2002. "Premiers' Council on Canadian Health Awareness: Backgrounder." 27 September. http://www. releases.gov.nl.ca/releases/2002/exec/0927n03.htm.

Prémont, M.-C. 2006. "Wait-Time Guaranteed for Health Services: An Analysis of Quebec's Approach." Translated by B. Chodos and S. Joanis. First published in French in *Les Cahiers de Droit* 47 (September 2006). http://www.healthcoalition. ca/archive/mcp2007-2.pdf.

Presse canadienne. 1995. "Listes d'attentes dans les hôpitaux: Rochon dévoile son plan d'action en trois volets." *Le Soleil,* 25 mars, A17.

Priest, L. 2005a. "A Boy's Plight, a Nation's Problem." *Globe and Mail,* 13 January, A1, A6.

—. 2005b. "After 2½ Years, Newfoundland Boy Gets MRI." *Globe and Mail,* 2 Feb- ruary, A7.

—. 2005c. "Newfoundland Boy's Case Highlights Shortage of MRIs." *Globe and Mail,* 14 January, A7.

Provincial and Territorial Ministers of Health. 2000. *Understanding Canada's Health Care Costs: Final Report.* August. Toronto: Ministry of Health and Long-Term

Care. http://www.health.gov.on.ca/en/common/ministry/publications/reports/ptcd/ptcd_mn.aspx.

Quebec. 1970. *Loi sur l'assurance maladie* (L.R.Q., chapitre A-29). Éditeur officiel du Québec.

——. 1971. *Loi sur les services de santé et les services sociaux* (L.R.Q., chapitre S-4.2). Éditeur officiel du Québec.

——. 1991. *Loi sur les services de santé et les services sociaux* (L.R.Q., chapitre S-4.2). Éditeur officiel du Québec.

——. 1996. *Loi sur l'assurance médicaments et modifiant diverses dispositions législatives, Projet de loi no. 33* (1996, chapitre 32). Éditeur officiel du Québec.

——. 1998. "Québec's Historical Position on the Federal Spending Power 1944–1998." Secrétariat aux Affaires intergouvernementales canadiennes: Direction des politiques institutionnelles et constitutionnelles Ministère du Conseil exécutif. July.

——. 2000. *Loi sur l'équilibre budgétaire du réseau public de la santé et des services sociaux, Projet de loi n.107* (2000, chapitre 17). Éditeur officiel du Québec.

——. 2001. *Loi modifiant la Loi sur les services de santé et les services sociaux et modifiant diverses dispositions législatives, Projet de loi no 28* (2001, chapitre 24). Éditeur officiel du Québec.

——. 2003. *Loi sur les agences de développement de réseaux locaux de services de santé et de services sociaux* (L.R.Q., chapitre A-8.1). Éditeur officiel du Québec.

——. 2004. 2004–2005 Budget Speech.

——. 2005. *Loi modifiant la Loi sur les services de santé et les services sociaux et d'autres dispositions législatives, Projet de loi no 83* (chapitre 32). Éditeur officiel du Québec.

——. 2006. *Loi modifiant la Loi sur les services de santé et les services sociaux et d'autres dispositions législatives, Projet de loi no 33* (chapitre 43). Éditeur officiel du Québec.

——. 2007. "Communiqué de presse de la présidente du Conseil du Trésor: Constitution du Groupe de travail sur le financement du système de santé." 27 juin. Accessed 29 January 2008. http://communiques.gouv.qc.ca/gouvqc/communiques/GPQF/Juin2007/27/c9896.html.

Rachlis, M. 1999. "A Paper Prepared for a Workshop on Intersectoral Action and Health." Sponsored by Health Canada (Alberta and NWT) in partnership with Alberta Health and Alberta Community Development. Unpublished manuscript, 26 March. http://www.michaelrachlis.com/publications.php.

——. 2002. "Beam Me Up, Tony: Who Will Cash In on Those Scans?" *Toronto Star*, 17 July.

Rae, B. 1996. *From Protest to Power: Personal Reflections on a Life in Politics.* Toronto: Viking Canada.

RAMQ (Régie de l'assurance maladie du Québec). 2004. "Les régimes privés." Accessed 29 January 2008. http://www.ramq.gouv.qc.ca/fr/citoyens/assurancemedicaments/regimesprives/regimesprives.shtml.

——. 2006. "Principales variables selon la catégorie de personnes assurées: régime public d'assurance médicaments, Québec." Accessed 29 January 2008. https://www.prod.ramq.gouv.qc.ca/IST/CD/CDF_DifsnInfoStats/CDF1_Cnsul InfoStatsCNC_iut/RappPDF.aspx?TypeImpression=pdf&NomPdf= CCB3R01A_AM06_2006_0_O.PDF.

Ramsay, C., and M. Walker. 1998. *Waiting Your Turn: Hospital Waiting Lists in Canada.* 8th ed. Vancouver: Fraser Institute.

Ramsay, C., M.A. Walker, and W. McArthur. 1996. *Healthy Incentives: Canadian Health Reform in an International Context.* Vancouver: Fraser Institute.

Redden, C.J. 2002. *Health Care, Entitlement, and Citizenship.* Toronto: University of Toronto Press.

Reid, T.R. 2009. *The Healing of America: A Global Quest for Better, Cheaper, and Fairer Health Care.* New York: Penguin Press.

Reinharz, D., L. Rousseau, and S. Rheault. 1999. "La place du médicament dans le système de santé du Québec." In *Le système de santé québécois: Un modèle en transformation,* edited by C. Bégin, P. Bergeron, P.-G. Forest, and V. Lemieux, 149-67. Montreal: Les Presses de l'Université de Montréal.

Rich, P. 1999. "Newfoundland Set for Major Primary Care Reform." *The Medical Post* 35 (26), 20 July.

Royal Commission on Health Services. 1964. Vol. 1, tabled in the House of Commons on 19 June. Ottawa: Queen's Printer. www.positivelivingbc.org/files/resources/hall-report.pdf.

Ruttan, S. 2009. "Supersized." *Alberta Views Magazine,* November.

Sabatier, P. 1988. "An Advocacy Coalition Framework of Policy Change and the Role of Policy-Oriented Learning Therein." *Policy Sciences* 21: 129-68.

Santé Canada. 2007. "À propos du Fonds pour l'adaptation des services de santé." Accessed 10 April 2008. http://www.hc-sc.gc.ca/hcs-sss/ehealth-esante/infostructure/finance/htf-fass/about-apropos/index_f.html.

Saskatchewan Commission on Directions in Health Care. 1990. *Future Directions for Health Care in Saskatchewan.* Chaired by R.G. Murray. Regina: Government of Saskatchewan.

Saskatchewan Health. 1992. *A Saskatchewan Vision for Health: A Framework for Change.* Regina: Government of Saskatchewan.

—. 2002. *The Action Plan for Saskatchewan Health Care.* Regina: Government of Saskatchewan.

—. 2004. *Medical Services Branch Annual Statistical Report, 2003/2004.* Regina: Government of Saskatchewan.

—. 2010. *Drug Plan and Extended Benefits Branch Annual Statistical Report 2009/10.* Regina: Government of Saskatchewan.

Saskatchewan Party. 2007. "Securing the Future: New Ideas for Saskatchewan." Election platform.

Schipper, H., M. Pai, and H. Swain. 2008. "Putting People First: Critical Reforms for Canada's Health Care System." Toronto. http://www.globalcentres.org/publicationfiles/Schipper%20Pai%20Swain%200708.pdf.

SECOR. 2000. "La pratique du médecin omnipraticien dans un réseau de services intégrés: Positionnement des cabinets privés – un cadre d'orientation." *Le médecin du Québec* 35 (3): 103-34.

Select Committee on the Election Act. 2005. Information booklet. Accessed 29 January 2008. http://www.assnat.qc.ca/eng/37legislature2/commissions/CSLE/infobooklet.htm.

Sinclair, D., M. Rochon, and P. Leatt. 2005. *Riding the Third Rail: The Story of Ontario's Health Services Restructuring Commission, 1996–2000.* Montreal: Institute for Research on Public Policy.

Sirois, A. 2000. "Québécois et Albertains: du pareil au même ... ou presque!" *La Presse,* 9 septembre, B5.

—. 2001. "Groupes de médecine familiale: Les médecins inquiets." *La Presse,* 19 décembre, A6.

Smith, N., and J. Church. 2008. "Shifting the Lens: The Introduction of Population-Based Funding in Alberta." *Healthcare Management Forum* 21 (2): 36-42.

Soroka, S.N. 2007. *Canadian Perceptions of the Health Care System.* A report to the Health Council of Canada, Toronto.

—. 2011. *Public Perceptions and Media Coverage of the Canadian Healthcare System: A Synthesis.* A report to the Canada Health Services Research Foundation, Ottawa. http://www.cfhi-fcass.ca/Libraries/Commissioned_Research_Reports/Soroka1-EN.sflb.ashx.

Spencer, C. 2010. "Health Care Top Concern of Canadians: Poll." *Toronto Sun,* 13 May. http://www.nanosresearch.com/news/in_the_news/Toronto%20Sun%20May%2013%202010.pdf.

St-Pierre, M.-A. 2001. *Le système de santé et de services sociaux du Québec: Une image chiffrée.* Direction des communications, Ministère de la Santé et des Services sociaux, Québec.

Standing Senate Committee on Social Affairs, Science and Technology. 2002a. *The Health of Canadians – The Federal Role.* Vol. 4, *Issues and Options.* Interim report. Chaired by the Hon. M.J.L. Kirby.

—. 2002b. *The Health of Canadians – The Federal Role.* Vol. 6, *Recommendations for Reform.* Final report. Chaired by the Hon. M.J.L. Kirby.

—. 2012a. "The Senate Standing Committee on Social Affairs, Science and Technology Tables Its Report on the Review of the 2004 Health Accord." News release, 27 March. http://www.parl.gc.ca/Content/SEN/Committee/411/soci/DPK/home-e.htm.

—. 2012b. "Time for Transformative Change: A Review of the 2004 Health Accord." http://www.parl.gc.ca/Content/SEN/Committee/411/soci/press/27mar12B-e.htm.

Starfield, B. 1994. "Is Primary Care Essential?" *The Lancet* 344 (8930): 1129-33.

Statistics Canada. 2012. "Employment, Health Care and Social Assistance, by Province and Territory." CANSIM Table 281-0024. Cat. No. 72-002-XIB. http://www.statcan.gc.ca/tables-tableaux/sum-som/l01/cst01/health22-eng.htm.

Steinbrook, R. 2006. "Private Health Care in Canada." *New England Journal of Medicine* 354 (20 April): 1661-64. http://www.nejm.org/doi/full/10.1056/NEJMp068064.

Sullivan, D.S. 2005. "Family Discouraged by Drug Decision." *The Telegram,* 29 March, A1, A2.

Supreme Court of Canada. 2005. *Chaoulli v. Quebec* (Attorney General). ([2005] 1 S.C.R. 791, 2005 SCC 35).

Taras, D., and A. Tupper. 1994. "Politics and Deficits: Alberta's Challenge to the Canadian Political Agenda." In *State of the Federation 1994,* edited by D.M. Brown and J. Hiebert, 61-83. Kingston: McGill-Queen's University Press.

Taylor, M.G. 2009. *Health Insurance and Canadian Public Policy: The Seven Decisions That Created the Health Insurance System and Their Outcomes.* 2nd ed. First printed 1987. Republished in Carleton Library Series 213. Montreal and Kingston: McGill-Queen's University Press.

Tomblin, S.G. 1995. *Ottawa and the Outer Provinces: The Challenge of Regional Integration in Canada.* Toronto: Lorimer Press.

Tomblin, S., and J. Braun-Jackson. 2005. "Health Budgeting Models and the Experience of Newfoundland and Labrador: Why We Haven't Moved to a Needs-Based System?" Project website.

Trypuc, J. 2001. *Cardiac Care Network of Ontario: Driven by Data, Consensus and Concern – Ten Years, 1990–2000.* Toronto: Cardiac Care Network of Ontario.

Tupper, A. 2001. "Debt, Populism and Cutbacks: Alberta Politics in the 1990s." In *Party Politics in Canada*, 7ᵗʰ ed., edited by H.G. Thorburn. Scarborough, ON: Prentice Hall Canada.

Tupper, A., L. Pratt, and I. Urquhart. 1992. "The Role of Government." In *Government and Politics in Alberta*, edited by A. Tupper and R. Gibbons. Edmonton: University of Alberta Press.

Tuohy, C.H. 1988. "Medicine and the State in Canada: The Extra-Billing Issue in Perspective." *Canadian Journal of Political Science* 21 (2): 267-95.

—. 1999. *Accidental Logics: The Dynamics of Change in the Health Care Arena in the United States, Britain, and Canada.* New York: Oxford University Press.

Tyler, T., and M. Maycheck. 1989. "Second Heart Patient Dies as Surgery Delayed 9 Times." *Toronto Star*, 6 January, A2.

Venne, M. 1995. "Le Québec divisé." *Le Devoir*, 31 octobre, A1.

Walkom, T. 1994. "Whatever the Motive, NDP Improves Drug Coverage." *Toronto Star*, 1 December, A31.

—. 1995. "Out of Crass Political Pressure, Drug Plan Is Born." *Toronto Star*, 2 February, A17.

Weller, G.R. 1977. "From 'Pressure Group Politics' to 'Medical-Industrial Complex': The Development of Approaches to the Politics of Health." *Journal of Health Politics, Policy and Law* 1 (4): 444-60.

White, G. 2005. *Cabinets and First Ministers.* Vancouver: UBC Press.

Wilson, G., and M. Zelder. 2000. *Waiting Your Turn: Hospital Waiting Lists in Canada.* 10ᵗʰ ed. Calgary, AB: Fraser Institute.

Wilson, M.G. 2004. "Health Care Reform in Ontario: Case Studies of the Trillium Drug Plan and the Cardiac Care Network Policy Decisions." Thesis submitted for a Bachelor of Health Sciences, McMaster University, Hamilton, Ontario.

Wright, L. 1995. "Grier Warned of Abuses as Drug Plan Takes Effect." *Toronto Star*, 6 April, A8.

CONTRIBUTORS

JEFF BRAUN-JACKSON, former lecturer in political science at Memorial University. He currently works with the Ontario Professional Firefighters Association in Burlington

JOHN CHURCH, associate professor, Department of Political Science, University of Alberta

JULIA DIAMOND, graduate student in public administration, University of Victoria

MICHAEL DUCIE, Alberta Health and Wellness

PIERRE-GERLIER FOREST, professor and director, Institute for Health and Social Policy, Bloomberg School of Public Health, Johns Hopkins University

JOHN N. LAVIS, professor, Department of Clinical Epidemiology and Biostatistics, McMaster University; director, McMaster Health Forum; associate director, Centre for Health Economics and Policy Analysis, McMaster University

HARVEY LAZAR, adjunct professor, School of Public Administration, University of Victoria; Fellow, Institute of Intergovernmental Relations, Queen's University

ELISABETH MARTIN, doctoral candidate in community health, Université Laval

TOM MCINTOSH, professor of political science and researcher at the Saskatchewan Population Health and Evaluation Research Unit, University of Regina

DIANNA PASIC, research coordinator, Centre for Health Economics and Policy Analysis, McMaster University

MARIE-PASCALE POMEY, associate professor, Department of Health Administration, Faculty of Medicine, Université de Montréal; researcher, Institut de recherche en santé publique de l'Université de Montréal

NEALE SMITH, Centre for Clinical Epidemiology & Evaluation, Vancouver Coastal Health Research Institute, University of British Columbia

STEPHEN G. TOMBLIN, professor of political science (cross-appointed in medicine), Memorial University

MICHAEL G. WILSON, assistant professor, McMaster University; assistant director, McMaster Health Forum

Queen's Policy Studies
Recent Publications

The Queen's Policy Studies Series is dedicated to the exploration of major public policy issues that confront governments and society in Canada and other nations.

Manuscript submission. We are pleased to consider new book proposals and manuscripts. Preliminary inquiries are welcome. A subvention is normally required for the publication of an academic book. Please direct questions or proposals to the Publications Unit by email at spspress@queensu.ca, or visit our website at: www.queensu.ca/sps/books, or contact us by phone at (613) 533-2192.

Our books are available from good bookstores everywhere, including the Queen's University bookstore (http://www.campusbookstore.com/). McGill-Queen's University Press is the exclusive world representative and distributor of books in the series. A full catalogue and ordering information may be found on their web site (**http://mqup.mcgill.ca/**).

For more information about new and backlist titles from Queen's Policy Studies, visit http://www.queensu.ca/sps/books.

School of Policy Studies

Building More Effective Labour-Management Relationships, Richard P. Chaykowski and Robert S. Hickey (eds.) 2013. ISBN 978-1-55339-306-1

Navigationg on the Titanic: Economic Growth, Energy, and the Failure of Governance, Bryne Purchase 2013. ISBN 978-1-55339-330-6

Measuring the Value of a Postsecondary Education, Ken Norrie and Mary Catharine Lennon (eds.) 2013. ISBN 978-1-55339-325-2

Immigration, Integration, and Inclusion in Ontario Cities, Caroline Andrew, John Biles, Meyer Burstein, Victoria M. Esses, and Erin Tolley (eds.) 2012. ISBN 978-1-55339-292-7

Diverse Nations, Diverse Responses: Approaches to Social Cohesion in Immigrant Societies, Paul Spoonley and Erin Tolley (eds.) 2012. ISBN 978-1-55339-309-2

Making EI Work: Research from the Mowat Centre Employment Insurance Task Force, Keith Banting and Jon Medow (eds.) 2012. ISBN 978-1-55339-323-8

Managing Immigration and Diversity in Canada: A Transatlantic Dialogue in the New Age of Migration, Dan Rodríguez-García (ed.) 2012. ISBN 978-1-55339-289-7

International Perspectives: Integration and Inclusion, James Frideres and John Biles (eds.) 2012. ISBN 978-1-55339-317-7

Dynamic Negotiations: Teacher Labour Relations in Canadian Elementary and Secondary Education, Sara Slinn and Arthur Sweetman (eds.) 2012. ISBN 978-1-55339-304-7

Where to from Here? Keeping Medicare Sustainable, Stephen Duckett 2012. ISBN 978-1-55339-318-4

International Migration in Uncertain Times, John Nieuwenhuysen, Howard Duncan, and Stine Neerup (eds.) 2012. ISBN 978-1-55339-308-5

Life After Forty: Official Languages Policy in Canada/Après quarante ans, les politiques de langue officielle au Canada, Jack Jedwab and Rodrigue Landry (eds.) 2011. ISBN 978-1-55339-279-8

From Innovation to Transformation: Moving up the Curve in Ontario Healthcare, Hon. Elinor Caplan, Dr. Tom Bigda-Peyton, Maia MacNiven, and Sandy Sheahan 2011. ISBN 978-1-55339-315-3

Academic Reform: Policy Options for Improving the Quality and Cost-Effectiveness of Undergraduate Education in Ontario, Ian D. Clark, David Trick, and Richard Van Loon 2011. ISBN 978-1-55339-310-8

Integration and Inclusion of Newcomers and Minorities across Canada, John Biles, Meyer Burstein, James Frideres, Erin Tolley, and Robert Vineberg (eds.) 2011. ISBN 978-1-55339-290-3

A New Synthesis of Public Administration: Serving in the 21st Century, Jocelyne Bourgon, 2011. ISBN 978-1-55339-312-2 (paper) 978-1-55339-313-9 (cloth)

Recreating Canada: Essays in Honour of Paul Weiler, Randall Morck (ed.), 2011. ISBN 978-1-55339-273-6

Data Data Everywhere: Access and Accountability? Colleen M. Flood (ed.), 2011. ISBN 978-1-55339-236-1

Making the Case: Using Case Studies for Teaching and Knowledge Management in Public Administration, Andrew Graham, 2011. ISBN 978-1-55339-302-3

Centre for International and Defence Policy

Afghanistan in the Balance: Counterinsurgency, Comprehensive Approach, and Political Order, Hans-Georg Ehrhart, Sven Bernhard Gareis, and Charles Pentland (eds.), 2012. ISBN 978-1-55339-353-5

Security Operations in the 21st Century: Canadian Perspectives on the Comprehensive Approach, Michael Rostek and Peter Gizewski (eds.), 2011. ISBN 978-1-55339-351-1

Institute of Intergovernmental Relations

Canada: The State of the Federation 2010, Matthew Medelsohn, Joshua Hjartarson and James Pearce (ed.), 2013. ISBN 978-1-55339-200-2

The Democratic Dilemma: Reforming Canada's Supreme Court, Nadia Verrelli (eds.), 2013. ISBN 978-1-55339-203-3

The Evolving Canadian Crown, Jennifer Smith and D. Michael Jackson (eds.), 2011. ISBN 978-1-55339-202-6

The Federal Idea: Essays in Honour of Ronald L. Watts, Thomas J. Courchene, John R. Allan, Christian Leuprecht, and Nadia Verrelli (eds.), 2011. ISBN 978-1-55339-198-2 (paper) 978-1-55339-199-9 (cloth)

The Democratic Dilemma: Reforming the Canadian Senate, Jennifer Smith (ed.), 2009. ISBN 978-1-55339-190-6